THE AROMATHERAPY ENCYCLOPEDIA

A CONCISE GUIDE TO OVER 385 PLANT OILS

CAROL SCHILLER & DAVID SCHILLER
ILLUSTRATED BY JEFFREY SCHILLER

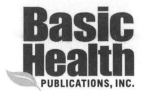

Basic Health
PUBLICATIONS, INC.

This book is for educational purposes only and is not intended to replace the services of a natural practioner. Before using any of the oils, please read the safety guidelines in Chapter 1 very carefully. The safe and proper use of the oils is the sole responsibility of the reader. The authors and publisher assume no responsibility or liability for anyone's misuse, carelessness, allergic reactions, skin sensitivity, or any other conditions arising directly or indirectly from the use of this book.

The publisher does not advocate the use of any particular healthcare protocol but believes the information in this book should be available to the public. The publisher and author are not responsible for any adverse effects or consequences resulting from the use of the suggestions, preparations, or procedures discussed in this book. Should the reader have any questions concerning the appropriateness of any procedures or preparation mentioned, the author and the publisher strongly suggest consulting a professional healthcare advisor.

Basic Health Publications, Inc.

28812 Top of the World Drive

Laguna Beach, CA 92651

949-715-7327 • www.basichealthpub.com

Library of Congress Cataloging-in-Publication Data

Schiller, Carol.
    The aromatherapy encyclopedia : a concise guide to over 385 plant oils /
Carol Schiller and David Schiller ; illustrated by Jeffrey Schiller.
        p. cm.
    Includes bibliographical references and index.
    ISBN 978-1-59120-228-8
    1. Aromatherapy—Encyclopedias. 2. Essences and essential oils—Encyclopedias.
I. Schiller, David II. Title.

    RM666.A68S3525   2008
    615'.321903—dc22

                                                            2008022199

Editor: Karen Anspach
Typesetting/Book design: Gary A. Rosenberg
Cover design: Mike Stromberg
Illustrations and front cover photographs: Jeffrey Schiller

Printed in the United States of America

10   9   8   7   6   5   4   3   2   1

Contents

INTRODUCTION
Aromatherapy Over the Years, 1

CHAPTER 1
Safety, Handling, and Selection of Oils, 3

CHAPTER 2
Vegetal Oils, Butters, and Waxes, 7

CHAPTER 3
Essential Oils, 67

CHAPTER 4
Infused Oils, 191

CHAPTER 5
Methods of Application, Dispersion,
and Inhalation of Essential Oils, 195

CHAPTER 6
Category Listing of Oil Properties, 197

Cross-Reference of Botanical Names to Common Names, 205

Plant Family Name Classification, 213

Glossary, 221

Bibliography, 224

Index, 227

About the Authors, 234

Aromas open the gateway of the mind
and bring forth memories, feelings, and emotions.
All of us are affected—some more so than others.
—DAVID SCHILLER

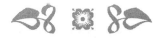

Acknowledgments

We'd like to thank the following people:

Dr. Karl Werner Quirin, the pioneer of CO_2 extractions, and founder and president of Flavex, a high-quality producer of CO_2 extracts in Germany.

Norman Goldfind, founder and publisher of Basic Health Publications.

Bernard Otremba-Blanc, Ph.D., for seeing the benefits of the essential oils and sharing the information so more people can learn about and experience their great and important value.

To Harvey Farber, John Wendel, Ken Goodger, David Beaver, Dieter Kuster, Ph.D., Alban Muller, and Xavier Ormancey, Ph.D., for providing quality education at the AromaHerb Conference and Trade Show that helped people in the trade become more knowledgeable of the industry.

Ann Albers, an exceptional person and dedicated teacher; always helping people.

Sharon Muir, for supporting the education of aromatherapy so that many people can learn and incorporate the essential oils into their lives.

Roslyn Blumenthal, for her valuable insight.

The libraries are the greatest institutions for learning. We extend our gratitude to the librarians and staff at the Phoenix Public Library, especially: Greg Hills, Doris Foose, Maritza Jerry, Kathleen Birtciel, Keith Cullers, Caren Lumley, Debbie Fincher, Nancy Madden, Karen Berner, Alex Latham, Louis Howley, Randle's Lunsford Jr., Delphine Snowden, Jonathan Cole, Rob Steele, and Rita Martinez.

The librarians and staff at the Glendale Public Library, especially: Joan Jensen, Anne Owen, and Stuart Levine.

INTRODUCTION

Aromatherapy Over the Years

Since the beginning of recorded history, aromatic plants have been used to scent, beautify, and heal the body. In ancient times, wealthy Egyptians luxuriated in the pleasures of bathing in scented waters, indulging in a delightful fragrant massage, and perfuming their bodies with enchanting oils and ointments. The priests were the first perfumers and healers to dispense aromatics by preparing blends for the kings, queens, and high dignitaries of temples and governments. During religious ceremonies, they used aromatic waters in the anointing rituals, burned incense in an effort to protect against evil spirits, and help the worshippers concentrate on their prayers. When the pharaohs died, their bodies were wrapped with fabric containing cinnamon, myrrh, cedarwood, and other resins and oils. This mummification method was confirmed to have been effective when modern-day archaeologists excavated the mummies and found them to be well preserved in their original burial chambers.

The ancient Romans lavishly perfumed their bodies and scented everything from military flags to the walls of their homes. Eventually Rome became the bathing capital of the world, with one thousand public bath houses located throughout the city for people to bathe, socialize, and afterwards enjoy a pampering massage with scented oils and unguents.

The art of extracting the volatile essences from plants was initiated by the Egyptians, who heated them in clay containers. Two centuries later, Greek alchemists invented the distillation process, which further developed the use of essences for religious and therapeutic purposes. By 1000 A.D., the Arabic physician, Avicenna, perfected the extraction method by introducing the cooling system into the distillation process, thereby creating the most potent essences with stronger fragrances.

During the fourteenth century, the Great Plague devastated Europe and Asia, killing millions of people. All aromatic substances available were used for their antiseptic properties to fight off the dreaded disease. Cedar, clove, cypress, pine, sage, rosemary, and thyme were burned in the streets, hospitals, and sickrooms in a desperate attempt to prevent the spread of the epidemic. It was reported that perfumers and those who handled and used aromatics of various kinds were virtually immune to the ravages of the plague and survived.

The study of the therapeutic effectiveness of essential oils was further advanced by René-Maurice Gattefosse, a French cosmetic chemist. In the early 1920s, while working in his laboratory, Gattefosse accidentally burned his hand and immediately immersed it into the nearest cold liquid, which happened to be a container of lavender oil. Surprisingly, the pain lessened and the reaction of redness, inflammation, and blistering was drastically reduced. In addition, the wound healed very quickly and no scar developed. After this incident, Gattefosse decided to dedicate the rest of his life to the study of the remarkable healing properties of the essential oils and coined the term "aromatherapy" in 1928.

Inspired by Gattefosse's work, Jean Valnet, a French medical doctor, exclusively used the essential oils to treat the battle wounds of the French soldiers during World War II. Dr. Valnet's extensive use of essences gained him official recognition in France and acknowledged aromatherapy as a true therapy. His book, *The Practice of Aromatherapy*, is a classic work on the subject.

About the same time as Dr. Valnet was practicing aromatherapy, Madame Marguerite Maury, a biochemist, pursued her study of the cosmetic and therapeutic uses of the essential oils. She was later awarded the Prix International for her work in natural skin care.

Today, the use of essential oils worldwide is steadily becoming more widespread as greater numbers of individuals become aware of the myriad life-enhancing properties of these remarkable substances. These precious essences help balance and put us in greater harmony with the natural world. They protect us with their antibacterial properties, reduce our stress, and give us comfort, reassurance, and pleasure.

Some of the oils can produce instantaneous results that are easily recognizable, while others perform their work at a slower pace in a relatively unnoticeable, subtle way. Only those people who use the oils on a regular basis can begin to understand and fully appreciate and respect their miraculous value.

Aromatherapy offers us a chance to reach out to our forgotten past. By looking to nature, with all of its benefits and beauty, we can take advantage of the valuable wisdom of the ages from our ancestors and benefit from this very precious gift of aromatic essential oils.

CHAPTER 1

Safety, Handling, and Selection of Oils

SAFETY AND HANDLING OF OILS

Essential oils can be extremely beneficial when used properly; therefore, please follow these guidelines:

- Essential oils are highly concentrated substances and should be diluted in a carrier oil such as almond (sweet), jojoba, macadamia nut, or sesame oil before being applied on the skin, in order to prevent skin irritation. (See Chapter 2 for proper blending.) If any skin irritation should occur as a result of using the essential oils, immediately apply additional carrier oil or lavender oil to the area. This will quickly soothe the skin.

- When applying essential oils on the skin, using a mist spray, or taking a scented bath, be careful not to get the oils into the eyes. If this should occur, flush the eyes with cool water.

- Care must be taken when using carrier and essential oils during pregnancy. Many of the oils have a stimulating effect on the uterus, which can be very helpful at the appropriate time to facilitate childbirth. However, if those oils are used prior to the time of childbirth, they can bring on premature labor. Even certain common foods, spices, and vegetable oils, such as celery, carrots, parsley, basil, bay leaves, marjoram, and safflower oil, can stimulate uterine contractions.

- Small amounts (two to three drops at one time) of the following essential oils are known to be safe during pregnancy: bergamot, coriander, cypress, frankincense, geranium, ginger, grapefruit, lavandin, lavender, lemon, lime, mandarin, neroli, orange, patchouli, petitgrain, sandalwood, tangelo, tangerine, tea tree, and temple orange. Sesame oil can be used as a carrier oil.

- A woman nursing her baby should exercise caution when using the essential oils as the effects of the oils will be readily passed on to the infant.

- If a person is highly allergic, a simple test can determine if there is any sensitivity to a particular oil. Rub a drop of carrier oil on the upper chest area, and in twelve hours, check if there is redness or any other skin reaction. If the skin is clear, dilute one drop of an essential oil in twenty drops of the same carrier oil and again apply to the upper chest area. If there is no skin reaction after twelve hours, both the carrier and the essential oil can be used.

- Do not consume alcohol, except for a small glass of wine with a meal, in the time period when using essential oils.

- Do not use essential oils while on medication as the oils might interfere with the medicine.

- After an essential oil blend is applied on the skin, avoid, for at least four hours, sunbathing, sauna/steam room, or a hot bath, in order to prevent the possibility of skin irritation. This precaution is especially important when using citrus, phototoxic, and other essential oils that can irritate the skin.

- There are people with extremely sensitive skin who cannot tolerate the essential oils without experiencing skin irritation. If this is the case, discontinue use.

- Many essential oils will remove the finish when spilled on furniture; therefore, be careful when handling the bottles.

- Light and oxygen cause oils to deteriorate rapidly. Refrigeration does not prevent spoilage, but diminishes the speed at which it occurs. Therefore, oils should be stored in brown glass bottles in a dark and cool place.

- Always use a glass dropper when measuring drops of essential oil.

- Keep all bottles tightly closed to prevent the oils from evaporating and oxidizing.

- Always store essential oils out of sight and reach of children.

METHODS OF EXTRACTION

The extraction process is a factor in determining the purity of the oil. Before purchasing carrier and essential oils, it is important to become knowledgeable of these methods.

Steam Distillation

Steam from boiling water is used to extract the essential oil from the plant material. The steam rises and passes through a cold coil, turning into a liquid. The essential oil floats on top of the water and is skimmed off. The leftover water contains water-soluble components and is used as floral water. Steam distillation is extensively used and produces a good quality essential oil.

Carbon Dioxide Gas Extraction

Expensive high-technology equipment is used to extract the essential oils. It employs carbon dioxide gas (CO_2), high pressure, and low temperature. This process produces an oil that retains a greater amount of aromatic components than oil derived by steam distillation. The scent of CO_2 extracted oil is more identical to that of the original plant.

There are two types of CO_2 extractions: Select and Total.

Select CO₂ Extraction

In the *select* method, the oil is extracted at a temperature of around 88°F (31°C). The plant material is placed in a chamber and then the compressed CO_2 gas is released. As the gas passes through the plant material, it draws the plant components into solution. When the process is completed the pressure is lowered, and the extracted materials precipitate out and are collected. The CO_2 gas is then recompressed and recycled to be used again, without leaving any residue in the extracted oil. The extracted oil contains selected components similar to oils that are steam distilled.

Total CO₂ Extraction

In the *total* method, the plant material is processed at a higher temperature. The extracted oil contains more plant components than the select method.

Cold Pressed Citrus Oils

The essential oil is produced from the citrus peel. The fruits are placed on a conveyor belt and then dropped into a cup with knives. As the cup closes, the knives puncture the fruit. The fruit is pressed for juice, and the peel is sprayed with water to create a slurry, which is collected and put through a centrifuge process to separate out the essential oil.

Maceration

Flowers, such as rose and jasmine, are soaked in hot oil to release their fragrant components into the oil.

Solvent Extraction

Solvents, such as hexane and other toxic chemicals, are used to extract the oil from the plant material. This method is less costly and more efficient in producing a greater amount of oil. However, toxic residues are left from the hexane, making it undesirable for those wanting pure oils. Absolute flower oils and a high percentage of commercial vegetable oils are extracted using this method.

Cold, Expeller, or Mechanically Pressed Extraction of Vegetal Oils

Seeds, nuts, fruits, and vegetables are pressed without using heat to preserve the components in the oil.

Cold pressed oils are produced by a mechanical batch-pressing process in which heat-producing friction is minimized, keeping temperatures below 120°F (49°C). The expeller-pressed method generates more heat to extract the oil, so in-line refrigerated cooling devices are added to the presses to keep the temperatures down to 185°F (85°C) during the pressing.

A large percentage of vegetal oils are usually refined after being pressed, using high heat and harsh chemicals. Therefore, it is important to check the label on the container to ensure that the oil is unrefined, containing all the valuable nutrients.

Refining Process for Vegetal/Carrier Oils

After the oil has been extracted from the plant material, it is usually put through a refining process that includes the following:

Degumming: Removes chlorophyll, vitamins, and minerals from the oil.

Refining: An alkaline solution called lye is added to refine the oil.

Bleaching: Fuller's Earth, a naturally occurring clay-like substance, is added as a bleaching agent and then filtered out, further removing nutritive substances. The oil at this stage becomes clear.

Deodorizing: The oil is deodorized by steam distillation at high temperatures over 450°F (232°C) for thirty to sixty minutes.

Winterizing: The oil is then cooled and filtered. This process prevents the oil from becoming cloudy during cold temperatures.

The finished product is nutrient deficient, with only fatty acids remaining.

SELECTION OF QUALITY OILS

It is unfortunate that a high percentage of oils commonly sold to the public are adulterated. This is done to increase profits without much concern for the consequences to the consumer. Some of the adulteration consists of adding cheaper oil to a more expensive oil to "stretch" it. Many other more serious adulterations take place by adding synthetic as well as fractionalized components, which contaminate the oils. This practice is common knowledge in the essential oil industry and is referred to as "making a soup." Each time the oil changes hands, the possibility increases for the original oil to become more diluted. A few common examples of adulteration are:

Essential Oil	Adulterated with
Lavender	Lavandin
Neroli	Petitgrain
Pimento berry	Clove
Rose	Palmarosa
Rosemary	Eucalyptus
Patchouli	Gurjun Balsam
Peppermint	Cornmint
Sandalwood	Amyris
Ylang-Ylang	Cananga

Synthetic oils and oils that are extracted by chemical or petroleum solvents should never be used. The man-made chemicals that replicate the aromas of natural oils do not contain the beneficial properties of the pure plant oils. As a matter of fact, many of these synthetic compounds can be very irritating to the nervous system and entire body. The oils that are solvent-extracted contain toxic residues from the solvent and can be harmful as well.

The highest-grade and most effective oils are produced from plants that are grown wild and away from polluted sources or are cultivated by natural farming methods without the use of pesticides, herbicides, or any other unnatural substances. It is important to select for purchase unrefined carrier oils that are cold, expeller, or mechanically pressed, and essential oils that have either been steam distilled, CO_2 extracted, or, in the case of citrus oils, cold pressed.

CHAPTER 2

Vegetal Oils, Butters, and Waxes

Vegetal oils are derived from seeds, nuts, fruits, and vegetables. Many of these oils are used as a carrier oil to dilute essential oils so that the blend can be applied safely on the skin. Vegetal butters and waxes are mainly used as ingredients in skin and hair care products.

The following oils, butters, and waxes are covered in this chapter:

Acai Fruit	Candelilla Wax	Hazelnut	Neem
Acai Seed	Canola (*Rapeseed*)	Hemp	Noni Seed
Almond (*Sweet*)	Carnauba Wax	Illipe Butter	Oat
Amaranth	Carob Pod	Jojoba*	Okra
Andiroba	Carrot Root*	Kalahari Melon Seed	Olive
Annatto	Cashew Nut*	Kapok Seed	Palm**
Apricot Kernel	Castor	Karanja	Palm Kernel
Argan	Chaulmoogra	Kiwifruit Seed*	Papaya Seed
Avocado*	Cherry Kernel	Kukui Nut*	Passion Fruit Seed
Babassu**	Chia Seed	Macadamia Nut	Pastel
Bacuri (*Bukuri*)	Chufa	Macauba	Pataua Fruit
Baobab	Cocoa Butter	Macauba Seed	Pataua Seed
Beechnut	Coconut**	Mafura Butter	Peach Kernel
Black Cumin	Coffee	Mango*	Peanut
Black Currant Seed*	Corn	Mango Butter	Peach Kernel
Black Raspberry Seed	Cottonseed	Mangosteen Butter	Pecan
Blackberry Seed	Cranberry Seed	(*Kokum Butter*)	Pequi
Blueberry Seed	Cucumber Seed	Manketti (*Mongongo*	Perilla Seed
Borage*	Cupuacu Butter	*Nut*)	Pine Nut
Boysenberry Seed	Cynara (*Cardoon*)	Marigold (*Calendula*)	Pistachio Nut
Brazil Nut	Echium	Marula	Pomegrante
Broccoli Seed	Evening Primrose*	Meadowfoam	Poppy Seed
Buriti Fruit	Fenugreek Seed	Mobola Plum	Pracaxi
Buriti Kernel	Flaxseed	(*Parinari Kernel*)	Prickly Pear
Calophyllum*	Grapeseed	Moringa (*Ben or Behen*)	Prickly Pear Seed
Camelina	Gromwell Root	Mowrah Butter	(*Opuntia*)
Camellia	Guanabana	Murumuru Butter	Prunus Kernel

Pumpkinseed*	Sal Butter (*Shorea Butter*)	Shikonin Seed	Tucuma Butter
Quinoa	Sapote	Sisymbrium*	Ucuuba Butter
Ramtil	Saw Palmetto	Soybean*	Walnut
Raspberry Seed	Sea Buckthorn Fruit*	Strawberry Seed	Watermelon Seed
Rhatany Root	Sea Buckthorn Seed*	Sunflower	Wheat Germ*
Rice Bran	Sesame	Tamarind Seed	Wolfberry
Rose Hip Seed	Shea	Tomato Seed	Ximenia Seed
Safflower	Shea Butter	Tucuma	Yangu

Vegetal/carrier oils denoted with one asterisk (*) in the list above can be combined with one of the other vegetal/carrier oils to comprise a percentage of the total mixture. This is usually done since some oils are best used in smaller amounts, as well as to create a blend that has a smooth texture and can be absorbed into the skin during a massage.

The vegetal/carrier oils denoted with two asterisks (**) harden at below room temperature and are appropriate as an ingredient when making an ointment or skin cream.

The specific percentage is indicated under the "Practical Uses" for each individual oil that has an asterisk. For example, a good formula for 1 ounce (30 ml) of a skin-rejuvenating facial oil would be:

Borage*	1 teaspoon (17 percent)
Pine Nut	5 teaspoons (83 percent)

When combining essential oils with the carrier oil(s), blend 12 to 30 drops of the essential oils into 1 ounce (30 ml) of carrier oil.

Thus, with the addition of specific essential oils, the formula for the skin-rejuvenating facial oil becomes:

Pine Nut	5 teaspoons
Borage*	1 teaspoon
Sandalwood	8 drops
Bois de Rose	7 drops
Patchouli	5 drops

An example of two massage oil blends for relaxation/stress reduction would be:

Massage Oil Blend One

Almond (*Sweet*)	4 teaspoons
Mandarin	5 drops
Lemongrass	5 drops
Lavender	5 drops
Ylang-Ylang	5 drops

Massage Oil Blend Two

Evening Primrose*	1 teaspoon
Hazelnut	5 teaspoons
Litsea Cubeba	8 drops
Sandalwood	8 drops
Chamomile (*Roman*)	5 drops
Vetiver	5 drops
Bergamot	4 drops

Helpful Measurement Equivalents

2 tablespoons	=	1 ounce
6 teaspoons	=	1 ounce
1 teaspoon	=	5 ml (milliliters)
1 tablespoon	=	15 ml
1 ounce	=	30 ml
1 teaspoon	=	100 drops
1 tablespoon	=	300 drops

ACAI FRUIT

ACAI SEED

Botanical Name: *Euterpe edulis, Euterpe oleracea*

Family: *Arecaceae*

The fruit oil is obtained from the fruit.

The seed oil is obtained from the seeds.

History and Information

- Acai is a palm tree native to Central and South America. The tree grows in swamps and reaches a height of about 90 feet (27 meters). The flowers are white and are followed by small purple berries with seeds. Acai belongs to a group of palm trees called cabbage palms and is also known as assai.

- The fruits and roots have been used for digestion problems.

- In Brazil, a tea made from the roots is taken as a blood purifier and to help strengthen the liver. The seeds are roasted and made into a drink similar to coffee.

- The fresh fruit has a short shelf-life, therefore products have to be produced from it rather quickly. The fruit is high in vitamin C.

Practical Uses

Skin regeneration, skin care

Hair care

Documented Properties

Antioxidant

ALMOND *(Sweet)*

Botanical Name: *Prunus amygdalus, Prunus dulcis*

Family: *Rosaceae*

The oil is obtained from the nuts.

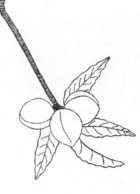

History and Information

- Sweet almond is native to Asia and the Mediterranean region, and is found in dry soils. The medium-sized tree grows to a height of about 35 feet (10.5 meters) and has pinkish-white flowers. There are approximately fifty species of the wild almond trees, but only a few varieties produce a sweet kernel. The cultivated types of almond trees require cross-pollination with another variety.

- Pliny, the Roman herbalist, listed the use of almonds as a treatment for many disorders.

- Throughout the years, women have used almond oil on their face to promote a nice complexion and massaged the oil into their skin to give it elasticity and to prevent wrinkles.

- In Ayurvedic medicine, almonds are taken as a laxative; and it is said they improve eyesight. The nuts and oil are considered aphrodisiacs.

- In Europe, before the eighteenth century, almonds were powdered, soaked in water, and made into a nutritional beverage as a substitute for milk.

- In China, almonds and brown rice are ground up into a powder and taken with water and honey to help or prevent dry throats and other dry conditions.

- In Asia, almonds are eaten to improve memory.

- Almonds are rich in calcium, potassium, magnesium, iron, and phosphorus, and have an oil content of 54 percent.

- Almost all almonds grown in the United States are produced in California, which supplies more than half of the world's production. The second largest producer is Spain. Almonds do poorly in tropical regions since high humidity during ripening may cause rancidity to develop in the kernels.

- Almonds are the most consumed of all the nuts.

Practical Uses

Skin care; moisturizing to the skin

Suntanning oil

The carrier/base oil is used to dilute essential oils in aromatherapy for massage oils and other formulations.

Documented Properties

Alterative, anti-inflammatory, antilithic, antipruritic, antitumor, astringent, carminative, demulcent, diuretic, emollient, galactagogue, laxative, nervine, tonic, vulnerary

Caution: The nuts contain cyanide. It is best to use small amounts of the oil at one time.

AMARANTH

Botanical Name: *Amaranthus candatus, Amaranthus cruentus, Amaranthus hypochondriacus*

Family: *Amaranthaceae*

The oil and CO_2 extract are obtained from the seeds.

History and Information

- Amaranth is an annual plant native to the Americas and India. The plant grows to about 3–5 feet (1–1.5 meters) with lance-shaped purple-green leaves and red flowers. Amaranth is also known as pigweed.

- The Aztecs believed the plant had supernatural powers and that the seeds, when eaten, would give them enormous strength.

- In Peru, the flowers have been used for toothaches and fevers. The flowers are also made into a tea to normalize the menstrual cycle.

- Amaranth has been used to heal wounds, stop nose bleeds, help mouth and throat sores, regulate excessive bleeding during menstruation, soothe inflammation, and for diarrhea.

- The seeds are eaten as a cereal. They contain a high protein content and many essential nutrients and amino acids. The leaves are used as a vegetable.

- The red pigment of the flowers is used to color foods and cosmetics.

- The oil is valued in skin care for moisturizing dry skin, improving elasticity, reducing wrinkles, slowing the skin aging process, and providing healing properties to damaged and itching skin.

- Quinoa is a close relative of amaranth.

- Amaranth isn't a grain.

Practical Uses

Skin care; moisturizing to the skin

Documented Properties

Astringent, cooling

ANDIROBA

Botanical Name: *Carapa guianensis*

Family: *Meliaceae*

The oil is obtained from the nuts.

History and Information

- Andiroba is native to South America. The tree grows in wet locations to a height of about 400 feet (122 meters) and has fragrant flowers, followed by a nut. The tree is also known as Brazilian mahogany.

- In South America, andiroba is used for wound and skin healing, lamp oil, and soap.

- The oil has a short shelf-life.

Practical Uses

Skin care

Documented Properties

Analgesic, anti-inflammatory, antiseptic, emollient, febrifuge, parasiticide, vermifuge

ANNATTO

Botanical Name: *Bixa orellana*

Family: *Bixaceae*

The oil is obtained from the seeds.

History and Information

- Annatto is native to tropical areas in America. The shrub grows to a height of about 20–30 feet (6–9 meters), has oval, leathery green leaves and pink blossoms resembling a rose, followed by a red fruit with small brown seed pods that are surrounded by a red powder. The shrub is also known as anatto, arnatto, and lipstick tree.

- In Latin America, the plant has been used to get rid of intestinal parasites, reduce inflammation, as a tonic, and to heal the skin.

- In Asia, the leaves and seeds are made into a tea to lower body temperature during fevers.

- The fruit produces a red juice that is used as a dye to color fabrics.

- The yellow-orange seed oil is the coloring agent permitted for butter and cheese, and is also used for coloring fabrics, cosmetics, and soaps. The oil is topically applied to treat skin ailments and leprosy.

Practical Uses

Skin care

Documented Properties

Antibacterial, anti-inflammatory, antioxidant, antiseptic, antitussive, astringent, depurative, diuretic, emollient, expectorant, febrifuge, hepatic, hypotensive, parasiticide, purgative, stomachic

APRICOT KERNEL

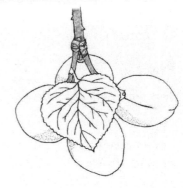

Botanical Name:
Armeniaca vulgaris,
Prunus armeniaca

Family: *Rosaceae*

The oil is obtained from the kernels.

History and Information

- Apricot is native to Asia. The tree grows to a height of about 35 feet (10.5 meters), has white to pink flowers and orange-yellow fruit.

- The Hunza women use the oil to maintain a nice complexion and wrinkle-free skin.

- In northern China, the apricot tree is primarily cultivated for its edible nuts, which are almost identical to almonds.

- The oil is similar in texture and properties to almond oil.

Practical Uses

Skin care; moisturizing to the skin

The carrier/base oil is used to dilute essential oils in aromatherapy for massage oils and other formulations.

Documented Properties

Analgesic, anthelmintic, anti-inflammatory, antioxidant, antirheumatic, antiseptic, antispasmodic, antitumor, antitussive, aphrodisiac, demulcent, emetic, emollient, expectorant, laxative, nourishing (skin), pectoral, sedative, vulnerary

Caution: The kernels contain cyanide. It is best to use small amounts of the oil at one time.

ARGAN

Botanical : *Argania sideroxylon, Argania spinosa*

Family: *Sapotaceae*

The oil is obtained from the nuts.

History and Information

- Argan is an evergreen tree native to Africa, and is found in dry soils. It is tolerant of drought and high heat. The shrubby tree reaches a height of about 30 feet (9 meters), has a thorny trunk, and small greenish-yellow flowers, followed by small yellow bitter fruits that contain brown nuts inside. The tree is also known as Moroccan ironwood tree.

- Argan has softening, protective effects on the skin, and revitalizes damaged skin.

- The nuts have an oil content of over 50 percent.

- The oil has a short shelf-life.

Practical Uses

Skin care; silky, nongreasy, absorbs easily into the skin

Documented Properties

Regenerator (skin)

AVOCADO

Botanical Name:
Persea americana,
Persea gratissima

Family: *Lauraceae*

The oil is obtained from the kernels.

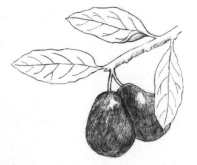

History and Information

- Avocado is an evergreen tree native to the Americas. The tree grows to a height of about 30–60 feet (9–18 meters), has dark-green oval leathery leaves and greenish-yellow flowers that develop into yellow, green, red, or purple, or black fruit. The pulp is soft and buttery with a large kernel inside. Avocado grows in many tropical regions.

- Avocados were highly esteemed by the Aztec and Maya Indians.

- The fruit was used for stomach upsets, ulcers, to regulate menstruation, and topically placed to heal skin bruises, burns, and irritations.

- In Latin America, the leaves are made into a tea and taken to abort a fetus, and to help with menstrual problems. A bark tea is also made for menstrual discomfort. The fresh kernels are eaten to help the liver and regulate blood sugar.

- In the country of Zaire, a beer is brewed from the avocado leaves.

- The unripe fruit is said to be poisonous. Its unripe powdered kernel is mixed with cheese to poison mice.

- Avocados have been recommended for a person to eat three to five fruits daily to help inflamed areas, muscle and joint problems, digestion, to regulate the bowels, as a liver and gall bladder cleanser, and contributes to the overall well-being of the body.

- Avocado oil is very nourishing to the skin, and is known to contain vitamins A, B, C, and E, and especially large amounts of vitamin D and potassium. The avocado has the highest protein content of any fruit. The oil is extensively used in cosmetics.

- The oil is very stable, having a shelf-life of more than ten years.

Practical Uses

Skin care; moisturizing, removes impurities from the skin

The carrier/base oil is used to dilute essential oils in aromatherapy for massage oils and other formulations. For massage oils, it is best to mix 20 percent of avocado oil with another carrier oil before adding the essential oils.

Documented Properties

Abortifacient, hepatic, rejuvenator, restorative, tonic, vulnerary

Comments: Poisoning of animals feeding on the leaves, bark, and fruit of the avocado tree has been reported. The leaves soaking in water have killed fish. However, the ripe fruit and oil, in moderate amounts, seem safe to humans.

BABASSU

Botanical Name: *Orbignya barbosiana*

Family: *Arecaceae*

The oil is obtained from the kernels.

History and Information

- Babassu is a wild and fast-growing palm tree in Brazil that reaches a height of about 66 feet (20 meters). The fruits are fleshy with a hard shell on the outside. Babassu tastes and smells like coconut but yields a higher amount of oil. The tree is also known as aguassu or babacu.

- The Amazonian people use every part of the tree for food, shelter, utensils, and clothing.

- The properties of the oil are similar to, and sometimes substituted for, coconut oil. Babassu oil is used in cooking, margarine, fuel, lubricants, detergents, soaps, and cosmetics. The oil has a longer shelf-life than other palm tree oils.

Practical Uses

Skin care; soothing to the skin; helps with stretch marks

The carrier/base oil is used to dilute essential oils in aromatherapy for massage oils and other formulations.

Documented Properties

Anthelmintic, antibacterial, antidote, antiseptic, aperient, aphrodisiac, astringent, emollient, depurative, diuretic, hemostatic, laxative, moisturizing, purgative, refrigerant, stomachic, vermifuge

BACURI *(Bukuri)*

Botanical Name: *Platonia esculenta, Platonia insignis*

Family: *Guttiferae; also Clusiaceae*

The oil is obtained from the seeds.

History and Information

- Bacuri is an evergreen tree native to Brazil. The tree grows to a height of about 70–125 feet (21–38 meters), has leathery dark-green leaves and reddish flowers that develop into a tart-sweet yellow-orange fruit with a thick rind, which contains seeds that taste like almonds.

- In the Amazon region, the fruits are highly valued.

- The seeds have a high oil content. The oil is used in soaps and candles. It is also known as bacury oil.

Practical Uses

Skin care; moisturizing to the skin

Documented Properties

Rejuvenator (skin)

BAOBAB

Botanical Name: *Adansonia digitata, Adansonia grandidieri*

Family: *Malvaceae;* also *Bombaceae*

The oil is obtained from the seeds.

History and Information

- Baobab is native to the African continent and Madagascar and is found in frost-free areas. The tree can reach as high as 50–60 feet (15–18 meters) and the trunk can be wider around. Baobab has a thick grey bark, sparse foliage, large dark-green leaves, and large white fragrant flowers with purple stamens. The edible green oval fruit has a thick covering and contains many black seeds inside.

THE AROMATHERAPY ENCYCLOPEDIA

The fruit can weigh several pounds. The trees are said to have a lifespan of 2,000–4,000 years. It is one of the longest-lived and most useful trees in Africa. Baobab is also known as monkey-bread tree. There are eight species of the tree.

- The seeds are surrounded by a white powder that is rich in vitamin C and other valuable nutrients. The powder is made into a cereal and a refreshing drink that is used to reduce fevers. The leaves and fruit also contain large amounts of vitamin C, and were used as a tonic and source of nutrition.

- The gum from the tree has anti-inflammatory properties.

- The large trees can store more than two hundred gallons of water inside the trunk. During droughts, people would access the water. The name "Tree of Life" was given for this reason.

- The bark was used for fevers and malaria. The leaves have been taken as a diuretic, to get rid of parasites, reduce fevers, infections, sweating, and for breathing congestion. The leaf extract has been topically applied to promote skin healing, relieve pain, and reduce bacterial infections and inflammation. The young leaves are eaten as salad.

- The seeds are high in protein and are eaten in a paste or made into oil.

- In Africa, the bark, wood, and fruit pulp are taken for fevers; the bark and leaves for urinary conditions; and the powdered seeds for hiccups.

- The wood yields a strong fiber to make cloth and other products.

Practical Uses

Skin care

The carrier/base oil is used to dilute essential oils in aromatherapy for massage oils and other formulations.

Documented Properties

Antifungal, antimicrobial, rejuvenator (sensitive skin)

BEECHNUT

Botanical Name: *Fagus grandifolia, Fagus sylvatica*
Family: *Fagaceae*
The oil is obtained from the nuts.

History and Information

- Beechnut is a deciduous tree native to the Northern Hemisphere. The tree grows to a height of about 80–150 feet (24–46.5 meters). The female flowers are green and the male flowers are yellow. The nuts are enclosed in prickly burrs. They open as the nuts mature in the fall season. There are ten species of the beechnut tree. The usual lifespan of the tree is about 300 years, but there are some that live to 500 years.

- Pliny, the Roman herbalist, praised the nuts as a food.

- The Greeks added the buds and young leaves to salads and in soups.

- North American Indians also valued the beechnuts as a food.

- In France, ground beechnuts have been made into a drink as a substitute for coffee.

- The bark tea was used as a remedy for fevers.

- The nuts are rich in nutrients, high in protein, and have an oil yield of about 50 percent. The oil is used as a salad oil or a substitute for butter. The nuts can be eaten fresh, dried, or roasted, but the fresh nuts spoil in a relatively short period of time.

- The wood of the tree is strong and hard, and is used for furniture.

Practical Uses

Skin care; soothing to the skin

The carrier/base oil is used to dilute essential oils in aromatherapy for massage oils and other formulations.

14

BLACK CUMIN

Botanical Name: *Nigella sativa*

Family: *Ranunculaceae*

The oil is obtained from the seeds.

History and Information

- Black cumin is native to Asia and the Mediterranean region. The plant grows to a height of about 1 foot (.5 meter), has greyish-green leaves, and white or blue flowers, followed by black seeds.

- The plant was cultivated by the ancient Egyptians. It was used as a spice and for medicinal purposes.

- The Romans used the seeds to flavor foods.

- The seeds have been used to expel intestinal worms, for stomach and liver conditions, to promote the flow of breast milk, relieve muscle and joint aches, help breathing conditions, and improve the appetite and digestion.

- In Europe and Asia, the seeds are used medicinally to raise body temperature, increase the pulse, stimulate the flow of urine, and promote perspiration.

- The French use black cumin as a substitute for pepper.

- The vegetal oil and essential oil are obtained from the seeds. However, the method of extraction is different for both oils. See Black Cumin essential oil in Chapter 3 on page 80.

- The essential oil is an ingredient in lipsticks and perfumes.

Practical Uses

Skin care

Documented Properties

Abortifacient, analgesic, anesthetic, anthelmintic, antibacterial, anticonvulsant, antidiabetic, antiedema, anti-inflammatory, antimicrobial, antioxidant, antiseptic, antispasmodic, antitumor, antitussive, cardiotonic, carminative, diaphoretic, digestive, diuretic, emmenagogue, galactagogue, hepatic, immune stimulant, laxative

BLACK CURRANT SEED

Botanical Name: *Ribes nigrum*

Family: *Grossulariaceae*

The oil and CO_2 extract are obtained from the seeds.

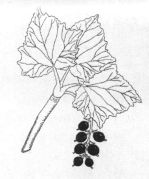

History and Information

- Black currant is a deciduous plant native to Europe and Asia. The plant grows to a height of about 7 feet (2 meters), has greenish flowers and edible black berries.

- Black currants have been cultivated since the beginning of the eighteenth century. They were considered a remarkable life-prolonging food, and the leaves were used as a tea.

- Black currant buds produce an essential oil that is an ingredient in expensive perfumes. The seeds are a valuable ingredient for body and hand creams, sun products, facial care, and hair care. The fruit pulp is added to facial masks. The berries are made into jam, syrup, wine, and liqueurs, and a fruit infusion is used to strengthen weak capillaries.

- Black currants are one of the richest sources of vitamin C.

- The oil contains gamma-linoleic acid (GLA), which is said to help slow down the skin's aging process. It has also has been reported to be helpful in reversing damage from multiple sclerosis, due to the gamma linolenic acid (GLA) content. A lack of GLA in the body prevents nerve cell membranes from functioning properly. GLA is needed for conduction of electrical impulses throughout the nervous system.

Practical Uses

Helps premenstrual stress

Relieves menstrual pain; reduces inflammation

Skin care; soothing and healing to the skin

The carrier/base oil is used to dilute essential oils in aromatherapy for massage oils and other formulations.

For massage oils, it is best to mix 20 percent of black currant seed oil with another carrier oil before adding the essential oils.

Documented Properties

Antibacterial, antidiarrhoeic, antilithic, antirheumatic, antisclerotic, antiscorbutic, diaphoretic, diuretic, hepatic

BLACK RASPBERRY SEED
BLACKBERRY SEED

See Raspberry Seed

BLUEBERRY SEED

Botanical Name:
Vaccinium myrtillus

Family: *Ericaceae*

The oil is obtained from the seeds.

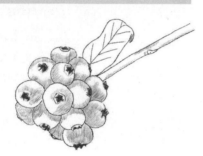

History and Information

- Blueberry is native to regions of the Northern Hemisphere in damp forest meadows. The shrub grows to a height of about 5 feet (1.5 meters), has green leaves and clusters of white flowers followed by round blue berries. The plant is also known as bilberry, huckleberry, and whortleberry.

- Herbalists in history used the leaves and berries to treat coughs, digestive problems, fever, muscle and joint pains, diarrhea, vision, and eye problems.

- The most valuable components in the fruits are flavonoids, which are powerful antioxidants.

- Blueberries are known to have antiaging properties.

Practical Uses

Skin care

The carrier/base oil is used to dilute essential oils in aromatherapy for massage oils and other formulations.

Documented Properties

Antioxidant

BORAGE

Botanical Name:
Borago officinalis

Family: *Boraginaceae*

The oil and CO_2 extract are obtained from the seeds.

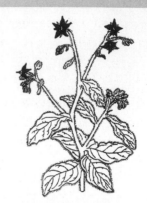

History and Information

- Borage is native to the Mediterranean region. The plant grows to a height of about 2–4 feet (.5–1.5 meters), has large pointed oval leaves, and star-shaped, sky-blue or purple flowers. The scent of the plant is similar to a cucumber.

- The ancient Celtic warriors drank a wine made with borage before battle to increase their courage. Roman soldiers also used borage for courage.

- Pliny, the Roman herbalist, and Dioscorides, the Greek physician, recommended borage for lifting one's spirits.

- In France, borage is used to lower fevers and for lung discomforts.

- The oil contains one of the highest amounts of gamma-linoleic acid (GLA), which is said to help slow down the skin's aging process. It has also been reported to be helpful in reversing damage from multiple sclerosis. A lack of GLA in the body prevents nerve cell membranes from functioning properly. GLA is needed for conduction of electrical impulses throughout the nervous system.

- The leaves of the plant contain alkaloids that may be harmful to the nervous system.

Practical Uses

Calming

Helps premenstrual stress

Relieves menstrual pain; reduces inflammation

Skin care; inflamed skin

The carrier/base oil is used to dilute essential oils in aromatherapy for massage oils and other formulations. For massage oils, it is best to mix 20 percent of borage oil with another carrier oil before adding the essential oils.

Documented Properties

Antidepressant, antidote, anti-inflammatory, anti-rheumatic, aperient, astringent, calmative, decongestant, demulcent, depurative, diaphoretic, diuretic, emollient, expectorant (mild), febrifuge, galactagogue, hepatic, hypotensor, nervine, refrigerant, regenerator (skin), regulator (menstrual), sedative, stimulant (mild) (bowels), sudorific, tonic

BOYSENBERRY SEED

See Raspberry Seed

BRAZIL NUT

Botanical Name: *Bertholletia excelsa*

Family: *Lecythidaceae*

The oil is obtained from the nuts.

History and Information

- Brazil nut is an evergreen tree that grows in the Amazon forests of South America. The tree reaches a height of 100–150 feet (30.5–45.5 meters), has leathery deep-green leaves and white to yellow flowers. The casing for the nuts contains up to approximately twenty nuts that take over a year to ripen on the tree. The nuts are opened with an ax.

- Brazil nuts tend to become rancid quickly unless they are stored in a closed container in a dry, dark, and cool place. The nut is also known as para nut, cream nut, and castanas nut.

- The nuts contain vitamin E and are one of the richest sources of selenium.

- The oil is an ingredient in soaps, creams, and hair products.

Practical Uses

Skin care; moisturizing and soothing to the skin

The carrier/base oil is used to dilute essential oils in aromatherapy for massage oils and other formulations.

Documented Properties

Antioxidant, emollient

BROCCOLI SEED

Botanical Name: *Brassica oleracea*

Family: *Brassicaceae*

The CO_2 extract is obtained from the seeds.

History and Information

- Broccoli is native to the Mediterranean region. The plant grows to about 4 feet (1.5 meters) and has green buds. The vegetable is also known as calabrese.

- Pliny, the Roman herbalist, wrote about the benefits of broccoli, and the Romans favored it as a food.

- Broccoli is a popular vegetable in the western world, where it is prized for its nutritional value. It contains high amounts of beta carotene, iron, folic acid, and vitamin C.

Practical Uses

Skin care

Hair care

Documented Properties

Emollient

BURITI FRUIT
BURITI KERNEL

Botanical Name: *Mauritia flexuosa*

Family: *Arecaceae*

The fruit oil is obtained from the fruit.

The kernel oil is obtained from the kernels.

History and Information

- Buriti is a palm tree native to South America; it is found along rivers, streams, and swamps. The tree grows to a height of about 90 feet (27.5 meters) and has large clusters of flowers that develop into red-brown fruit. There are male and female trees. Buriti is also known as mauriti palm and tree-of-life.

- The fruit and seeds are of great value to the people of Brazil. The fruit is eaten fresh, fermented into an alcoholic beverage, made into flour, and expressed into an edible oil. The leaves are made into ropes and cloth.

Practical Uses

Skin care

Documented Properties

Laxative

CALOPHYLLUM

Botanical Name: *Calophyllum inophyllum*
Family: *Guttiferae*
The oil is obtained from the kernels.

History and Information

- Calophyllum is an evergreen tree commonly found in moist soils in tropical Asia. It is very sensitive to extreme changes in temperature. The tree grows to a height of about 10–50 feet (3–15 meters), has glossy grey leaves, and white flowers that emit a sweet fragrance. The flowers develop into clustered green or yellow fruits that turn light brown when mature. The fruits have a thin pulp and taste similar to an apple. The tree is also known as Borneo mahogany and Alexandrian laurel. The genus has 180 species of plants.

- The ancient Polynesians considered the calophyllum tree sacred because of its valuable medicinal properties. Calophyllum is still used by hospitals in Tahiti and surrounding areas.

- The bark has been used for its diuretic properties

and to stop bleeding. The seeds produce a dark-green oil that has been used for severe skin problems, muscle and joint pains, to remove intestinal parasites, and repel insects.

- The calophyllum kernels are dried in the sun and yield approximately 75 percent oil. The oil has a thick consistency similar to olive oil and is also known as pinnay, dillo, domba, foraha, or tamanu oil. The seeds are called punnai nuts.

- The tree also produces a resin.

Practical Uses

Skin care; healing to the skin

The carrier/base oil is used to dilute essential oils in aromatherapy for massage oils and other formulations. For massage oils, it is best to mix 10 percent of calophyllum oil with another carrier oil before adding the essential oils.

Documented Properties

Analgesic, anti-inflammatory, antiviral, emmenagogue, diuretic, insecticide, regenerator (skin)

CAMELINA

Botanical Name: *Camelina sativa*
Family: *Brassicaceae*
The oil is obtained from the seeds.

History and Information

- Camelina is found in poor soils and produces a large crop. The plant is native to Europe and has been grown there for over 3,000 years.

- In Europe, camelina was an important oil seed plant until the 1940s.

- The seeds contain 40 percent oil, which is also known as gold of pleasure and false flax. The oil is applied to the scalp to protect the hair from dryness, and improves the elasticity of the skin.

- The oil is stable and has an extended shelf-life.

Practical Uses

Skin care; moisturizing to the skin

Documented Properties

Antiaging, antioxidant, emollient

CAMELLIA

Botanical Name: *Camellia japonica, Camellia sinensis*
Family: *Theaceae*
The oil is obtained from the seeds.

History and Information

- Camellia grows wild in the mountains of Japan and China. The plant reaches a height of about 6–20 feet (2–6 meters), has dark-green glossy leaves and snowy white or light pink blossoms with yellow stamens that develop into seeds. Camellia belongs to a family of eighty species of evergreen trees and shrubs. The plant thrives in the colder climates of Asia, blooming in the winter and even when it snows.

- Since recorded history, camellia has been taken as a tea in China.

- White tea comes from the new buds that are steamed or dried. Green tea leaves are steamed and dried. Black tea leaves are rolled, fermented, and dried. The oolong tea leaves are partially fermented and dried.

- Green tea has been taken for its antioxidant properties, as well as its beneficial effect on the cardiovascular system, circulation, breathing, and digestion, for mental clarity, and to heal wounds.

- The oil has been applied topically for centuries by Japanese women for skin and hair care.

- Camellia oil is also known as tsubaki oil. It is used for cooking, frying, to season salads, and in skin care products.

- The seeds contain 40 percent oil.

- The oil oxidizes rapidly when exposed to air.

Practical Uses

Skin care; soothing to the skin

Hair care

The carrier/base oil is used to dilute essential oils in aromatherapy for massage oils and other formulations.

Documented Properties

Analgesic, antimicrobial, antioxidant, astringent, cardiotonic, demulcent, diuretic, expectorant, galactagogue, nervine, stimulant, stomachic

CANDELILLA WAX

Botanical Name: *Euphorbia antisyphilitica, Euphorbia cerifera*
Family: *Euphorbiaceae*
The vegetable wax is obtained from the wax-covered stems and leaves.

History and Information

- Candelilla is native to Texas and Mexico and is found in the desert. The cactus-like plant grows to about 3 feet (1 meter) and has branches covered with a hard wax.

- The wax is an ingredient in cosmetics, ointments, and polishes. It is used instead of beeswax.

Practical Uses

Skin care formulas

Used in making candles, lipsticks, lip balms, and polishes

CANOLA *(Rapeseed)*

Botanical Name: *Brassica napus*
Family: *Brassicaceae*
The oil is obtained from the seeds.

History and Information

- The rape plant belongs to the same family as cabbage and is also known as cole or coleseed. The plant grows to a height of about 3 feet (1 meter) and has rows of yellow flowers.

- In Indonesia, the roots of the plant are used for sore throats and coughs.

Practical Uses

The carrier/base oil is used to dilute essential oils in aromatherapy for massage oils and other formulations.

Comments: The original rape seeds contained 40 percent erucic acid, which is known to be harmful to the thyroid, kidneys, heart, and adrenals. The genetically altered plant variety contains 1 percent of the toxic substance.

CARNAUBA WAX

Botanical Name: *Copernicia cerifera, Copernicia prunifera*

Family: *Arecaceae*

The vegetable wax is obtained from the leaves.

History and Information

- Carnauba is a palm tree native to Brazil, and is found along rivers and in low lying wet areas. The tree grows to a height of about 50 feet (15 meters) and has small greenish-white or brown-yellow flowers, followed by round black fruit. The leaves are coated with wax on both sides. Carnauba is also known as wax palm. There are thirty trees in this species.

- The wax is extracted by shaking the leaves, then boiling them in water.

- The wax was mainly used for candles in the nineteenth century.

- Carnauba is the hardest wax, and raises the melting point of oils and waxes when it is combined with them.

- In the cosmetic industry the wax is used for lipsticks, deodorants sticks, and depilatory waxes. It is also used in polishes and as an emulsifier for cosmetics.

Practical Uses

Skin care formulas

Used in making candles, lipsticks, lip balms, and polishes

CAROB POD

Botanical Name: *Ceratonia siliqua*

Family: *Fabaceae*, also *Caesalpiniaceae*

The oil is obtained from the pods.

History and Information

- Carob is an evergreen tree native to the Mediterranean region, and has been cultivated for as long as 4,000 years. The tree is slow-growing and drought resistant. It reaches a height of about 40–50 feet (12–15 meters), has glossy leaves, and small red or greenish-purple flowers, followed by many leathery pods containing a sweet pulp and five to fifteen seeds. The tree does not bear fruit for the first fifteen years. Once it begins to produce, thousands of pounds of pods can be harvested in a year. Carob is also referred to as locust and St. John's bread.

- In ancient Egypt, a wine was made from the beans.

- Dioscorides, the Greek physician, recommended carob to help digestion.

- Over the years, carob has been useful as a remedy for diarrhea.

- The pod pulp was fermented and made into an alcoholic drink, and the pods were roasted and ground to make flour. The powdered pods are added to foods as a thickener and stabilizer and used as a substitute for cocoa.

- In Europe, the roasted seeds are used as a beverage instead of coffee.

- In the Middle East, the seeds are sweetened and taken for loose bowels, and also applied to warts.

- The seeds are high in protein and fiber.

Practical Uses

Skin care

Documented Properties

Antibacterial, antioxidant, antiseptic, antitumor, antitussive, astringent, demulcent, digestive, laxative, purgative

CARROT ROOT

Botanical Name:
Daucus carota

Family: *Apiaceae*

The oil and CO_2 extract are obtained from the roots.

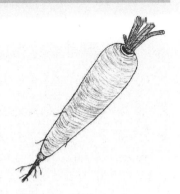

History and Information

- Carrots are native to Afghanistan and the Mediterranean region. The plant grows to a height of about 1 foot (.5 meter) and has white flower heads.

- Carrots were used in medicinal remedies during Roman and Grecian times, and only became recognized as an important food in the sixteenth century.

- The Greeks valued carrots as a tonic for the stomach.

- Initially carrots came from the Middle East, and they were purple and black. Wild carrots have a white root, but they are too tough to be edible.

- In Central and South America, the roots are used as an antifertility agent and to improve skin problems.

- Carrots help to bring on menstruation and stimulate lactation; the seeds are used to eliminate intestinal worms and relax the muscles.

- Carrots are a rich source of valuable nutrients and contain a high amount of vitamin A compared to other commonly eaten vegetables. It has been said that the juice helps neutralize stomach acidity and is important for good vision.

- The root oil is very high in beta carotene and vitamin A. It is used as a yellow food coloring and as a sunscreen in tanning lotions.

- The seed oil is used in perfumes, soaps, detergents, and lotions and as a coloring and flavoring for food, beverages, candy, baked goods, soups, and desserts.

Practical Uses

Skin care; moisturizing to the skin

Hair care; brittle and dry hair

The carrier/base oil is used to dilute essential oils in aromatherapy for massage oils and other formulations. For massage oils, it is best to mix 20 percent of carrot root oil with another carrier oil before adding the essential oils.

Documented Properties

Anthelmintic, antilithic, antioxidant, antipruritic, antisclerotic, aperitive, astringent, carminative, diuretic, emmenagogue, galactagogue, hemostatic, hepatic, laxative, parasiticide, rejuvenator (skin cells), stimulant (uterine), tonic, vasodilator, vermifuge, vulnerary

CASHEW NUT

Botanical Name: *Anacardium occidentale*

Family: *Anacardiaceae*

The oil is obtained from the nuts.

History and Information

- Cashew nut is an evergreen tree native to tropical areas of Latin America. The tree grows to a height of about 20–40 feet (6–12 meters), has leathery leaves and small fragrant pink flowers that develop into edible fruits known as cashew apples. The shell of the nut contains an oily liquid called cardol that is caustic and can cause inflammation and blistering when it comes in contact with a person's skin. Therefore the shells are either soaked in water or roasted before removing the nuts.

- Cashew consists of about sixty species and belongs to the same family as the poison ivy, poison oak, poison sumac, mango, and pistachio. Cashew is also referred to as cajueiro.

- In Ayurvedic texts dating back to the sixteenth century, cashews were mentioned as a skin rejuvenator and appetizer.

- In Latin America, the leaves were applied to the

skin to soothe burns. The bark was made into a tea and taken to relieve congestion, breathing difficulties, regulate blood sugar, and as a gargle for sore throats and inflammation. The fruit juice was used for colds and flu and the leaves, bark, and fruits were made into a tea for digestive problems, urinary disorders, breathing congestion, muscle and joint aches, skin conditions, and as a mouthwash. A tea from the nuts is consumed to help uterine problems. The nuts are said to have an aphrodisiac effect. The oil has been used to treat leprosy and syphills.

- In Brazil, a leaf tea is taken to balance blood sugar levels.

- The bark tea is used to stop bleeding and for diarrhea. A leaf tea is also made for diarrhea.

- In Asia, the young shoots, leaves, and buds are eaten raw.

- The cashew tree excretes a gum that can be substituted for gum arabic. The tree only excretes the gum in abundance when it is infested with parasites.

- India is the largest grower of cashew nuts.

- Cashew apple is a rich source in vitamin C. It can be eaten fresh, added to desserts, or made into jam. The juice is extracted to make a liquor, wine, or fruit juice.

- The nuts yield approximately 45 percent oil. The shell of the nut also yields an oil that is used as an insecticide.

Practical Uses

Skin care

The carrier/base oil is used to dilute essential oils in aromatherapy for massage oils and other formulations. For massage oils, it is best to mix 20 percent of cashew nut oil with another carrier oil before adding the essential oils.

Documented Properties

Anthelmintic, antidiabetic, anti-inflammatory, antitussive, aperitif, astringent, diuretic, febrifuge, hypotensive, purgative, rejuvenator (skin), stomachic, tonic

CASTOR

Botanical Name: *Ricinus communis*
Family: *Euphorbiaceae*
The oil is obtained from the beans.

History and Information

- Castor is native to India. The plant grows to a height of about 5–12 feet (1.5–3.5 meters) and has clusters of yellow or red flowers.

- Castor was one of the first medicinal plants known to humans. The beans were found in an ancient Egyptian tomb.

- The Egyptians added castor oil to beer and drank it as a purgative for cleansing their system. The oil was also used as a cosmetic for the skin and hair, to heal wounds, and induce labor.

- The oil has been applied to the breasts of nursing mothers to increase milk, relieve inflammation, and soften the mammary glands. It has also been used externally for abscesses, itching, dandruff, and hemorrhoids.

- Folk medicine in the 1700s used castor for intestinal parasites, fever, swellings, aching muscles and joints, as a laxative, and for skin conditions.

- The castor beans contain ricin, which is a deadly toxin. The ingestion of one to five seeds can be fatal to a child, and ten seeds can kill an adult. In order to extract a ricin-free oil, the beans must be hulled and crushed at temperatures below 100°F (38°C). After the oil is extracted from the seeds, the ricin remains in the seed cake.

- The oil has a long shelf-life and is added to many food products.

Practical Uses

Blackheads

Hair and scalp care; dandruff

Documented Properties

Analgesic (hot packs for pain and inflammation, recommended by Edgar Cayce), anti-inflammatory, galactagogue, laxative, vermifuge (tapeworms)

CHAULMOOGRA

Botanical Name: *Hydnocarpus anthelmintica, Hydnocarpus kurzii, Hydnocarpus laurifolia, Hydnocarpus wightiana, Oncoba echinata, Taraktogenos kurzii*

Family: *Flacourtiaceae*

The oil is obtained from the seeds.

History and Information

- Chaulmoogra is an evergreen tree native to Asia. The tree grows to a height of about 35–55 feet (10.5–16.5 meters), has long, thin leaves and greenish or white flowers that produce a fruit with seeds. There are forty varieties of chaulmoogra trees. The *Oncoba echinata* variety is known as the gorli shrub.

- Chaulmoogra oil has been used in Hindu medicine for many centuries for skin problems, wounds, leprosy, and muscle and joint aches.

- Chaulmoogra nuts are popular in Asia.

- The oil is also referred to as gynocardia oil, hydnocarpus oil, and krabao's tree seed.

Practical Uses

Skin care

Documented Properties

Analgesic, restorative (skin)

Comments: The botanical species of *Hypnocarpus laurifolia* is safer to use than the other varieties of chaulmoogra, which have been found to be toxic.

CHERRY KERNEL

Botanical Name:
*Prunus avium,
Prunus serotina*

Family: *Rosaceae*

The oil is obtained from the kernels.

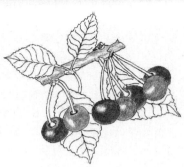

History and Information

- Cherry is native to North America. The tree grows to a height of about 60–80 feet (18–24 meters), has an aromatic bark, green leaves, and clusters of fragrant white flowers that turn into red to purple-black fruits with a round kernel inside. Cherry is also known as black choke, wild black cherry, choice cherry, rum cherry, and bird cherry.

- In folk medicine, the bark was brewed into a tea to ease coughs, colds, breathing congestion, and sore throats; calm nerves and digestive problems, reduce fever, diarrhea, headaches, and help childbirth. A syrup was also made for the same purpose; and the roots were used for intestinal parasites.

- Cherry has been an ingredient to flavor liqueurs, including rum.

- Cherries are said to have a component that cleanses the artery walls of calcium and other deposits when the fruit is eaten fresh.

- The fruit is rich in nutrients and is an antioxidant.

- Over the years, many individuals have stated that cherries and the juice are an effective remedy for muscle and joint aches and gout.

Practical Uses

Skin care; moisturizing to the skin

The carrier/base oil is used to dilute essential oils in aromatherapy for massage oils and other formulations.

Documented Properties

Antioxidant, antitussive, astringent, sedative

Caution: The kernels contain cyanide. It is best to use small amounts of the oil at one time.

CHIA SEED

Botanical Name: *Salvia chia, Salvia hispanica*

Family: *Lamiaceae*

The CO_2 extract is obtained from the seeds.

History and Information

- Chia is native to the Americas. The plant grows to about 2 feet (.5 meter) high.

- Before the Spanish settlers arrived in Mexico, the plant was cultivated there as a food grain to a greater extent than corn.

- The seeds were used for stomach upsets, breathing congestion, fevers, eye problems, and skin complaints.

- Chia seeds have good nutritional value, containing a high amount of protein, amino acids, vitamins, minerals, omega-3, and omega-6.

- The CO_2 extract is a valuable ingredient for skin and hair care. It helps to maintain moisture, prevent drying and scaling, as well as being beneficial for antiaging.

Practical Uses

Calming

Improves mental clarity

Loosens tight muscles

Skin care; moisturizing to the skin

Hair care

Documented Properties

Antiaging, anti-inflammatory, antioxidant

CHUFA

Botanical Name: *Cyperus esculentus*

Family: *Cyperaceae*

The oil is obtained from the tubers.

History and Information

- Chufa is native to Asia and the Mediterranean area. The grasslike sedge plant grows to a height of about 1–3 feet (.5–1 meter) and has underground tubers that have a sweet nutlike flavor. Chufa is also known as earth almond, earth nut, zulu nut, tiger nut sedge, chufa sedge, and yellow nut sedge.

- The tubers have been found in Egyptian tombs dating back to 2400 B.C.

- Theophrastus, the father of botany, described the plant in his writings.

- The tubers have been used as a substitute for coffee in various European countries. The cooked tubers are also used as a vegetable in India, Thailand, and Europe. In Africa, the tubers are chewed to help digestion, sweeten the breath, and encourage the onset of the menstrual period.

- The tubers contain about 30 percent oil content. The oil produced is edible, used in salads and cooking.

Practical Uses

Skin care

Documented Properties

Carminative, emmenagogue

COCOA BUTTER

Botanical Name: *Theobroma cacao*

Family: *Sterculiaceae*

The butter is obtained from the beans.

History and Information

- Cocoa is an evergreen tree native to Central America, where it thrives along riverbanks. The tree grows to a height of about 24 feet (7 meters), has large glossy green leaves and small yellow flowers that grow directly on the trunk and develop into large yellow or red fruits with seeds.

- Cocoa was first introduced to Europe by Christopher Columbus, who learned of its use from the Aztecs.

- In South America, miners were given cocoa leaves to chew to increase their energy level and enable them to work long hours. Today, the leaves are used as a heart tonic.

- In folk medicine, cocoa butter was a remedy for muscle and joint aches, coughs, dryness of the skin, wrinkles, hair loss, burns, and wounds.

- In Europe, cocoa is used to help the nervous system, reduce mental fatigue, and improve digestion and inflammation.

- The beans are used in products such as skin lotions, creams, lipsticks, soaps, suppositories, and in the manufacturing of chocolate. The butter is a base for ointments and salves to soothe the skin. An essential oil known as theobroma oil is produced from the fruit and beans of the tree.

- Theobromine is an alkaloid component of the cocoa bean, which is responsible for its stimulating effect.

Practical Uses

Stimulant

Skin and hair moisturizer

Documented Properties

Antioxidant, antiseptic, diuretic, emmenagogue, emollient, moisturizer, stimulant, tonic

COCONUT

Botanical Name: *Cocos nucifera*

Family: *Arecaceae*

The oil is obtained from the nuts.

History and Information

- Coconut is a large evergreen palm tree found growing along the seashore in the tropics. The tree reaches a height of about 100 feet (30.5 meters), has green fronds, and small sweet-scented flowers that produce fruits protected by a hard shell. One tree can produce forty coconuts annually. The tree is indispensable to the survival of millions of people, who rely on it as a primary source of food, drink, clothing, and shelter. The coconut fruit is regarded as one of the most important foods to one-third of the world's population.

- In Latin America, nursing mothers rub coconut milk on their breasts to reduce inflammation. It is also taken as a diuretic. The flesh of the nut assists to expel intestinal parasites; the root decoction reduces excessive bleeding during the menstrual cycle. It is also used for toothaches and as a mouthwash. The oil softens the skin.

- In recent years, much information has been presented about the role coconut plays for attaining good health. Dr. Bruce Fife is one of the world's leading research experts on coconut and other edible oils. In his book, *Coconut Cures,* published by Piccadilly Books, he provides very credible evidence of how unrefined, organic coconut oil prevents heart disease, enhances the immune system, protects against cancer, strengthens the skin and body against free radical damage that causes premature aging, balances blood sugar, and more.

- Coconut has an oil content of 35 percent. It is used in foods, body care, and industrial products.

Practical Uses

Skin care; soothing to the skin, helps with stretch marks

The carrier/base oil is used to dilute essential oils in aromatherapy for massage oils and other formulations. Coconut oil is generally solid at room temperature and, therefore, is useful for making ointments.

Documented Properties

Anthelmintic, antibacterial, antidote, antiseptic, aperient, aphrodisiac, astringent, depurative, diuretic, hemostatic, laxative, purgative, stomachic, vermifuge

COFFEE

Botanical Name:
Coffea arabica

Family: *Rubiaceae*

The oil is obtained
from the beans.

History and Information

- Coffee is a tropical evergreen tree native to Ethiopia. The tree has glossy dark-green leaves and small fragrant white flowers with a jasminelike fragrance. The flowers develop into sweet-tasting purple fruits with two beans inside. In the wild, the tree grows to a height of about 26–33 feet (8–10 meters). When cultivated, it only reaches about 14–20 feet (4–6 meters), but the trees are usually pruned to 4–6 feet (1.2–1.5 meters). There are more than twenty-five species of the coffee tree.

- Prior to being made into a hot beverage drink, coffee was used as a food, wine, and medicine.

- The Muslims highly prized coffee and drank it during prayers, even in the Holy Temple in Mecca.

- By the thirteenth century, coffee became a mainstay of Arabian life. Coffee houses emerged everywhere and became a meeting place where people gathered to discuss events of the day. Until the end of the seventeenth century, practically all coffee was produced in Arabia.

- Coffee drinking was condemned by the clergymen of the church until the seventeenth century, when Pope Clement VIII enjoyed the taste of it so much that he sanctioned its use for all of his followers. After his approval, coffee gained in popularity and coffee houses thrived in Europe.

- In Turkey, a wife could once be legally granted a divorce if her husband failed to furnish her with the daily allotment of coffee.

- In Latin America, the leaves are boiled and used in baths for muscle and joint aches. The leaves are also made into a poultice and placed on painful areas.

- Coffee is the world's favorite beverage. The United States consumes about 20 percent of all coffee grown. Brazil is the largest grower of coffee and produces about 25 percent of the world's supply.

- The oil has been used in anticellulite formulas.

- The leaves contain methyl salicylate, the same component as aspirin.

Practical Uses

Warming

Increases appetite

Stimulant

Mood uplifting, energizing, improves mental clarity

Skin care

Documented Properties

Diuretic, stimulant

Caution: Coffee is an adrenal gland and nervous system stimulant. In large amounts, it can be deleterious to a person's health.

CORN

Botanical Name: *Zea mays*

Family: *Poaceae*

The oil is obtained from the kernels.

History and Information

- Corn is native to the Americas and belongs to the grass family. The plant can reach a height of up to 18 feet (5.5 meters). The vegetable is a very important food staple to many people around the world.

- Corn was first cultivated in Mexico around 3400 B.C.

- In Europe, the corn silk has been used to treat kidney and urinary problems.

- In Latin America, the silk is used as a treatment for hepatitis, in addition to urinary problems, menstrual discomfort, and to stop the flow of breast milk. The husks are made into a tea to stop excessive menstrual bleeding. The powdered kernels are made into a plaster to help skin inflammations and tumors.

- The ground-up corncob and silk are used in China to relieve water retention and urinary stones.

- Corn, corn meal, and corn oil rank among the most consumed foods in the world. The silk is a flavoring for soft drinks, baked goods, ice cream, and candy. Alcohol is made from the corn kernel.

- Corn only has an oil content of 4 percent; therefore, most of the oil produced is extracted through the use of toxic solvents and high temperatures.

- The color of the unrefined oil is dark gold, with a popcorn scent. It is high in unsaturated fatty acids.

Practical Uses

Skin care; moisturizing and soothing to the skin

The carrier/base oil is used to dilute essential oils in aromatherapy for massage oils and other formulations.

Documented Properties

Diuretic, tonic, vulnerary

COTTONSEED

Botanical Name: *Gossypium species*
Family: *Malvaceae*
The oil is obtained from the seeds.

History and Information

- There are many different varieties of cotton plants cultivated throughout the world. The plant grows to a height of about 3 feet (1 meter), has a purple base, heart-shaped leaves, and yellow flowers.

- Cottonseed oil is extracted from the small seeds of the cotton plant and used in shortenings, margarine, salad, and cooking oil.

- Because cotton is generally not considered a food crop, few precautions are taken by growers on the use and selection of pesticides and defoliants.

Caution: The oil should be considered unsafe for consumption or skin use. The seed, stem, and root of the cotton plant produce a substance called gossy-pol, which suppresses sperm production in men. It has been used as an antifertility agent in China. The antifertility effect may become permanent. Twelve months after discontinuing the intake of gossypol, more than 50 percent of the males still showed a sperm count of zero. Female animals were also affected by having aborted pregnancies (Huang, Kee Chang. *The Pharmacology of Chinese Herbs.* CRC Press, 1993. p. 255).

CRANBERRY SEED

Botanical Name: *Vaccinium macrocarpon*
Family: *Ericaceae*
The oil is obtained from the seeds.

History and Information

- Cranberry is an evergreen shrub native to North America, Europe, and Asia. The shrub grows in swampy areas to a height of about 3 feet (1 meter), has dark-green oval leaves and clusters of pink flowers that turn into red berries.

- Native American Indians used the berries to help the digestion, ease nausea; for liver, kidney, and urinary tract problems; and as a dressing for wounds.

- English sailors ate cranberries to help prevent scurvy.

- The pilgrims in the United States ate cranberries during the first Thanksgiving celebrations.

- In the early 1900s, U.S. researchers found cranberries to be beneficial for urinary infections.

- People with kidney stones are advised not to exceed drinking a maximum of thirty-two ounces a day of the juice, since high amounts of oxalic acid contained in cranberries can irritate this condition.

Practical Uses

Skin care

Documented Properties

Antimicrobial, antioxidant, astringent, diuretic

CUCUMBER SEED

Botanical Name: *Cucumis sativus*

Family: *Cucurbitaceae*

The oil is obtained from the seeds.

History and Information

- Cucumber is native to Asia. The spreading plant has yellow flowers, followed by long green fruits containing many seeds inside.

- In ancient civilizations, cucumber was applied to the skin for its skin healing properties, in addition to being eaten as a food.

- Cucumber has been used mostly as a remedy for its diuretic properties and as a blood pressure balancer.

- Cucumber juice has been used to help heal the skin and for cosmetic purposes.

- In Latin America, the sliced fruit is placed topically for eye problems and inflammations.

- In the Middle East, cucumber is applied to help heal skin conditions and sunburn.

- The fruit pulp and seeds are used in cosmetics for face masks and as an ingredient in skin lotions and shampoos.

Practical Uses

Skin care; facial masks

Documented Properties

Anthelmintic, antibacterial, anti-inflammatory, antiseptic, demulcent, diuretic, febrifuge, purgative, vermifuge

CUPUACU BUTTER

Botanical Name: *Theobroma grandiflorum*

Family: *Sterculiaceae*

The butter is obtained from the seeds.

History and Information

- Cupuacu is native to Central and South America.

The tree grows to a height of about 25–60 feet (7.5–18 meters). The flowers are dark red or purple; the reddish-brown fruit weighs approximately one to eight pounds, has a tough skin, and contains around fifty seeds inside. The tree is also known as cupuassu.

- The pulp is made into beverages, baked goods, candies, jams, and ice cream. The seeds produce a chocolate and oil.

- The seeds yield about 50 percent of an oily butter.

Practical Uses

Skin care; moisturizing to the skin

Documented Properties

Anti-inflammatory, antioxidant, emollient, hydrating (skin)

CYNARA *(Cardoon)*

Botanical Name: *Cynara cardunculus*

Family: *Asteraceae*

The oil is obtained from the seeds.

History and Information

- Cardoon is native to the Mediterranean region. The plant grows to about 4 feet (1 meter) high, has grey-green leathery leaves and thistlelike lavender-colored flowerheads. The plant is closely related to the globe artichoke and the sunflower, but it resembles celery.

- Cardoon was known as edible thistle as far back as biblical times. The Romans praised it as a vegetable. Cultivated plants spread to different parts of the world as people moved to new locations and brought the plant with them.

- The plant has been used to help with muscle and joint pain and improve liver and gall bladder function.

- The vegetable has been popular in Europe since the seventeenth century, eaten in salads and cooked in stews.

- Cardoon was considered an unwanted weed by farmers, and expensive eradication efforts were waged to eliminate the plant.

Practical Uses

Skin care

Documented Properties

Antirheumatic, cholagogue, digestive, diuretic, hepatic

ECHIUM

Botanical Name: *Echium plantagineum*

Family: *Boraginaceae*

The oil and CO_2 extract are obtained from the seeds.

History and Information

- Echium is an annual plant native to the Mediterranean region, where it is found on grassland. The plant grows to a height of about 1–3 feet (.5–1 meter), has long green leaves and large blue-purple, sometimes pink, or white, flowers. The name of the plant is purple viper's bugloss, but it is also known as blueweed and wild borage.

- The leaves were used to relieve headaches and promote sweating to lower fevers.

- The oil is a rich source of gamma-linolenic acid (GLA), and omega 3 and omega 6 fatty acids. The GLA is important to regulate prostaglandin levels in humans. A lack of GLA occurs when people grow older and their bodies aren't able to produce it in sufficient amounts. This deficiency prevents nerve cell membranes from functioning properly. GLA is said to help slow down the skin's aging process. It has also been reported to be helpful in reversing damage from multiple sclerosis. GLA is needed for conduction of electrical impulses throughout the body.

- The oil helps improve skin problems, reduce inflammations, and is used in antiwrinkle applications and overexposure to the sun.

Practical Uses

Helps premenstrual stress

Relieves menstrual pain; reduces inflammation

Skin care

Documented Properties

Anti-inflammatory, antioxidant, antiwrinkle, cardiotonic, rejuvenative (skin)

Comments: The plant itself is poisonious to grazing animals, however, the oil from the seeds is said to be nontoxic.

EVENING PRIMROSE

Botanical Name: *Oenothera biennis*

Family: *Onagraceae*

The oil and CO_2 extract are obtained from the seeds.

History and Information

- Evening primrose grows to a height of about 1–8 feet (.5–2.5 meters) and has many fragrant yellow flowers that open at dusk to attract night flying insects for pollination. The plant originated in North America and was exported to Europe during the seventeenth century. Evening primrose is also known as evening star and king's cure-all.

- The American Indians made a preparation from the roots and applied it on their muscles to improve their strength and heal bruises. The roots were also used to treat obesity and hemorrhoids. The flowers were applied externally to heal bruises and skin problems.

- The seeds, flowers, leaves, and roots can be eaten cooked or raw, or in a salad. The roots taste similar to turnips.

- Evening primrose oil contains gamma-linoleic acid (GLA), which is said to help slow down the skin's aging process. It has also been reported to be helpful in reversing damage from multiple sclerosis. A lack of GLA in the body prevents nerve cell membranes from functioning properly. GLA is needed for conduction of electrical impulses throughout the nervous system.

- The oil contains a high amount of essential fatty acids.

- The ground-up flowers are an ingredient in cosmetic face masks.

Practical Uses

Helps premenstrual stress

Relieves menstrual pain; reduces inflammation

Skin care; moisturizing and soothing to the skin

The carrier/base oil is used to dilute essential oils in aromatherapy for massage oils and other formulations. For massage oils, it is best to mix 20 percent of evening primrose oil with another carrier oil before adding the essential oils.

Documented Properties

Analgesic, antiarthritic, anti-inflammatory, antiscorbutic, antispasmodic, antitoxic, astringent (mild), calmative, depurative, diuretic, febrifuge, hepatic, hypotensor, nervine, stimulant, tonic, uplifting

FENUGREEK SEED

Botanical Name: *Trigonella foenum-graecum*

Family: *Fabaceae*

The CO_2 extract is obtained from the seeds.

History and Information

- Fenugreek is an herbaceous plant that grows up to 2 feet (.5 meter) and has fragrant white flowers that turn into a pod with yellow seeds.

- In writings from 1000 B.C., there is evidence to show that fenugreek was cultivated in the Middle East and the seeds were used by the Egyptians for embalming.

- Dioscorides, the Greek physician, wrote that fenugreek was an active component in his ointments. He recommended it for women's problems.

- Emperor Charlemagne ordered cultivation of the plant in the ninth century.

- Chinese medicine began using fenugreek in the eleventh century.

- In folk medicine, the herb was taken for breathing congestion, to increase the flow of breast milk, and lower blood sugar levels; a poultice made from the herb was applied to reduce inflammations.

- In Africa, the seeds have been used to balance blood sugar; for digestion, coughs, muscle and joint aches; and as a general tonic.

- The herb has been used as a tonic to strengthen the body for those with physical debilitation, to relieve menstrual irregularities, and to reduce inflammation of swollen glands.

- In the Middle East, the seeds are taken for fevers, bone fractures, blood sugar imbalances, and heart-lung problems. The fresh leaves are added to stews and the seeds flavor foods.

- Fenugreek is used in perfumes, soaps, detergents, lotions, and in foods as an ingredient in curry powder and other blends of spices. The powder makes skin-nourishing cosmetic face masks.

- The seeds are used to make a yellow dye.

Practical Uses

Warming

Improves digestion, soothes the intestines

Calming, reduces stress

Helps premenstrual stress

Loosens tight muscles

Skin care

Documented Properties

Alterative, anthelmintic, antiatherosclerotic, antidiabetic, anti-inflammatory, antioxidant, antiseptic, antispasmodic, antitumor, antiviral, aperient, aphrodisiac, astringent, cardiotonic, carminative, contraceptive, demulcent, digestive, emmenagogue, emollient, estrogenic, expectorant, febrifuge, galactagogue, hepatic, hypotensor, immunostimulant, nutritive, restorative, tonic, vulnerary

FLAXSEED

Botanical Name:
Linum usitatissimum

Family: *Linaceae*

The oil is obtained
from the seeds.

History and Information

- Flax has been cultivated from before recorded history and, therefore, its place of origin is uncertain. The plant grows to a height of about 2 feet (.5 meter), has sky-blue flowers and brown seeds.

- Flax was one of the first crops to be cultivated by Mesopotamians and Egyptians. Cloths made of flax fiber were found in Egyptian burial chambers.

- In Switzerland, archaeologists discovered flaxseed and flax fiber cloth, with an estimated date of about 5000 B.C. For at least two centuries, the flax plant was one of the main sources of fabric for American clothing.

- Hippocrates mentioned the use of flaxseed to relieve inflammation of mucous membranes and abdominal pains.

- Emperor Charlemagne considered flaxseed so important to health that he issued a decree requiring its consumption.

- The oil was a folk remedy for lung congestion and tumors.

- Throughout history, flax has been used to maintain the health of animals. Farmers have reported that pregnant cows fed flaxseed gave birth to healthier calves. When flaxseeds are added to the diets of pets, their fur coat improves.

- In Europe, flaxseed was used as a laxative, to help congestion of the breathing passages, and for the urinary tract. Flax poultices were applied to swellings, skin problems, and aching muscles and joints.

- Ayurvedic medicine uses flax leaves to help breathing congestion and coughs.

- In the Middle East, the seeds in water are taken to relieve constipation, digestive upsets, and urinary inflammations.

- In Germany, Dr. Johanna Budwig, a world-renowned holistic doctor who studies and researches the effect of vegetable oils on the body, treats seriously ill patients by adding freshly pressed flaxseed oil to their diet.

- The unrefined fresh flax oil is a rich food source of both essential fatty acids. It contains 15 to 25 percent linoleic acid and 50 to 60 percent linolenic acid, which are necessary for good health. In addition, the oil is rich in lecithin and contains all of the essential amino acids and almost every known trace mineral. The oil spoils easily; therefore, to preserve the valuable properties, it is best stored in the freezer.

- The seed has an oil content of 35 percent.

Practical Uses

Skin care

The carrier/base oil is used to dilute essential oils in aromatherapy for massage oils and other formulations.

Documented Properties

Anti-inflammatory, antirheumatic, antiseptic, antitumor, antitussive, astringent, cardiotonic, demulcent, digestive, emmenagogue, emollient, laxative, purgative

GRAPESEED

Botanical Name:
Vitis vinifera

Family: *Vitaceae*

The oil is obtained
from the seeds.

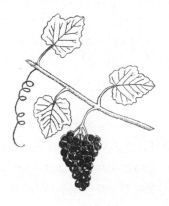

31

History and Information

- The grape is a climbing vine native to Asia. The vine grows to about 30 feet (9 meters) and has green flowers that develop into sweet green or purple-red fruits.

- The Egyptians made wine as far back as 3500 B.C., and dried grapes to make raisins before that time.

- References to the healing properties of grapes can be found in the writing of ancient Egyptians, Hippocrates, and the other Greek and Roman physicians.

- Grapeseed oil is produced from the residue of grapes that were pressed for wine. The oil is widely used in creams, massage oils, and on people who are allergic to other oils.

Practical Uses

General skin care

The carrier/base oil is used to dilute essential oils in aromatherapy for massage oils and other formulations. Grapeseed is a light oil and has a smooth texture.

Documented Properties

Anti-inflammatory, antimutagenic, antioxidant, cardiotonic

Comments: The majority of grapeseed oil is extracted with the use of solvents.

GROMWELL ROOT

See Shikonin Seed

GUANABANA

Botanical Name: *Annona muricata*

Family: *Annonaceae*

The oil is obtained from the fruit.

History and Information

- Guanabana is an evergreen tree native to Central America and the West Indies. The tree grows to a height of about 20 feet (6 meters), has glossy, fragrant, dark-green leaves and large yellow-green flowers that develop into kidney-shaped dark-green prickly fruits with leathery skins and soft spines. The white flesh is aromatic and juicy, containing black seeds inside. The edible fruit, also known as soursop, can weigh five or more pounds. Other names for guanabana are guanba and catoche.

- In Latin America, the leaf tea is taken to lower blood pressure, overcome nervousness, for pain relief, fevers, childbirth delivery, and to increase breast milk. The juice is consumed for liver conditions.

- The leaves are used for colds, congestion, and liver problems. The bark, roots, and leaves are made into a tea, which is taken to balance blood sugar, as a relaxant, for nervousness, and to promote sleep. The fruit is made into ice cream.

- A sweet-sour juice is extracted from the fruit for a cooling drink.

- Both the seeds and leaves contain alkaloids that can be harmful to the body. The seeds, known to be toxic, are used to get rid of topical parasites and as a fish poison and insecticide. The seed oil is applied to the scalp to kill lice.

Practical Uses

Skin care

Documented Properties

Antibacterial, antifungal, antispasmodic, galactagogue, hepatic, sedative

HAZELNUT

Botanical Name:
Corylus avellana

Family: *Betulaceae*

The oil and CO_2 extract are obtained from the nuts.

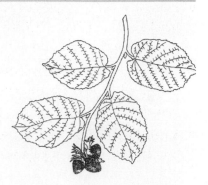

History and Information

- Hazelnut is a deciduous tree native to Europe and Asia. The tree grows to a height of about 12–30 feet (3.5–9 meters), has green leaves, light-yellow catkins, and red female flowers that develop into nuts. Hazelnut is also known as filbert nut and cob nut.

- The American Indians used the bark for hives, fevers, and wounds, and used the twigs to expel intestinal parasites.

- The nut is rich in oil, containing a 62 percent content.

- The powdered nuts are used as an ingredient in cosmetic face masks. The oil is rich in vitamin E and easily absorbs into the skin.

Practical Uses

Skin care; moisturizes, softens, repairs dry and damaged skin

The carrier/base oil is used to dilute essential oils in aromatherapy for massage oils and other formulations.

Documented Properties

Antilithic, aphrodisiac, astringent (mild), parasiticide, stomachic, tonic

HEMP

Botanical Name: *Cannabis indica, Cannabis sativa*
Family: *Cannabaceae*
The oil is obtained from the seeds.

History and Information

- Hemp is native to Asia. The plant grows to a height of about 10 feet (3 meters), has green flowers and small green fruit that contain seeds.

- The hemp plant is one of the oldest crops to be cultivated in Asia for fiber, food, oil, herbal use, and as a tranquilizer.

- Since ancient times, hemp was used for digestive problems, headaches, pain relief, and restful sleep.

- In ancient China, the seeds were added to the daily cuisine.

- Folk medicine used the herb for blood poisoning, snakebites, pain reliever, menstrual cramps, sleeplessness, and depression.

- In the Middle East, hemp was used as incense.

- In Asia and Africa, hemp was used in religious services and magic. The seeds were burned to create a calming smoke. The juice from the plant was helpful for earache.

- In the United States, hemp was sold over the years by physicians to relieve pain until it became illegal in the 1930s.

- Hemp was legalized in Canada in 1998.

- The herb has been used as an appetite stimulant.

- In China, hemp seeds are toasted and eaten as a snack. In Japan, the seeds are used as a seasoning to flavor foods. The seeds contain 20 percent protein, essential amino acids, valuable nutrients, and a balanced ratio of essential fatty acids.

- Hemp oil is used topically on the hair to stop hair loss, for wound healing, and skin care. It is said that the oil is helpful to the immune system.

- The fiber from the hemp plant is used in clothing, rope, cloth, shoes, paper, and fiberboard. Hemp fibers are strong and durable.

Practical Uses

Skin care

The carrier/base oil is used to dilute essential oils in aromatherapy for massage oils and other formulations. For massage oils, it is best to mix 20 percent of hemp oil with another carrier oil before adding the essential oils.

Documented Properties

Analgesic, anesthetic, anthelmintic, antiemetic, anti-inflammatory, antimicrobial, antispasmodic, cholagogue, demulcent, diuretic, emmenagogue, emollient, febrifuge, hallucinogen, intoxicant, laxative, moisturizing, sedative, tonic, vermifuge

ILLIPE BUTTER

Botanical Name: *Shorea stenoptera*

Family: *Dipterocarpaceae*

The butter is obtained from the nuts.

History and Information

- Illipe is native to Malaysia. The tree grows to a height of about 50–70 feet (15–21 meters) and produces nuts that have an acornlike covering. The nuts are known as borneo tallow nut.

- The nuts yield an edible fat that has a high melting point.

- The butter is used in lip balms, lipsticks, deodorant sticks, and soaps.

Practical Uses

Skin care; moisturizing to the skin

Documented Properties

Rejuvenator (skin and skin elasticity)

JOJOBA

Botanical Name: *Simmondsia chinensis*

Family: *Buxaceae*

The vegetable wax/oil is obtained from the beans.

History and Information

- Jojoba is an evergreen shrub native to the southwestern United States and northern Mexico. The plant grows to a height of about 3–18 feet (1–5.5 meters) and has small leathery leaves. There are male and female plants. The male flowers are yellow; the female flowers are green and develop into olive-shaped, dark-brown, nutlike fruits containing seeds. The seeds are called goat nuts. Jojoba plants can live up to 200 years.

- Historically, jojoba oil has been used as a hair restorer.

- The American Indians used jojoba oil for cooking and applied it to soothe the skin. The seeds were

made into a beverage and consumed instead of coffee.

- The oil is similar to, and can be used as a substitute for, sperm-whale oil. The wax is used to make candles, furniture polish, and floor wax, and in industry to lubricate machinery because it can withstand high temperatures. The oil is added as an ingredient in shampoos, moisturizers, sunscreens, and hair conditioners. Jojoba oil is stable and, if stored properly, can last for many years without spoiling.

Practical Uses

Skin care; moisturizes and softens dry skin, helps with stretch marks

Suntanning oil for those who burn easily in the sun

Scalp and hair care

The carrier/base oil is used to dilute essential oils in aromatherapy for massage oils and other formulations. For massage oils, it is best to mix 50 percent of jojoba oil with another carrier oil before adding the essential oils.

Documented Properties

Anti-inflammatory, antiseptic, emollient

KALAHARI MELON SEED

See Watermelon Seed

KAPOK SEED

Botanical Name: *Ceiba pentandra*

Family: *Malvaceae;* also *Bombacaceae*

The oil is obtained from the seeds.

History and Information

- Kapok is native to the Central and South America. The tree grows to a height of about 75–150 feet (23–46 meters) and has large white, yellow, or pink flowers that open at night for the purpose of pollination, followed by a leathery brown fruit capsule with a thick skin and many brown seeds surrounded by thick fibers similar to cotton.

- The fibers, called silk cotton, are many times lighter than cotton and are used to stuff pillows.

- The root extract helps with blood sugar problems. The gum has been used to treat stomach upsets, the bark to lower fevers, and the fruit to alleviate headaches. The bark and leaves help improve breathing congestion and are applied externally for sprains and wounds.

- The edible seeds yield about 25 percent oil, which is said to be almost identical to cottonseed oil.

Practical Uses

Skin care

Documented Properties

Astringent, diuretic, hemostatic

KARANJA

Botanical Name: *Pongamia glabra, Pongamia pinnata*
Family: *Fabaceae*
The oil is obtained from the seeds.

History and Information

- Karanja is a deciduous tree native to India. The tree grows to a height of about 40–80 feet (12–24 meters), has glossy green leaves and fragrant white to pink flowers that develop into a thick leathery oblong pod containing a seed. The tree is also known as Indian beech, poonga-oil tree, and karum tree.

- In Asia, the fruits and seeds have been used for tumors.

- The bark has been used to strengthen the nerves.

- In Ayurvedic medicine, the oil is widely used to treat skin problems.

- The juice from the leaves is taken for colds, coughs, and stomach problems.

- Karanja oil is also known as hongay oil, and is an ingredient in soaps and candles.

Practical Uses

Skin care

Documented Properties

Anthelmintic, antibacterial, carminative, depurative, febrifuge, insecticidal, styptic, tonic, vulnerary

KIWIFRUIT SEED

Botanical Name:
Actinidia chinensis

Family:
Actinidiaceae

The oil and CO_2 extract are obtained from the fruit and seeds.

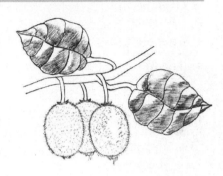

History and Information

- Kiwi is a climbing vine native to China. The vine can reach 25 feet (8 meters), has large heart-shaped green leaves, and white flowers, followed by an egg-shaped brown fruit with many tiny, soft, edible seeds inside. The male and female flowers are on different plants. The plant is also known as Chinese gooseberry.

- The largest producers of kiwifruit are New Zealand and France. Kiwi plants were brought to New Zealand from China in the early 1900s and were named after a bird whose appearance and color looked similar to the fruit.

- In China, kiwi leaf decoction has been used for mange in dogs.

- The fruit was used for the treatment of scurvy, heart and circulatory conditions, urinary tract stones, and to cleanse the liver.

- It has been recommended for a person to eat three to six kiwis daily to benefit the circulatory system, for healthy gums, and to promote good health.

- The kiwi fruit provides an excellent source of nutrients and vitamin C. It contains up to eight times more vitamin C than citrus. They are among the highest sources of antioxidants and an excellent provider of nutrients. The fruit also contains carotenoids that are beneficial to good health and eyesight.

- The seeds contain a rich amount of vitamin E.

- The young leaves of the plant are edible and are added to salads or cooked in soups.

- The oil is unsuitable as a cooking oil because it becomes unstable when heated.

Practical Uses

Skin care

The carrier/base oil is used to dilute essential oils in aromatherapy for massage oils and other formulations. For massage oils, it is best to mix 20 percent of kiwifruit seed oil with another carrier oil before adding the essential oils.

Documented Properties

Antimicrobal, antioxidant, antiscorbutic, astringent, cardiovascular protection, regenerator (skin), tonic

KUKUI NUT

Botanical Name: *Aleurites moluccana*

Family: *Euphorbiaceae*

The oil is obtained from the nuts.

History and Information

- Kukui nut is an evergreen tree native to Asia. The tree grows to a height of about 70 feet (21 meters), has glossy heart-shaped leaves and small clusters of white flowers that develop into nuts. The kukui nut tree is also referred to as varnish tree, candlenut tree, and candleberry tree. Kukui is the official tree of the State of Hawaii.

- The Polynesian people use the nuts as a food source and fuel for their torches. The oil is taken

as a laxative; and the wood of the tree is made into canoes.

- In Indonesia, the oil is used to treat hair loss and soften calluses.

- In China, the oil is massaged into the scalp to stimulate hair growth.

- Kukui nuts are also known as candlenuts because they are used as candles.

- The nuts are roasted and eaten. For some people, they act as a strong purgative.

- The nuts yield 60 percent oil, which is also known as lumbag oil.

Practical Uses

Skin care; balances, rejuvenates, and softens the skin

The carrier/base oil is used to dilute essential oils in aromatherapy for massage oils and other formulations. For massage oils, it is best to mix 20 percent of kukui nut oil with another carrier oil before adding the essential oils.

MACADAMIA NUT

Botanical Name: *Macadamia integrifolia, Macadamia ternifolia, Macadamia tetraphylla*

Family: *Proteaceae*

The oil is obtained from the nuts.

History and Information

- Macadamia is an evergreen tree native to Australia. Macadamia integrifolia grows to about 60 feet (18 meters) tall and has glossy oblong leaves. Macadamia tetraphylla reaches 40–50 feet (12–15 meters) and has dark-green leaves. Macadamia ternifolia grows to a height of about 15 feet (4.5 meters) and has dark-green glossy leaves. Depending on the variety, the trees have clusters of white, pink, or pale brown flowers that produce hardshelled brown nuts. The nuts are also known as Queensland nut, Australian nut, bauple nut, and bopple nut.

- Macadamia was first domesticated in Australia in the mid-1800s.
- The nuts have an oil content of 71 percent.

Practical Uses

Skin care; softens and restores the skin

The carrier/base oil is used to dilute essential oils in aromatherapy for massage oils and other formulations.

MACAUBA

MACAUBA SEED

Botanical Name: *Acrocomia aculeata, Acrocomia sclerocarpa, Bactris globosa*

Family: *Arecaceae*

The pulp oil is obtained from the fruit.

The seed oil is obtained from the seeds.

History and Information

- Macauba is a palm tree native Central and South America. The tree grows to a height of about 30–50 feet (9–15 meters), has a grey trunk, long leaves, and yellow flowers that develop into green fruits that contain seeds. The tree is also known as macaw palm, gru gru, and corozo.
- The seeds are hard and have to be roasted to be eaten.
- The sweet sap of the tree is fermented to make a wine.
- The edible fruits and seeds each contain oil. The seeds yield 50 percent oil that is semisolid, fragrant, and sweet tasting. It is used as an ingredient in making soaps.
- The leaves are used to make rope.

Practical Uses

Skin care

Hair care

MAFURA BUTTER

Botanical Name: *Trichilia emetica, Trichilia roka*

Family: *Meliaceae*

The butter is obtained from the seeds.

History and Information

- Mafura is a fast-growing evergreen tree native to Africa, and is found in rich soils around river banks and coastal forests. The tree grows to a height of about 30–65 feet (9–20 meters), has narrow, leathery deep-green leaves, and fragrant white or green flowers. The male and female flowers are on different trees. The edible fruit is green-brown or red and pear shaped with soft black seeds inside. The tree is known as natal mahogany, cape mahogany, woodland mahogany, and bitterwood.
- In Africa, the butter has been used for leprosy, aching muscles and joints, and applied to fractures to quicken healing time.
- The bark has been used for intestinal problems, as a purgative, and applied to the skin to get rid of parasites.
- The seeds and aril produce two different oils. The seeds yield up to 65 percent butter, which is solid at cold temperatures. The butter has a bitter taste and is used by the native people for cooking. The seeds are reported to be poisonous, but the poison is located only in the outer coating. When the skins are removed from the seeds, it is considered permissible to eat. The butter is said to be safe to use. The aril oil is sweet and is used to make a drink and added to foods.

Practical Uses

Skin care

Hair care

Documented Properties

Anti-inflammatory, antimicrobial, antirheumatic, purgative, vulnerary

MANGO
MANGO BUTTER

Botanical Name: *Mangifera indica*

Family: *Anacardiaceae*

The oil and butter are obtained from the kernels.

History and Information

- Mango is a fast-growing evergreen tree native to Asia. The tree reaches a height of about 65–100 feet (20–30.5 meters), has shiny, dark-green leathery leaves and small fragrant clusters of pinkish-white or light-green flowers that develop into smooth-skinned edible fruits with a large kernel inside. The mango has 210 varieties and is often referred to as the "queen of tropical fruits."

- The tree has been cultivated since 2000 B.C. in India.

- In Asia, the fruit is eaten to increase circulation. The seeds are taken to expel parasites and for diarrhea; the powdered leaves are used to remove warts and stop bleeding.

- The seeds have been used for colds and persistent coughs.

- In Latin America, the ripe fruit is eaten as a laxative. The leaves are rubbed on the teeth to clean them and strengthen the gums. The leaf tea is taken for coughs and breathing problems, for fevers, to lower high blood pressure, and for diabetes.

- The leaves provide a sour flavoring for foods, and the fruit is eaten fresh, dried, or pickled.

- The trunk, branches, and unripe fruit contain a sap that is a skin irritant.

- Consumption of large amounts of the fruit can cause serious problems in the digestive tract.

- Grazing on the leaves for a prolonged period of time has caused animal fatalities.

Practical Uses

Skin care

Hair care

The carrier/base oil is used to dilute essential oils in aromatherapy for massage oils and other formulations. For massage oils, it is best to mix 20 percent of mango oil with another carrier oil before adding the essential oils.

Documented Properties

Anthelmintic, antidiabetic, astringent, emollient, laxative, moisturizing (very dry skin), vermifuge

MANGOSTEEN BUTTER
(*Kokum Butter*)

Botanical Name: *Garcinia indica choisy, Garcinia mangostana*

Family: *Guttiferae*, also *Clusiaceae*

The butter is obtained from the kernels.

History and Information

- Mangosteen is a slow-growing evergreen tree native to Asia. The tree grows to a height of about 30–50 feet (9–15 meters), has large, leathery, thick, glossy dark-green leaves, large pink flowers, and an edible, thin-skinned, reddish-purple fruit containing seeds. The fruit is about the size of an orange, and has a thick hard rind with white flesh inside. The male and female flowers are on separate trees. The tree can yield more than one thousand fruits in a season. Mangosteen is also known as black kokam, kokum butter tree, and mangosteen oil tree.

- In Asia, the tea from the leaves and bark is taken for fevers and mouth ulcers.

- In China, the dried fruits are made into an ointment for skin problems.

- The fruit is said to strengthen the circulatory and immune systems.

Practical Uses

Skin care; moisturizing and soothing to the skin

Documented Properties

Anthelmintic, antimicrobial, antiscorbutic, astringent, cardiotonic, demulcent, diuretic, rejuvenator (skin elasticity)

MANKETTI (Mongongo Nut)

Botanical Name: *Schinziophyton rautanenii*

Family: *Euphorbiaceae*

The oil is obtained from the nuts.

History and Information

- Manketti is native to Africa; it is found in high elevations. The tree grows to a height of about 45 feet (14 meters), has dark-green leaves and small light-yellow or white flowers, followed by round, tough-skinned, brown fruits the size of small plums. The flesh is sweet and contains an edible kernel inside. The outer shell is hard to open. The male and female flowers are on different trees. It can be twenty-five years before the tree produces its first crop. Many trees are nonbearing. Manketti is also known as featherweight tree.

- The nuts are among the most popular foods consumed by the native people. They are highly nutritious and have been eaten, raw or roasted, for thousands of years.

- The oil from the kernels is highly valued for helping restore skin tissue to a healthy state.

- The oil contains a substantial amount of vitamin E that keeps it stable, for a good shelf-life.

Practical Uses

Skin care

Hair care

The carrier/base oil is used to dilute essential oils in aromatherapy for massage oils and other formulations.

Documented Properties

Emollient, skin protectant

MARIGOLD (Calendula)

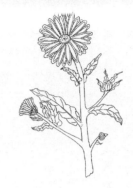

Botanical Name:
Calendula officinalis

Family: *Asteraceae*

The oil and CO_2 extract are obtained from the flowers.

History and Information

- Marigold is native to Central America and Europe. The plant grows to a height of about 3 feet (1 meter), has leathery leaves and large yellow-orange or reddish flowers with a strong scent. There are about fifty species of the marigold plant.

- South American Incas planted marigolds together with other plants to reduce insect damage.

- Since the earliest times, calendula has been grown throughout Europe to flavor soups and stews.

- In folk medicine, marigold was used for dry skin, bee bites, inflammatory conditions of the intestines, constipation, intestinal parasites, coughs, cramps, fevers, and liver problems.

- During the Civil War, European settlers came to America and used the plant to stop bleeding and promote the healing of wounds.

- A tea from the flowers is taken for menstrual problems, coughs, liver conditions, fevers; and applied externally on skin eruptions and inflammations.

- The Arabs feed marigold flowers to their thoroughbred ponies to keep their circulatory vessels healthy. These ponies are highly esteemed all over the world.

- A powder made from the dried flowers is used to season foods and as a coloring agent. The flowers and leaves are eaten in salads and made into an herbal tea.

Practical Uses

Skin care; skin eruptions, bruises, boils, corns, eczema, acne, damaged skin and tissue, burns, sunburns;

chapped, sensitive, rough, inflamed skin, insect bites and stings

Documented Properties

Analgesic, anthelmintic, antibacterial, antifungal, anti-inflammatory, antiseptic, antispasmodic, antiviral, aperient, astringent, blood purifier, carminative, cholagogue, depurative, diaphoretic, digestive, diuretic, emmenagogue, febrifuge, healing, hemostatic, hepatic, laxative, stimulant (mild) (circulatory system), stomachic, styptic, sudorific, tonic, tonifying (skin), vermifuge, vulnerary

MARULA

Botanical Name: *Sclerocarya birrea, Sclerocarya caffra*

Family: *Anacardiaceae*

The oil is obtained from the nuts.

History and Information

- Marula is native to Africa; it is found in drier soils. The tree grows to a height of about 40–60 feet (12–18 meters), has thin grey-green leaves and green-white, white-pink, or red flowers followed by clusters of yellow plum-like fruit with leathery tough skins, juicy flesh, and a large seed containing two or more edible kernels inside. The kernels are hard to remove, requiring pounding with rocks to crack the hard shell. The tree produces a prolific amount of fruit that fall to the ground when green and then ripen to yellow. The male and female flowers are on different trees. The tree plays a vital role in providing sustenance to the people living where it grows.

- Archeological evidence shows that the marula fruit was consumed around the time of the ancient Egyptians.

- In Africa, the leaves and root bark have been used as a remedy for snakebites. The bark infusion was used for inflammation, malaria, and to strengthen the heart. The natives preserve meats for up to a year by putting the nut oil on it and then storing the meat in a cool place.

- Zulu women in Africa boil the fruit and seeds in water until it yields an oily residue. It is then applied to the skin for beauty treatments. The fruit is added to bathwater and rubbed on animals that are infested with insects.

- In folk medicine, marula was used for muscle and joint aches, cramps, stomach upsets, as a relaxant, and to improve sleep.

- The bark has been used for fevers and to improve circulation.

- A beer and liqueur, as well as jams, are made from the fruit.

- The fruits are high in vitamin C.

- The bark is a source of a red dye.

- The nuts contain 60 percent oil and are high in protein.

- The oil has been an ingredient in soaps, skin- and sun-care products, and for insect bites.

Practical Uses

Skin care; hydrating and soothing, absorbs easily into the skin.

Documented Properties

Anti-inflammatory, antioxidant, cardiotonic, depurative, hydrating (skin), sedative

MEADOWFOAM

Botanical Name: *Limnanthes alba, Limnanthes douglasii*

Family: *Limnanthaceae*

The oil is obtained from the seeds.

History and Information

- Meadowfoam is an annual plant native to the United States; it is found in wet areas. The spreading plant grows to about 1 foot (.5 meter) and has shallow, cup-shaped, fragrant yellow-white flowers that produce seeds.

- The oil yield from the seeds is about 30 percent and has a very stable shelf-life.

Practical Uses

Skin care

The carrier/base oil is used to dilute essential oils in aromatherapy for massage oils and other formulations.

Documented Properties

Emollient

MOBOLA PLUM
(Parinari Kernel)

Botanical Name: *Parinari curatellifolia*

Family: *Chrysobalanaceae*

The oil is obtained from the kernels.

History and Information

- Mobola plum is an evergreen tree native to Africa, and is found in low lying areas. The tree grows to a height of about 35–60 feet (10.5–18 meters), has dark-grey-green leathery leaves and sweet-scented white or yellow-green flowers that develop into small yellow-red or orange-yellow fruit. Some trees bear fruit once every two years. The tree is said to give off an unpleasant scent, especially in hot weather. It is also known as cork tree and sand apple.

- The bark was used to heal fractures, treat fevers, and for chest congestion.

- The fruits are pleasant tasting and are eaten fresh, made into syrup, or used to make beer. The seeds are eaten raw or pressed into oil. The kernel has a high oil content.

- The oil is used for dry skin, hair care, and lip balms.

Practical Uses

Skin care

Hair care

Documented Properties

Rejuvenator (skin)

MORINGA (Ben or Behen)

Botanical Name: *Moringa oleifera, Moringa pterygosperma*

Family: *Moringaceae*

The oil is obtained from the seeds.

History and Information

- Moringa is a fast-growing deciduous tree native to Asia and Africa. The tree grows to a height of about 25–35 feet (7.5–10.5 meters), has large pale-green leathery leaves, white or yellow fragrant flowers, and long brown pods containing many brown seeds. Moringa is also known as the drumstick tree, horseradish tree, and benzolive tree. The genus moringa has fourteen species.

- The plant has been used as a remedy for throat problems; the leaves for nervous conditions, wound healing, to normalize blood pressure, for nervous system problems, constipation, and to improve sleep; the roots for fever, aching muscles and joints, breathing congestion, ear infections, and to stimulate the nerves.

- In folk medicine, the oil was used for skin problems.

- In India, the roots have been used for nervous conditions, epilepsy, a tonic for the heart and circulatory system, and as a stimulant for paralysis.

- In Ayurvedic medicine, the leaves are used to relieve congestion and as a poultice for injuries and swellings. The flowers are used as an aphrodisiac and the oil is used for gout and painful joints.

- In Africa, the liquid extract from the roots, bark, leaves, and flowers, combined with honey, is used to strengthen the nervous system. The leaves have also been used to soothe animal and snakebites.

- It is said that the juice from the leaves helps to eliminate intestinal parasites. The fruit strengthens the liver and pancreas. The gum from the bark is used for diuretic purposes.

- The seed oil is rubbed on the skin to ease muscle and joint discomforts.

- The roots are fleshy and smell like horseradish.

41

The fruit, leaves, and flowers are edible. The seeds yield approximately 40 percent oil and are used in salads, foods, artist paints, lubricants, soaps, cosmetics, and perfumery. The oil is scentless, colorless, and tasteless; it is resistant to oxidation and has a high melting point.

Practical Uses

Skin care

Documented Properties

Antibacterial, antidote, anti-inflammatory, antimicrobial, antioxident, antiseptic, antispasmodic, cholagogue, depurative, diuretic, emetic, emollient, estrogenic, expectorant, galactagogue, purgative, rubefacient, stimulant, tonic, vermifuge

MOWRAH BUTTER

Botanical Name: *Bassia latifolia, Madhuca indica, Madhuca latifolia*

Family: *Sapotaceae*

The butter is obtained from the seeds.

History and Information

- Mowrah is native to India. The tree grows to a height of about 60 feet (18 meters), has large leaves and fragrant, small clusters of white flowers that develop into green fruit containing seeds. The tree is also known as Indian butter tree.

- The flowers are eaten and made into a drink. They are taken to help strengthen the heart, ease coughs, and for ear problems. The bark is used for leprosy.

- The oil is used in cooking and as an ingredient in soaps.

Practical Uses

Skin care

Documented Properties

Antiwrinkle, cardiotonic, hydrating (skin), rejuvenator (skin and hair)

MURUMURU BUTTER

Botanical Name: *Astrocaryum murumuru*

Family: *Arecaceae*

The butter is obtained from the seeds.

History and Information

- The palm tree grows on the riverbanks within the flood plain. The large fruit has a yellow fleshy-oily pulp with seeds.

- The fruit contains over twice the amount of beta-carotene than carrots.

- The seeds contain 40 percent oil that is edible.

Practical Uses

Skin care

Documented Properties

Emollient, mosturizing (skin and hair)

NEEM

Botanical Name: *Azadirachta indica*

Family: *Meliaceae*

The oil is obtained from the seeds.

History and Information

- Neem is native to Asia. The tree is an evergreen, except in freezing temperature regions. It grows to a height of about 100 feet (30.5 meters), has dark-green leaves and white or yellow fragrant flowers that produce yellow or purple fruit with a seed inside. Neem is also known as nim or margosa tree.

- The neem tree is considered sacred in India.

- The first reported use of neem was by the ancient Indian Harappa culture around 2500 B.C. For centuries, the oil has been used in Asia for skin and hair care, the bark extract for mouth and gum inflammations, and the leaves as an insecticide.

- In countries where the neem grows, every part of the tree is used. A resin is produced when the trunk is wounded. The leaves are added to animal feed for their high protein content, and the seeds and leaves yield an insect repellent. The fruits are sweet tasting and have an olivelike appearance.

- In Africa, neem has been used for malaria.

- The flowers and leaves are edible. The flowers are taken as a tonic, and the oil is made into a preparation for liver and digestive problems.

- The tree contains the chemical component azadirachtin, which interferes with the metamorphosis of insect larvae, preventing the larvae from developing further into pupae. Many leaf-chewing insects find the tree leaves so repulsive that they would rather die of starvation than eat the leaves (*Neem, a Tree for Solving Global Problems.* National Academy Press, 1992).

- Farmers and food merchants add neem to grains in storage to prevent insect infestation.

- The seeds yield approximately 40 percent oil. The oil is an ingredient in toothpastes, lotions, and soaps. The unrefined oil contains sulfur compounds, which contribute to a pungent odor that is similar to garlic.

Practical Uses

Skin care

Documented Properties

Antibacterial, antifungal, anti-inflammatory, antiseptic, insecticide, tonic

NONI SEED

Botanical Name: *Morinda citrifolia*

Family: *Rubiaceae*

The oil is obtained from the seeds

History and Information

- Noni is native to Asia; it is found in forests and off coastal shores. The tree grows to a height of about 30 feet (9 meters), has large leaves and small yellowish-white flowers followed by a white ined-

ible fruit with many seeds. Noni is also known as Indian mulberry.

- The fruit is most commonly used for juice, but the leaves, flowers, seeds, roots, and bark also have therapeutic benefits.

- The Polynesian people applied the large leaves to painful inflamed areas for relief. The juice of the fruit and leaf infusion has been taken for balancing blood sugar, to soothe the digestive system, relieve muscle and joint aches, help breathing problems, relieve headaches, lower fevers, and as a blood purifier.

Practical Uses

Skin care

Hair care

Documented Properties

Analgesic, antibacterial, antidiabetic, anti-inflammatory, antioxidant, astringent, decongestant, depurative, digestive, febrifuge, hepatic, hypotensor, laxative, sedative, tonic

OAT

Botanical Name: *Avena sativa*

Family: *Gramineae*

The oil and CO_2 extract are obtained from the grain.

History and Information

- Oat grass grows to a height of about 4 feet (1 meter).

- Oats were cultivated in 500 B.C. At first, oats were used for medicinal purposes, then later as a food. It is used internally to calm and relax, and topically to heal the skin.

- In Europe, oat straw is put into baths to improve health.

- Oats were recommended to people convalescing from illness to help them recover quicker. It was also used to bring an individual out of nervous exhaustion and depression, as well as to help get a restful sleep and strengthen the female reproductive system.

- Athletes who were on an oat diet had increased endurance.

- Oats have a high content of silica and are beneficial for healthy skin, bones, teeth, hair, and nails. Oats are added to bathwater to soften the skin.

- The oil is hydrating to the skin and added to skin care and baby care products.

Practical Uses

Skin care

The carrier/base oil is used to dilute essential oils in aromatherapy for massage oils and other formulations.

Documented Properties

Antidepressant, antioxidant, antispasmodic, demulcent, diaphoretic, diuretic, emollient, febrifuge, hydrating (skin), laxative, moisturizing (skin), nervine, nutritive, restorative, stimulant, tonic, vulnerary

OKRA

Botanical Name:
Abelmoschus esculentus,
Hibiscus esculentus

Family: *Malvaceae*

The oil is obtained from the seeds.

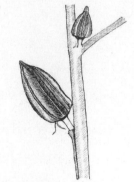

History and Information

- Okra is native to Africa. The plant grows to about 7 feet (2 meters) and has large yellow flowers with a red spot at the base followed by green pods up to twelve inches long, with numerous seeds. The plant is also known as ladies-finger and gumbo.

- The okra mucilage has been used to treat urinary problems, rashes, and other skin conditions.

- The leaves and unripe fruits are applied as a poultice to ease pain.

- The seeds are brewed into a beverage as a coffee substitute.

- The vegetable is highly mucilaginous and is added to soups as a thickener.

- The oil content of the seeds is about 40 percent.

- The fruit is rich in nutrients and vitamin C.

Practical Uses

Skin care; moisturizing to the skin

Documented Properties

Antiaging, diuretic

OLIVE

Botanical Name:
Olea europaea

Family: *Oleaceae*

The oil is obtained from the fruit.

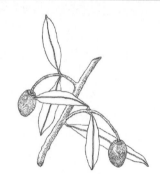

History and Information

- Olive is an evergreen tree native to the Mediterranean region. The tree reaches a height of about 25–40 feet (7.5–12 meters), has a smooth grey bark, leathery greenish-grey leaves, and fragrant clusters of white flowers. Olive trees are slow to mature, requiring ten years to start to bear fruit, and thirty years for a sizable crop to be produced. The trees may reach an age of 1,500 years.

- The first historical mention of the olive occurred in Egypt in the seventeenth century B.C.

- Olive oil was part of religious ceremonies since biblical times.

- The olive was an ancient symbol of peace and prosperity.

- Kings were anointed with olive oil.

- Throughout history, olive oil was the most important of all the vegetable oils. Italy, Spain, Greece, and France produce the finest quality olive oil.

- As a folk remedy, the leaves were used to lower blood pressure and blood sugar levels.

- In Africa, the leaves are taken to regulate blood sugar and blood pressure, relieve muscle and joint aches, and reduce fevers. The leaves are also used in Latin America to normalize blood pressure.

- The leaves have been known to have relaxant properties on muscles and improve circulation.

- The first pressing of the finest selected olives is called extra virgin oil, which is considered the top grade. Virgin oil is considered the second-best grade, and pure olive oil is the third. The pure olive oil is extracted from the pulp and pits left over from the other pressings; it is generally produced by the use of heat and high pressure, solvents, bleaching, and deodorizing.

- Olives yield an oil content of 20 percent. The oil oxidizes less rapidly than other oils and, therefore, has a longer shelf-life.

Practical Uses

Skin care

The carrier/base oil is used to dilute essential oils in aromatherapy for massage oils and other formulations. For massage oils, it is best to mix 20 percent of olive oil with another carrier oil before adding the essential oils, due to its thickness.

Documented Properties

Antipruritic, cholagogue, demulcent, emollient, laxative, relaxant, vulnerary

PALM
PALM KERNEL

Botanical Name: *Elaeis guineensis*
Family: *Arecaceae*
Palm fruit oil is obtained from the fruit.
Palm kernel oil is obtained from the kernels.

History and Information

- Palm is native to Africa. The tree grows to a height of about 70 feet (21 meters), has green fronds and clusters of two hundred to three hundred flowers. The red or black fruits are plumlike in appearance and contain a hard black nut with a white kernel.

- Palm oil has been used for more than 5,000 years.

- A sap exudes from the tree; it is used in Africa as a laxative. The fermented sap is made into a wine taken by nursing mothers to increase lactation.

- The tree yields more oil per acre than any other vegetable oil plant. Two types of oil are produced from the palm tree; both are quite similar to coconut oil and are used in soaps, candles, ointments, margarine, shortenings, and cooking. Palm oil is the second most produced oil in the world—the first being soybean oil.

- During the 1700s, palm oil was used in Britain as a hand cream.

- Both the fruit and seed have an oil content of 35 percent and are especially rich in carotene. Palm oil is solid at room temperature.

- Palm kernel oil is yellowish in color. The pulp oil is reddish-orange.

- Dr. Bruce Fife, one of the world's leading research experts on edible oils, writes about palm oil in his book, *The Palm Oil Miracle,* published by Piccadilly Books. The book states that the virgin red palm oil can protect against many common health problems. Some of the health benefits are: protection against heart disease and cancer, improved blood circulation, blood sugar control, increased nutrient absorption, healthy liver-function support, and more.

Practical Uses

Skin care

The carrier/base oil is used to dilute essential oils in aromatherapy for massage oils and other formulations. For massage oils, it is best to mix 20 percent of palm oil with another carrier oil before adding the essential oils.

Documented Properties

Analgesic, antidote, aphrodisiac, diuretic, galactagogue, laxative, vulnerary

PAPAYA SEED

Botanical Name: *Carica papaya*

Family: *Caricaceae*

The oil is obtained from the seeds.

History and Information

- Papaya is an evergreen tree native to Central and South America; it is found in warm climates. The tree grows to a height of about 25 feet (7.5 meters), has yellow-green leaves and white flowers that turn into sweet, pear-shaped, yellow-orange fruits with many small black edible seeds that taste peppery. Male and female flowers are produced on separate trees. The tree only lives five to six years. Papaya is also known as paw paw.

- In warm climates the trees can produce fruit when they are under a year old. The trees only bear fruit for three to four years.

- In Africa, the root infusion has been used for venereal illnesses; the unripe fruits applied topically for ringworm; the ripe fruits used for digestion and the leaves smoked to help ease breathing congestion.

- In Japan, eating papaya is believed to prevent muscle and joint pains.

- In Latin America, the flowers are brewed into a tea to help with breathing, menstrual problems, and fevers. The unripe fruit is taken for high blood pressure and is made into a poultice and placed on inflammations, ringworm, and skin problems. The ripe fruit is eaten to alleviate constipation. The leaves are placed on cuts or wounds to stimulate healing. The seeds are used to help digestion and act as a laxative. The latex of the plant is taken to expel intestinal parasites and is topically applied for ringworm and warts. When consumed, the latex and unripe fruit can cause pregnant women to abort the fetus. The sap of the tree is used externally to heal skin wounds and for bacterial infections.

- In Brazil, a tea is made from the flowers to strengthen the heart and liver.

- The unripe fruits are eaten to bring on menstruation and also to induce childbirth labor. The flowers help liver problems.

- The juice has been used to remove skin growths and freckles. The leaves, wrapped around wounds and open skin tissue, promote healing. The seeds improve liver and spleen conditions, and are topically applied for ringworm. The fruit and seeds assist in digestion and help expel intestinal parasites.

- Papaya fruits are sweet and contain a large amount of an enzyme, papain, that assists in the digestion of protein. They also contain caroteinoids, which are vital for maintenance of good eyesight, in addition to valuable minerals and vitamins.

Practical Uses

Skin care

Documented Properties

Abortifacient, antibacterial, antifungal, anti-inflammatory, antimicrobial, antioxidant, cardiotonic, carminative, decongestant, diaphoretic, digestive, diuretic, emmenagogue, expectorant, laxative, stomachic, tonic, vermifuge

PASSION FRUIT SEED

Botanical Name: *Passiflora incarnata*

Family: *Passifloraceae*

The oil is obtained from the kernels and fruit.

History and Information

- Passion fruit is a climbing vine native to South America. The vine reaches a height of about 30 feet (9 meters) and has flowers approximately two inches wide with white or lavender petals. Passionflower bears an edible, egg-shaped yellow fruit that is about three inches long. There are over two hundred species of passion flower.

- Native Americans used the flowers to heal bruises

and wounds, calm and encourage sleep, and help settle the nerves.

- Throughout the years, the herb was most commonly used for nervous conditions.

- The American Indians used the leaves and the root as a poultice for injuries and boils and made a tea to calm the nerves.

- In the Americas, the leaves were used for headaches, pain, digestive upsets, to calm the nerves, relax spasms, promote sleep, ease menstrual discomfort, expel intestinal parasites, and heal skin abrasions. The fruit has been used as a heart tonic. The juice has a gentle diuretic effect and is taken to help the urinary tract and to soothe coughs.

- The leaves of the plant are an ingredient in many European medicines for nervous disorders.

Practical Uses

Skin care; soothing to the skin

The carrier/base oil is used to dilute essential oils in aromatherapy for massage oils and other formulations.

Documented Properties

Analgesic, anticonvulsant, antidepressant, anti-inflammatory, antioxidant, antispasmodic, cardiotonic, diuretic, nervine, rejuvenator (skin elasticity), sedative, vermifuge

PASTEL

Botanical Name: *Isatis tinctoria*

Family: *Brassicaceae*

The oil is obtained from the leaves.

History and Information

- The plant grows to about 3 feet (1 meter) and has yellow flowers. Pastel is also known as dyer's woad.

- A blue dye has been made from the leaves since ancient Roman times. The Romans also used the plant to stop bleeding and for wounds.

Practical Uses

Skin care

Documented Properties

Anti-inflammatory, moisturizing

PATAUA FRUIT

PATAUA SEED

Botanical Name: *Jessenia bataua, Jessenia polycarpa, Oenocarpus bataua*

Family: *Arecaceae*

The fruit oil is obtained from the fruit.

The seed oil is obtained from the kernels.

History and Information

- Pataua is a palm tree native to South America. The tree grows 80–90 feet (24–27.5 meters) tall in the rainforest, in areas ranging from wet lowlands to mountainous regions of over 3,000 feet elevation. The tree bears an edible fruit.

- In Central America, the oil is used to alleviate lung congestion.

- The fruit contains over 50 percent oil and is used for hair, skin, and as a laxative. The kernels yield an edible oil that has a good shelf-life and is similar to olive oil. Both oils are used in soaps and cosmetic skin care products.

Practical Uses

Skin care

PEACH KERNEL

Botanical Name:
Prunus persica

Family: *Rosaceae*

The oil is obtained
from the kernels.

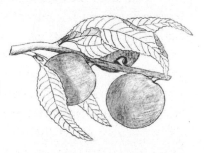

History and Information

- Peach is native to China. The tree grows to a height of about 16–25 feet (5–7.5 meters) and has light-pink to red flowers, followed by juicy yellow, orange, or red fruits with a seed inside.

- Peach leaves have been used for chest congestion, incontinence, as a laxative, and to calm and heal wounds.

Practical Uses

Skin care; moisturizing to the skin

The carrier/base oil is used to dilute essential oils in aromatherapy for massage oils and other formulations.

Documented Properties

Diuretic, expectorant, laxative, sedative

Caution: The kernels contain cyanide. It is best to use small amounts of the oil at one time.

PEANUT

Botanical Name: *Arachis hypogaea*

Family: *Fabaceae*

The oil and CO_2 extract are obtained from the "nuts."

History and Information

- Peanut is native to Central and South America; it is found in warm climates. The plant grows to a height of about 1 foot (.5 meter) and has yellow flowers. After becoming pollinated, the stalk bearing the flowers pushes the pods into the soil. The pods remain there until maturity. The peanut is a legume, not a nut. It is also known as groundnut.

- The peanut has been known as a food since 1500 B.C.

- In China, peanuts are used to stop bleeding and increase lactation in nursing mothers.

- Peanuts are more popular in the United States than any nut.

- About 50 percent of the peanuts grown in the United States are made into peanut butter.

Practical Uses

Skin care

Documented Properties

Galactagogue, hemostatic

PECAN

Botanical Name: *Carya illinoinensis*

Family: *Juglandaceae*

The oil is obtained from the nuts.

History and Information

- Pecan is native to North America and belongs to the walnut family. The tree grows to a height of about 100–170 feet (30.5–52 meters) and has yellow-green flowers followed by a thin-shelled nut. The tree takes over ten years to produce nuts. When it matures, it bears about 200 pounds of pecans.

- Pecan is the official tree in Texas.

- The nuts were a food staple of the American Indians in the southern states.

- The United States is the largest producer, claiming about 80 percent of the world's pecan market.

- Pecans have a high oil content of 71 percent.

Practical Uses

Skin care

The carrier/base oil is used to dilute essential oils in aromatherapy for massage oils and other formulations.

PEQUI

Botanical Name: *Caryocar brasiliense*

Family: *Caryocaraceae*

The oil is obtained from the seeds.

History and Information

- Pequi is an evergreen tree native to South America; it requires a tropical climate. The tree grows to a height of about 60 feet (18 meters) and has flowers that produce a grey-green fruit containing a brown kernel similar to brazil nuts. The fruit can weigh up to six pounds and have up to four nuts inside, also known as souari nuts. The outer shell of the seed has many sharp thorns that face inward. When the shells are opened, these thorns splinter and can penetrate a person's skin.

- The fruit is made into a liquor and the kernels are eaten.

Practical Uses

Skin care

PERILLA SEED

Botanical Name: *Perilla frutescens, Perilla ocimoides*
Family: *Lamiaceae*
The oil is obtained from the seeds.

History and Information

- Perilla is native to Asia. The plant grows to a height of about 3 feet (1 meter) and has green or purple leaves and pink or red flowers. It is also known as shiso.

- In folk medicine, perilla was used for calming, breathing congestion, coughs, colds, flu, fevers, nausea, muscle and joint aches, pain, spasms, and digestive upsets.

- The seed oil has been a remedy in China since the sixth century.

- According to He-Ci Yu, author of the book *Perilla,* published by Harwood Academic Publishers, the seed oil enhances brain activity and nerve systems and suppresses cancer development, thrombosis, and allergic reactions.

- In Japan, the plant has been used to relieve congestion in the breathing passages, nausea, and con-

stipated bowels. The leaves and seeds are eaten, made into tea, and used as a food coloring. The seeds are an ingredient in confectionaries. The seed oil is called egoma.

- The seeds yield about 45 percent oil, which is edible.

- The paint, varnish, and printing industries use the oil because it dries quickly.

Practical Uses

Skin care; moisturizing to the skin

Documented Properties

Analgesic, anti-inflammatory, antioxidant, antiseptic, antispasmodic, antitussive, carminative, diaphoretic, expectorant, febrifuge, sedative, stomachic, tonic

PINE NUT

Botanical Name: *Pinus edulis, Pinus pinea*
Family: *Pinaceae*
The oil is obtained from the nuts.

History and Information

- The Pinus pinea species is native to the Mediterranean region and is also known as Italian stone pine. The tree grows to a height of about 80 feet (24 meters) and has needlelike leaves and nuts inside the cones. Generally, the tree does not bear any edible nuts until its fifteenth year when cultivated and about the twenty-fifth year when growing in the wild. The nuts take approximately three years to ripen. The species of Pinus edulis is native to America; it grows to a height of about 50 feet (15 meters).

- Pine nuts are found in the cones of certain pine trees. They are also referred to as pignolia, pine seed, Indian nuts, and piñons. More than one hundred seeds may be in a single cone.

- Archeological evidence shows the nuts were eaten by the Romans and Greeks.

- The nuts have been prized as a delicacy over the

years, especially in China and Japan. Many Mediterranean dishes contain pine nuts.

- Pine nuts served as an important food staple for Native Americans.

- In the Middle East, the oil is topically applied for skin injuries.

- The nut has an oil content of 55 percent and contains the highest amount of protein of all the nuts.

- Most of the production of the nuts come from Italy and Spain.

Practical Uses

Skin care; soothing and healing to the skin tissues

The carrier/base oil is used to dilute essential oils in aromatherapy for massage oils and other formulations. For massage oils, it is best to mix 20 percent of pine nut oil with another carrier oil before adding the essential oils.

The oil is light in texture and absorbs readily into the skin.

Documented Properties

Antiseptic, hemostatic, purgative, tonic

PISTACHIO NUT

Botanical Name: *Pistacia officinarum, Pistacia reticulata, Pistacia vera*

Family: *Anacardiaceae*

The oil is obtained from the nuts.

History and Information

- Pistachio nut is native to Asia. The tree grows to a height of about 20–40 feet (6–12 meters), has shiny green leaves and red fruit containing edible green or yellow nuts. The male and female flowers are produced on different trees. The tree does not bear fruit until about ten years old. The tree can live to approximately 1,500 years. Pistachio is related to the poison ivy, poison oak, poison sumac, mango, and the cashew nut tree.

- Pistachios have been cultivated for 3,000 years.

- In Asia, the oil is taken to help with stomach problems.

- The nut contains an oil content of 54 percent and is rich in iron. The oil is used in food flavorings and cosmetics.

Practical Uses

Skin care; moisturizing to the skin

The carrier/base oil is used to dilute essential oils in aromatherapy for massage oils and other formulations.

Documented Properties

Analgesic, anticoagulant, antiseptic, antitoxic, aphrodisiac, astringent, demulcent, digestive, hepatic, sedative, tonic

POMEGRANATE

Botanical Name:
Punica granatum

Family: *Punicaceae*

The oil and CO_2 extract are obtained from the seeds.

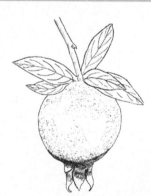

History and Information

- Pomegranate is native to Asia. The shrub grows to a height of about 16–23 feet (5–7 meters), has glossy green narrow leaves and red flowers followed by dark-red fruits with thick skins containing several chambers of many seeds.

- The shrub was cultivated before 2000 B.C.

- In ancient times, a wine was produced from the seeds and mixed with grape wine. In modern day Egypt, pomegranate wine is still made.

- In Chinese medicine, pomegranate was used for intestinal parasites and to stop bleeding. It is listed in the pharmacopoeia in China and Japan.

- In the Arabic countries, the dried fruit peel is made into a tea and taken as a contraceptive.

- In Africa, a tea from the roots or leaves is taken for intestinal parasites and menstrual problems. A tea from the fruit peel is consumed to regulate blood sugar.

- In Latin America, a tea made from the fruit is applied topically to wounds, bruises, lesions, and skin abrasions.

- In Indonesnia, a tea from the fruit peel or root bark is consumed to abort a fetus.

- In Mexico, a flower decoction is made as a gargle to relieve throat inflammation.

- The fruit and rind have been taken for diarrhea. The dried, pulverized flower buds were used to help with congested breathing passages. The bark and root contain alkaloids, which are active against tapeworms. The juice is considered beneficial for leprosy and stomach upset.

- The seed oil is used in skin care to promote skin tissue regeneration, improve elasticity, reduce wrinkles, and provide healing to dry skin.

- Pomegranate fruit contains valuable nutrients including estrone, an estrogen hormone, vitamin B, vitamin C, potassium, magnesium and phosphorous.

Practical Uses

Warming

Calming

Skin care

Documented Properties

Abortifacient, analgesic, anthelmintic, antiaging, antibacterial, antifertility, anti-inflammatory, antioxidant, antiseptic, antispasmodic, antitumor, antiviral, aphrodisiac, astringent, cardiotonic, contraceptive, diuretic, emmenagogue, febrifuge, hemostatic, hypotensive, rejuvenator (skin elasticity), stomachic

POPPY SEED

Botanical Name: *Papaver somniferum*

Family: *Papaveraceae*

The oil is obtained from the seeds.

History and Information

- Poppy is native to the Mediterranean region. The plant is an annual herb that grows to about 4 feet (1.5 meters) high and produces beautiful large flowers, followed by dark seeds.

- Archaeological excavations reveal that the Sumerians used the poppy seeds over 6,000 years ago.

- The plant has been cultivated in the Middle East region for over 3,000 years. The seeds were used by the Egyptians, Greeks, and Romans.

- Poppy was used medicinally as a relaxant and to relieve pain. Physicians in Europe recommended poppy to relieve menstrual cramps, calm the nerves, and improve sleep.

- In the early 1800s, morphine and codeine were isolated from the poppy, which created huge problems with their addictive properties.

- In the Middle East, the seeds are used to stop nosebleeds and relieve pain.

- The seeds are ground and made to thicken and flavor food. The flower petals are used as a food-coloring agent.

- The oil is a food ingredient, as well as being used in soaps, paints, and varnishes.

Practical Uses

Skin care

Hair care

Documented Properties

Abortifacient, analgesic, antibacterial, antidiarrhea, anti-inflammatory, antispasmodic, antitussive, astringent, calmative, carminative, decongestant, demulcent, diaphoretic, emollient, expectorant, febrifuge, hemostatic, hypotensor, narcotic (mild), nervine, sedative, sudorific, tonic, tranquilizer

PRACAXI

Botanical Name: *Pentaclethra filamentosa, Pentaclethra macroloba*

Family: *Fabaceae*

The oil is obtained from the seeds.

History and Information

- Pracaxi is native to Central and South America; it is found on riverbanks around wetlands. The tree grows to a height of about 30–130 feet (9–39.5 meters) and has glossy dark-green leaves with white or yellow flowers that develop into a large pod that changes from green to brown and contains seeds.

- The wood is used as a fish poison.

- The tree has a sap that acts as a blood coagulant.

Documented Properties

Antibacterial, antifungal, antioxidant

Caution: It is said that the seeds contain an alkaloid that is toxic.

PRICKLY PEAR

PRICKLY PEAR SEED *(Opuntia)*

Botanical Name: *Opuntia ficus-indica, Opuntia streptacantha*

Family: *Cactaceae*

The oil is obtained from the fruit.

The seed oil is obtained from the seeds.

History and Information

- Prickly pear is native to the Americas. The cactus grows to a height of about 18 feet (5.5 meters), has spiny leaves, pink flower buds, and yellow to orange flowers; however, the flowers can also be other colors. The red-purple fruits are pear shaped and contain edible seeds. The cactus is also known as nopal, tuna, Indian fig, Indian pear, mission cactus, and barberry pear. The opuntia genus consists of 250 species.

- The cactus has been cultivated by the indigenous people for many centuries, well before the Spainards arrived to the Americas.

- Native American Indians highly regarded prickly pear juice for its diuretic and anti-inflammatory benefits.

- Before childbirth, women ate the fruits to facilitate delivery.

- The fruit juice was put on warts to remove them and taken as an anti-inflammatory. The flowers helped to heal wounds.

- Prickly pear fruit is an important food for many people. The fruits and powdered leaves have been used to balance blood sugar levels. The flowers settled the stomach.

- The juice from the fruit makes a red dye. The pulp is used for face and body creams and hair care products.

Practical Uses

Skin care

Documented Properties

Anti-inflammatory, astringent, laxative, pectoral, vermifuge

PRUNUS KERNEL

Botanical Name: *Prunus domestica*

Family: *Rosaceae*

The oil is obtained from the kernels.

History and Information

- Prunus is native to China, America, and Europe. The tree grows to a height of about 20–35 feet (6–10.5 meters) and has white flowers followed by round or oval fruits. Prunus is also known as plum.

- The seeds are ground up and used for cosmetic face masks.

- Throughout the years, many immigrants who came to the United States from Europe considered prunes a staple food. These people kept their kitchen cupboard stocked with this valuable dried fruit. The prunes would be soaked overnight in a bowl of water. The hydrated plump fruit and water were consumed upon awaking the first thing in the morning. Prunes assured regular bowel movements and helped to avoid constipation. Even back then, people knew the importance of keeping the colon clean.

Practical Uses

Skin care; moisturizing to the skin

The carrier/base oil is used to dilute essential oils in aromatherapy for massage oils and other formulations.

Caution: The kernels contain cyanide. It is best to use small amounts of the oil at one time.

PUMPKINSEED

Botanical Name: *Cucurbita pepo*

Family: *Cucurbitaceae*

The oil is obtained from the seeds.

History and Information

- The pumpkin is native to the Americas. The climbing plant reaches a length of about 30 feet (9 meters), has large leaves, fragrant yellow-orange flowers, and orange fruits. Pumpkins are the largest fruits in the plant kingdom.

- Pumpkins were a staple in the Native American diet.

- In Oriental medicine, a tea made from the seeds, taken over a period of time, is said to help reduce swellings of the legs, ankles, and abdomen.

- In Latin America, Africa, and India, the seeds are used to expel intestinal worms. Some European physicians recommend pumpkin seeds to prevent prostate problems in men. The seeds contain nutrients known to be components of the male hormone testosterone.

- In China, the roasted seeds are eaten to promote longevity.

- The seeds contain up to 40 percent protein and valuable minerals and nutrients.

- The seed has an oil content of 46 percent. Most of the oil is produced in Austria and popularly used to flavor food.

Practical Uses

Skin care

The carrier/base oil is used to dilute essential oils in aromatherapy for massage oils and other formulations. Due to the pumpkinseed oil's sticky nature, it is best to mix 20 percent of the oil with another carrier oil.

Documented Properties

Anthelmintic, anti-inflammatory, diuretic, stomachic, tonic, vermifuge, vulnerary

QUINOA

Botanical Name: *Chenopodium quinoa*

Family: *Chenopodiaceae*

The oil is obtained from the seeds.

History and Information

- Quinoa is native to South America. The plant grows to a height of about 5 feet (1.5 meters).

- Quinoa has been used since 3000 B.C.

- In Latin America, the seeds are a staple food.

- Quinoa is cooked as a cereal. It is rich in protein, amino acids, and other nutrients.

Practical Uses

Skin care

RAMTIL

Botanical Name: *Guizotia abyssinica, Guizotia oleifera*

Family: *Asteraceae*

The oil is obtained from the seeds.

History and Information

- Ramtil is native to Africa. The leafy plant grows to about 3 feet (1 meter) and higher. The flowers are yellow and produce black seeds.

- The seeds are edible and yield up to 50 to 60 percent oil. The oil has a sweet taste and is used as a food condiment. Ramtil oil is mainly used to extend sesame oil. It is also known as ramtilla and warinnua oil.

Practical Uses

Skin care

RASPBERRY SEED
BLACK RASPBERRY SEED
BLACKBERRY SEED
BOYSENBERRY SEED

Botanical Name:
Rubus fruticosus
(Blackberry), *Rubus idaeus* (Raspberry),
Rubus occidentalis
(Black Raspberry
Seed), *Rubus urisinus*
(Boysenberry)

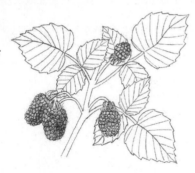

Family: *Rosaceae*

The oil is obtained from the seeds.

Raspberry CO_2 extract is obtained from the seeds.

History and Information

- Raspberry is native to Asia and North America. The shrub grows to a height of about 6 feet (2 meters) and has white flowers that develop into red berries.

- Blackberry is a shrub that grows to about 6 feet (2 meters) tall and has white flowers followed by black berries with seeds.

- Boysenberry is a hybrid, related to the blackberry.

The plant reaches about 6 feet (2 meters) high, and has white flowers.

- The tea from the blackberry leaves is used as a blood purifier, for childbirth, sores in the mouth and skin, and helps a sluggish liver. The leaves have been used for bleeding gums and other bleeding problems, due to their astringent property.

- Raspberry leaf tea has been made for many centuries by pregnant women to reduce chances of miscarriages, ease morning sickness, as a tonic for the stomach, to make childbirth easier, and to help lactation afterwards.

- The raspberry leaf tea has been used as a mouthwash, for skin rashes and skin wounds, and to stop diarrhea.

- The raspberry leaves and fruit are said to be helpful to balance blood sugar levels and strengthen connective tissue.

- Raspberries have a high content of vitamin C.

- Raspberry has been used as a tissue decongestant in cosmetic face masks.

Practical Uses

Skin care; moisturizing to the skin

The carrier/base oil is used to dilute essential oils in aromatherapy for massage oils and other formulations.

Documented Properties

Antimutagenic, antioxidant, astringent, cardiotonic, laxative

RHATANY ROOT

Botanical Name: *Krameria lappacea, Krameria triandra*

Family: *Krameriaceae;* also *Polygolaceae*

The CO_2 extract is obtained from the roots.

History and Information

- Rhatany is an evergreen tree native to South America; it is found in dry hilly areas and mountain slopes. The shrub grows to a height of about 3 feet (1 meter), has a deep root and large red flowers that develop into red fruit.

- In South America, the root has been used for stomach upsets, urinary incontinence, coughs, and diarrhea. It is also used to stop bleeding and discomfort due to inflammation, and is especially helpful for infected gums, bleeding gums, and sore throats. The dried roots are added to oral health products in toothpastes, mouthwashes, and gargles.

- Rhatany CO_2 extract is used in toothpastes and oral care products, hair care, skin care, for antiaging, and to support the skin repair system.

Practical Uses

Calming, relieves tension

Mood uplifting, euphoric; improves mental clarity

Skin care, sun care

Oral care

Hair care

Documented Properties

Abortifacient, antibacterial, anti-inflammatory, antimicrobial, antioxidant, antitussive, antiviral, astringent, diuretic, styptic, tonic

RICE BRAN

Botanical Name: *Oryza sativa*

Family: *Poaceae*

The oil is obtained from the grains.

History and Information

- Rice is native to Asia. The plant grows to a height of about 2–6 feet (.5–2 meters), has narrow blade-like leaves and grains encased in husks.

- Rice has been a food staple since 2500 B.C.

- Rice bran is said to contain a substance that helps prevent deposits in the arteries.

- The bran has an oil content of only 10 percent.

- Rice flour is used in cosmetics as a face powder.

Practical Uses

Skin care; soothing to the skin

The carrier/base oil is used to dilute essential oils in aromatherapy for massage oils and other formulations. The oil has a light texture and readily absorbs into the skin.

Documented Properties

Antidiarrhoeic, depurative, hypotensive, tonic

ROSE HIP SEED

Botanical Name: *Rosa eglanteria, Rosa rubiginosa*

Family: *Rosaceae*

The oil and CO_2 extract are obtained from the hips and seeds.

History and Information

- Rose is native to the Mediterranean region. There are many varieties of the rose bush that grow to various heights and produce fragrant flowers in varying colors.

- Since the beginning of recorded time, the rose has been considered the most valuable flower for beautifying and restoring health to the skin.

Practical Uses

Skin regeneration, skin care; moisturizing, reduces wrinkles

The carrier/base oil is used to dilute essential oils in aromatherapy for massage oils and other formulations. For massage oils, it is best to mix 20 percent of rose hip seed oil with another carrier oil before adding the essential oils.

Documented Properties

Rejuvenator (skin scars and stretch marks)

SAFFLOWER

Botanical Name:
Carthamus tinctorius

Family: *Asteraceae*

The oil is obtained
from the seeds.

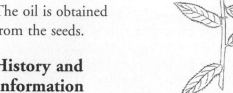

History and Information

- Safflower is native to India. The plant grows about 3 feet (1 meter) high and has orange-yellow flowers.

- The historical use of safflower oil dates back to the ancient times when it was used by the Egyptian pharaohs for cooking.

- During the Middle Ages, the juiced safflower seeds mixed with sweetened water was a recommended drink when suffering from respiratory ailments and constipation.

- The plant was found to have antifertility properties (*Medicinal Plants of China* by James A. Duke, Reference Publications, Inc., page 158).

- Safflower oil was introduced experimentally in the United States as an oil crop in 1925.

- The flower heads yield a red and yellow dye, the seeds produce an oil, and the leaves are eaten as a vegetable. The red dye has been used since ancient times to color cloth, especially silk, and in make-up, such as rouge. The yellow dye is used as a food coloring agent. The seed has an oil content of 59 percent. Approximately 75 percent of the oil consists of linoleic acid, which is an essential fatty acid that plays an important nutritional role in the body. Because it is rich in unsaturated fatty acids, safflower is one of the most popular oils used as a salad and cooking oil. It has also been noted for its ability to slow down digestion and allow the food to combine with the digestive enzymes for proper assimilation.

Practical Uses

Skin care

The carrier/base oil is used to dilute essential oils in aromatherapy for massage oils and other formulations.

Documented Properties

Analgesic, depurative, diaphoretic, digestive, diuretic, febrifuge, hypotensor, regenerator, stimulant (uterine), tonic

SAL BUTTER *(Shorea Butter)*

Botanical Name: *Shorea robusta*

Family: *Dipterocarpaceae*

The butter is obtained from the seeds.

History and Information

- Sal is native to India. The tree grows 90 feet (28 meters) tall and has yellow flowers that develop into yellow-green to red fruits with a seed inside.

- Aromatic gum collected from the stem is called sal dammar, from which chua oil is distilled.

- The bark is used to make a black dye.

- The seeds are eaten mainly during famine times, since consuming too many can be injurous to one's health.

- The seeds yield about 20 percent oil.

- Sal butter is used as substitute for cocoa butter.

Practical Uses

Skin care

SAPOTE

Botanical Name: *Pouteria sapota*

Family: *Sapotaceae*

The oil is obtained from the kernels.

History and Information

- Sapote is native to South America; it thrives in tropical low elevation areas where there is an abundance of moisture and warm weather. The tree grows to a height of about 65–130 feet (20–39.5

meters), has broad leaves and clusters of small greenish-white or yellow flowers that turn into large fruits with a shiny black seed inside.

- Sapote has been used to stop hair loss and promote hair growth, as well as for skin problems.

- In Central America, the oil from the seeds is used for the hair.

- A tea from the bark and leaves is used in Latin America to remove deposits from the blood vessels and balance blood pressure. The white gummy latex from the tree is applied to warts and other growths.

- The seeds have been used for a food flavoring, but are said to be moderately toxic.

Practical Uses

Skin care

Hair care

SAW PALMETTO

Botanical Name: *Sabel serulata, Serenoa repens, Serenoa serrulata*

Family: *Arecaceae*

The CO_2 extract is obtained from the berries.

History and Information

- Saw palmetto is a low-growing palm tree native to the United States, and is found in coastal regions. The tree reaches a height of about 16–20 feet (5–6 meters), has fan-shaped yellow-green leaves with thorny teeth and clusters of small, sweet-scented white flowers that develop into black berries. The tree is also known as cabbage palm, sabal, and shrub palmetto.

- The Native Americans and early settlers used the berries for digestive disorders, urinary tract problems, coughs, inflammation, to open the breathing passages, and as a tonic. An alcoholic drink was made from the fruits, and the seeds were eaten.

- In folk medicine, a remedy was made from saw

palmetto for irritated mucus membranes in the sinus passages and throat.

- The powdered berries are taken by women to stop abnormal hair growth on the body and for menopause.

- The herb is used as a remedy for prostate inflammation and tumors. It is also said to be helpful for urinary and reproductive disorders, as well as hair loss.

- The CO_2 extract is made into a nutritional supplement to help with prostate problems.

Practical Uses

Warming

Reduces stress, relieves tension

Loosens tight muscles, lessens inflammation

Hair care

Documented Properties

Anti-inflammatory (prostate), antimutagenic, antiseptic, antispasmodic, aperient, decongestant, digestive, diuretic, expectorant, galactagogue, nutritive, rejuvenator, restorative, sedative, tonic

SEA BUCKTHORN FRUIT
SEA BUCKTHORN SEED

Botanical Name: *Hippophae rhamnoides*

Family: *Elaeagnaceae*

The fruit oil is obtained from the berries.

The seed oil is obtained from the seeds.

The CO_2 pulp extract is obtained from the berries.

The CO_2 seed extract is obtained from the seeds.

History and Information

- Sea buckthorn is native to Europe and Asia. The thorny shrub grows to a height of about 30 feet (9 meters), has greyish-green narrow leaves and clusters of small yellow flowers that develop into small orange or red berries. There are male and female flowers on different plants.

- Herbal healers in Russia have used the oil for its anti-inflammatory and skin healing properties.

- Sea buckthorn is said to help prevent scarring and has been used to heal wounds as well as damage from radiation.

- The people of Nepal eat the berries raw or preserved.

- The berries are made into jams and are high in vitamin C.

- It is said that the berries help vascular elasticity and stops bleeding.

- The red dye from the fruit is used by women in Asia to color their face and lips. A yellow dye is made from the plant and roots.

Practical Uses

Warming; improves circulation

Relaxing

Mood uplifting

Loosens tight muscles

Softens and heals the skin

Documented Properties

Analgesic, antiaging, antibacterial, anticoagulant, anti-inflammatory, antimicrobial, antioxidant, anti-wrinkle, cardiotonic, hepatic (liver protectant), regenerator (skin)

SESAME

Botanical Name: *Sesamum indicum, Sesamum orientale*

Family: *Pedaliaceae*

The oil is obtained from the seeds.

History and Information

- Sesame is native to Africa and Asia. The plant grows to a height of about 3–6 feet (1–2 meters) and has white or pink tubular flowers with purple spots. The color of the seeds can be white, yellow, red, brown, or black. There are thirty-seven species of the plant. Sesame is also referred to as sim-sim.

Sesame oil is also known as benne oil, gingle oil, and teel oil.

- The seeds and leaves have been eaten in Africa and India since ancient times. It is probably the oldest crop grown for its oil. Records of the production of sesame seeds date back to 1600 B.C.

- The name sesame was included on a list of Egyptian medicinal preparations recorded on papyrus dated about 1550 B.C.

- Women in ancient Babylonia used sesame seeds and honey to increase their vitality for lovemaking and fertility.

- Sesame has been the primary cooking oil in Africa and Asia.

- In Africa, the powdered leaves have been used for coughs and congestion.

- In Oriental medicine, a tea from the seeds is consumed two to three times daily to promote an abundant supply of milk in nursing mothers, improve eyesight, and darken the hair. In China, the seeds are cooked in water and made into a soup to relieve toothaches and swollen gums. A paste from the seeds is recommended for hemorrhoids and to heal sores. The flower and leaf infusions are said to improve hair growth.

- In Latin America, the powdered seeds made into a tea is taken to help nursing women with the flow of breast milk. A leaf tea is used as an eye wash and rubbed into the scalp to stop the hair from falling out. The oil is taken as a nerve tonic and to relieve muscle and joint aches.

- The seed has an oil content of 49 percent. It is more stable and oxidizes less than other oils when heated. The oil has a shelf-life of several years. The raw seeds produce a light-colored oil and the roasted seeds yield a darker-colored oil.

Practical Uses

Skin care; moisturizing and soothing to the skin

Hair and scalp care

The carrier/base oil is used to dilute essential oils in aromatherapy for massage oils and other formulations.

Documented Properties

Demulcent, diuretic, emmenagogue, emollient, galactagogue, laxative, sun protectant, tonic

SHEA

SHEA BUTTER

Botanical Name: *Butyrospermum parkii*

Family: *Sapotaceae*

The oil and butter are obtained from the kernels.

History and Information

- Shea is native to Africa. The tree grows to a height of about 70 feet (21 meters) and has white flowers with a sweet fragrance. The fruit is brown with a large white kernel inside. Generally the trees do not produce fruit until they are twenty years old.

- In Africa, the bark has been used to help ease childbirth delivery. The leaves are taken for headaches. The seeds help with digestive upsets. The butter is used for food and in body care products. It is also employed as a massage oil for sore muscles and applied to heal burns and bruises.

- In Japan, shea butter is consumed as a substitute for dairy butter.

- The seeds contain 50 percent fat content. The bark yields a reddish gum called gutta shea. Shea oil is made from the raw kernels, while shea butter is produced from the roasted kernels that are put through a process. The butter is also known as African butter and karite butter.

Practical Uses

Skin and hair moisturizer; suntan cream

SHIKONIN SEED

GROMWELL ROOT

Botanical Name: *Lithospermum erythrorhizon*

Family: *Boraginaceae*

The seed oil is obtained from the seeds.

The root oil is CO_2 extracted from the roots.

History and Information

- The oils of shikonin seed and gromwell root are extracted from the same plant.

- Native Americans used the plant as a contraceptive. The user was rendered sterile after six months of taking the herb. Gromwell was also taken to purify the system to help with skin conditions and used as a body paint and dye.

- The herb was used to stimulate circulation, clear toxins, and lower fevers.

- The plant has a long history of being used in Chinese medicine.

- The root yields a reddish-purple dye and is extensively used in cosmetics and skin care products.

- The shikonin seed oil contains gamma-linoleic acid (GLA), which is said to help slow down the skin's aging process. It has also been reported to be helpful in reversing damage from multiple sclerosis. A lack of GLA in the body prevents nerve cell membranes from functioning properly. GLA is needed for conduction of electrical impulses throughout the nervous system.

- The leaves of the plant contain alkaloids that may be harmful to the body.

- The seed oil is used to heal burns, wounds, and other skin conditions.

Practical Uses

Skin care

Hair care

The root is used as a red coloring.

Documented Properties of Shikonin Seed Oil

Anti-inflammatory, vulnerary

Documented Properties of Gromwell Root Oil

Antibacterial, antifungal, anti-inflammatory, antipyretic, antitumor, cardiotonic, depurative, febrifuge, vulnerary (burns and wounds)

SISYMBRIUM

Botanical Name: *Erysimum officinale, Sisymbrium officinale*
Family: *Brassicaceae*
The oil is obtained from the seeds.

History and Information

- Sisymbrium is native to North America and Europe. The plant is also known as hedge mustard, which is a common weed that grows up to about 4 feet (1.5 meters) high and has small yellow flowers followed by seeds that resemble mustard seeds.

- Sisymbrium is known for its beautifying properties. Roman women had their servants massage rose and sisymbrium oil on their bodies after bathing.

- In some areas of India, sisymbrium seed infusions are used to treat many skin conditions. In other countries, the seeds are used in facial masks to improve the skin's complexion.

- Sisymbrium was given to people who lost their voice to help them regain it.

- The herb is high in vitamin C and is a tonic.

- In Britain, the plant is eaten as a vegetable.

Practical Uses

Skin care; softens the skin, improves the complexion, reduces wrinkles

The carrier/base oil is used to dilute essential oils in aromatherapy for massage oils and other formulations. For massage oils, it is best to mix 20 percent of sisymbrium oil with another carrier oil before adding the essential oils. Sisymbrium oil absorbs into the skin very quickly, leaving no oily residue.

Documented Properties

Decongestant, diuretic, expectorant, laxative, stomachic, tonic

SOYBEAN

Botanical Name: *Soja hispida*
Family: *Fabaceae*
The oil is obtained from the beans.

History and Information

- Soybean is native to Asia. The bushy plant grows to a height of about 6 feet (2 meters) and has small white or purple flowers.

- The soybean plant was first cultivated in China around the eleventh century B.C. Today, it is one of the world's most important sources of protein.

- The beans are rich in estrogen and could inhibit fertility or help replace estrogen in postmenopausal women.

- Since soy foods have become so popular in recent years in the western world, controversy has developed in the health food field whether these foods are beneficial or harmful to the body. *The Whole Soy Story* by Kaayla Daniel, Ph.D., published by New Trends Publishing, presents evidence of the detrimental effects of soy foods, countering many of the claims by the industry that soy foods are healthy. In addition, most soy beans now grown are genetically modified, posing further dangers to health, according to the experts in the organic food industry.

- Soybean oil contains 2 percent lecithin and essential fatty acids. Choline, found in lecithin, is needed for the proper function of the brain and liver. In addition, choline enables the body to utilize cholesterol and fats, and it prevents deposits of cholesterol in the arterial linings.

- Since the beans only contain 17 percent oil, high temperatures and toxic solvents are commonly used to extract the oil. Soybean oil is used in cooking, margarine, shortening, salad dressing, and for industrial products.

Practical Uses

The carrier/base oil is used to dilute essential oils in aromatherapy for massage oils and other formulations. For massage oils, it is best to mix 10 percent of soybean oil with another carrier oil before adding the essential oils.

Documented Properties

Detoxifier, diuretic, estrogenic, febrifuge, stimulant, tonic

STRAWBERRY SEED

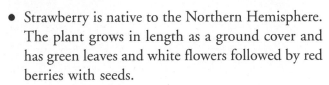

Botanical Name:
Fragaria ananassa,
Fragaria vesca

Family: *Rosaceae*

The oil is obtained from the seeds.

History and Information

- Strawberry is native to the Northern Hemisphere. The plant grows in length as a ground cover and has green leaves and white flowers followed by red berries with seeds.

- A tea made from the leaves was used by Native Americans for diarrhea.

- The dried leaves have been used for liver problems, congestion in breathing passages, muscle and joint pain, nervous tension, and sore throat.

- In Latin America, the leaves are mainly taken to help the kidneys. The leaves act as a diuretic. Both the leaves and roots are used for urinary inflammations and to break up calcifications.

- The berries are very high in vitamin C and are said to help with mouth ulcers and be beneficial to teeth and gums.

Practical Uses

Skin care

Documented Properties

Antioxidant, astringent, diuretic, galactagogue, purgative

SUNFLOWER

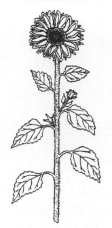

Botanical Name: *Helianthus annuus*

Family: *Asteraceae*

The oil and butter are obtained from the seeds.

History and Information

- Sunflower is native to America. The plant grows to a height of about 6–15 feet (2–4.5 meters), has a tall hairy stem and red to purple rays with large orange-yellow flower petals that look similar to a large daisy. The flower disc produces many edible seeds. There are 110 varieties of sunflower plants, and they belong to the daisy family.

- Sunflowers were first grown as an oil crop in Bavaria in 1725, then in France in 1787.

- Gypsies used the fresh leaves and flowers of the plant to treat malaria.

- The Inca Indians of Peru worshipped the sunflower. The American Indians highly regarded the plant. They used the oil as a tonic for the hair and brewed the flowers to relieve congestion and as a remedy for malaria.

- In Europe, a tea was brewed from the flowers and taken as a remedy for chest congestion and coughs.

- The czars of Russia fed their soldiers two pounds of sunflower seeds as part of their daily food rations.

- Chickens lay more eggs when sunflower seeds are added to their diet.

- The burnt stems are used for potash, and the leaves for an herbal tobacco.

- The seeds have an oil content of 47 percent and contain high amounts of essential fatty acids. The oil is used to make candles and soaps.

Practical Uses

Skin care

The carrier/base oil is used to dilute essential oils in aromatherapy for massage oils and other formulations.

Documented Properties

Antisclerotic, antiseptic, aphrodisiac, diuretic, emollient, expectorant, insecticidal, sudorific

TAMARIND SEED

Botanical Name: *Tamarindus indica*

Family: *Caesalpiniodeae*

The oil is obtained from the seeds.

History and Information

- Tamarind is an evergreen tree native to Africa; it is found in dry locations. The tree grows to a height of about 40–85 feet (12–26 meters), has green leaves and large yellow and red flowers followed by long, curved, brown fruits that are sweet and sour with many brown seeds inside. The tree is also known as Indian tamarind, tamarindo, and rilytree.

- Tamarind pulp was mentioned in the Vedic texts written in the thirteenth century.

- In Africa, the leaves have been used for fevers, as a laxative, and for wounds.

- In Latin America, the major use for the fruit is as a laxative. It is also taken to reduce water retention, lower fevers, and to abort a fetus. The leaves and bark are taken for liver ailments, and the bark to move the bowels. In Brazil, the bark tea was used to alleviate parasites.

- The tree offers many medicinal remedies. It has been used for intestinal parasites, aching muscles and joints, to normalize blood sugar, ease sore throats, and soothe the skin.

- The fruit is a highly nutritive tonic and has been taken in China as a laxative and to remedy nausea during pregnancy.

- The leaves and flowers have been used for inflammation of the joints and sprains.

- The leaves are made into a tea to soothe the skin.

- The pulp is a diuretic and has been said to be helpful with urinary infections.

- The seeds can be toasted or ground into flour. The flowers and leaves are eaten in salads or made into soups.

- The fruit is high in vitamin C and has antiscorbutic properties. Sailors ate the fruit to prevent scurvy.

- The fruit is made into jams and added as an ingredient to beverages and candy.

Practical Uses

Skin care

Documented Properties

Abortifacient, anthelmintic, diuretic, febrifuge, laxative

TOMATO SEED

Botanical Name: *Lycopersicon esculentum*

Family: *Solanaceae*

The oil is obtained from the seeds.

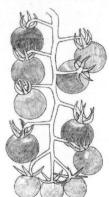

History and Information

- Tomato is native to Latin America. The plant grows to a height of about 6–10 feet (2–3 meters), has green leaves and yellow flowers that develop into reddish round edible fruits.

- In the sixteenth century, tomato was known as apple of Peru.

- In Turkey and Italy, the fruit is applied topically to scorpion stings and insect bites.

- The leaves and fruit are used to stop bleeding.

- Tomatoes are a popular food eaten raw in salads or made into a sauce or paste to flavor meals. They are a great source of beta-carotene, vitamin C, vitamin K, minerals, lycopene and other nutrients.

Practical Uses

Skin care

Hair care

Documented Properties

Antibacterial

TUCUMA
TUCUMA BUTTER

Botanical Name: *Astrocaryum tucuma*

Family: *Cocoideae*

The pulp oil is obtained from the fruit.

The butter is obtained from the seeds.

History and Information

- Tucuma is a palm tree native to South America. The tree grows to a height of about 50 feet (15 meters) and has yellow-orange fruit.

- The fruit is eaten fresh and is a good source of vitamins A, B, and C.

- The kernel oil is solid. The pulp oil is orange colored.

Practical Uses

Skin care

UCUUBA BUTTER

Botanical Name: *Virola sebifera*

Family: *Myristicaceae*

The butter is obtained from the seeds.

History and Information

- Ucuibeira is native to South America; it is found in swampy areas. The tree grows to a height of about 120 feet (36.5 meters) and has small flowers, followed by a green fruit with brown seeds. It is also known as tallow tree.

- In folk medicine, liniments made from the tree were used for tumors, muscle and joint aches, and pains.

- The seeds have a short shelf-life and turn rancid quickly.

- The oil has a high melting point and is used to make candles and soaps.

Practical Uses

Skin care

Documented Properties

Balancing (oily skin), emollient, moisturizing (dry, sensitive skin), nourishing (skin)

WALNUT

Botanical Name:
Juglans regia

Family: *Juglandaceae*

The oil is obtained
from the nuts.

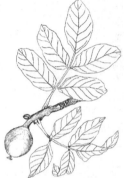

History and Information

- Walnut is a deciduous tree native to America, Europe, and Asia. The tree grows to a height of about 100 feet (30.5 meters), has aromatic dark-green, glossy, oval-shaped leaves, green female flowers, and yellowish-green male flowers in catkins. The nuts are hard shelled. There are twenty species of walnut trees.

- Walnut was one of the most popular trees in the Middle East in early times for the nuts and timber.

- In an ancient Chinese herbal, walnut was described as promoting circulation, darkening the hair, and making the skin smooth. It was used to relieve stomach acid and excessive urination.

- The Romans made a wine from walnuts.

- In Africa and the Middle East, walnut shells were burned and the smoke inhaled to soothe breathing congestion and repel insects. The leaves are heated in water and made into a shampoo for hair growth, as well as an insect repellent.

- The American Indians juiced the hulls as a remedy

to rid their animals of parasites. The crushed green hulls were also used to stupefy fish so they could be easily caught.

- Until the end of the eighteenth century, European households drank walnut milk as a substitute for dairy milk. The nuts were finely powdered and soaked in water to create this nourishing drink.

- Gypsies have traditionally used the nut hulls and tree roots to make dyes; theatrical performers have also used them to stain their skin dark brown.

- In Asia, walnut oil has been recommended to help improve vision.

- In Ayurvedic medicine, walnuts are considered to be a brain tonic.

- Many Europeans substitute olive oil with walnut oil. In southern Europe, walnut oil has long been popular for cooking. France is said to make the finest-quality oil, which accounts for approximately 33 percent of the country's total oil production.

- In Germany, a tea made from walnut leaves is given daily to children for two to six months to alleviate skin problems.

- In China, the nuts are used as a laxative and pain reliever.

- When the bark is tapped in the spring, it yields a sweet sap similar to maple syrup.

- The green rind of the walnut has been used in many applications, such as a fungicide for agriculture, a poultice for ringworm, and a source of iodine for individuals deficient in it. The inner bark and leaves have been used for skin problems, gout, colic, impotence, and to expel worms.

- The bark extract is antibacterial and is added to personal care products.

- The nut has a rich oil content of 60 percent. The oil is used in tanning lotions.

- A red dye is produced from the bark, and the husks yield a light- to dark-brown dye. The wood is manufactured into valuable furniture.

Practical Uses

Skin care

The carrier/base oil is used to dilute essential oils in aromatherapy for massage oils and other formulations.

Documented Properties

Analgesic, anthelmintic, antibacterial, antidepressant, antigalactagogue, anti-inflammatory, antilithic, antioxidant, antiseptic, antispasmodic, antitumor, aperitive, astringent, cardiotonic, carminative, chologogue, depurative, digestive, diuretic, emollient, expectorant, hemostatic, immunostimulant, laxative, moisturizing (lungs), parasiticide, stimulant (kidneys and lungs), tonic, vasoconstrictor, vermifuge, vulnerary

WATERMELON SEED
KALAHARI MELON SEED

Botanical Name: *Citrullus lanatus, Citrullus vulgaris*
Family: *Cucurbitaceae*
The oil is obtained from the seeds.

History and Information

- Watermelon is native to Asia and Africa. The spreading plant has green leaves and yellow flowers, followed by large red-fleshed fruits with seeds.

- Kalahari is an African watermelon plant that produces red-, orange-, or yellow-fleshed fruits.

- Native Americans used the seeds for kidney and urinary problems.

- In Asia, the fruit and rinds are eaten for diabetes, liver problems, sore throat, and mouth sores.

- In Latin America, the seeds are highly esteemed for their diuretic property. A tea is made for urinary problems. The crushed seeds in water are taken to get rid of worms, and the rind is placed topically for headaches.

- Watermelon has been consumed to help with heat exhaustion and dehydration, to balance blood pressure, help liver problems, reduce swelling of the ankles, and relieve digestive upsets. The fruits and seeds have been used as a tonic, for urinary problems, and intestinal parasites.

- Cosmetic face masks are made from the pulp of the melon-rind.

- Eating the unripe melons can cause serious illness, and even death (*Atlas of Medicinal Plants of Middle America,* by Julia F. Morton, Charles C. Thomas Publisher, page 885).

- The seeds contain up to 50 percent oil.

Practical Uses

Skin care

The carrier/base oil is used to dilute essential oils in aromatherapy for massage oils and other formulations.

Documented Properties

Anthelmintic, antiaging, antiseptic, antitumor, demulcent, diuretic, emollient, febrifuge, hypotensor, moisturizing, purgative, vermifuge

WHEAT GERM

Botanical Name: *Triticum vulgare*

Family: *Poaceae*

The oil is obtained from the grains.

History and Information

- Wheat has been one of the most important food staples worldwide. The plant belongs to the grass family and grows to a height of about 2–4 feet (.5–1 meter).

- Wheat germ oil contains valuable essential fatty acids; the linoleic acid content is approximately 58 percent. It is also a rich source of vitamins, especially vitamin E, a natural antioxidant that helps prolong the shelf-life of any blend to which it is added.

- The wheat germ has an oil content of only 10 percent.

- Many people consuming wheat products unknowingly may have a gluten intolerance to the grain. The book *Dangerous Grains,* written by Dr. James Braly, published by Penguin Group, is an important read.

Practical Uses

Skin care

The carrier/base oil is used to dilute essential oils in aromatherapy for massage oils and other formulations. For massage oils, it is best to mix 10 percent of wheat germ oil with another carrier oil before adding the essential oils.

Documented Properties

Galactagogue, tonic

WOLFBERRY SEED

Botanical Name: *Lycium barbarum, Lycium chinese*

Family: *Solanacae*

The CO_2 extract is obtained from the seeds.

History and Information

- Wolfberry is native to Europe and Asia. The spreading vine has narrow green leaves and clusters of pinkish or purplish flowers, followed by little red berries. It is also known as goji berry.

- In China, the berries have been used for 2,000 years. The people believed that the nutrients from the wolfberries promoted a longer life. They are taken as a tonic for the blood, liver, and kidneys to protect against damage caused by toxins and to improve the circulation and absorption of nutrients by the cells. In addition, the berries are considered to be valuable for eyesight and to strengthen the immune system. The root is used to lower fevers, relax the muscles, improve the circulatory system, and reduce thirst.

- The berries are edible raw or cooked and are considered a highly nutritional superfood, having a large amount of trace minerals. They are known to be beneficial to nourish the skin and hair.

Practical Uses

Skin care; absorbs easily into the skin

Hair care

Documented Properties

Cooling, febrifuge, hepatic, hyptensor, tonic

XIMENIA SEED

Botanical Name: *Ximenia americana*

Family: *Olacaceae*

The oil is obtained from the seeds.

History and Information

- Ximenia is native to Africa; it is found in moist soils. The small tree grows to a height of about 15 feet (3.5 meters), has a black bark with sharp spines, highly fragrant dark-green leathery leaves, and scented greenish-white flowers that develop into oval yellow-orange fruit with a sour flesh and bitter rind containing a kernel. The tree is also known as seaside plum, wild plum, sour plum, wild lime, wild oliver, limoncilla, citron de mer, monkey plum, and tallow wood.

- In Africa, a tea brewed from the leaves has been used to reduce fevers and inflammations, and to soothe abdominal discomforts.

- The powdered roots are used for leprosy, mental disorders, impotence, and edema. A preparation of the leaves, bark, and roots is used for toothaches and headaches.

- The powdered bark is placed on wounds for healing.

- The fruits eaten in large quantities help expel intestinal parasites.

- The fruits are a rich source of vitamin C. They are made into preserves and beer. When dehydrated, it is powdered and made into porridge.

- The wood is heavy and scented and serves as a substitute for sandalwood.

- The seed contains up to 75 percent oil and has a high amount of hydrocyanic acid content. The oil is also known as wild olive seed oil and is said to be edible.

- The oil is semisolid and is used in hair care, shampoos, soaps, and lipsticks.

Practical Uses

Skin care

Hair care

Documented Properties

Febrifuge, laxative, vermifuge

Caution: The kernels contain cyanide. It is best to use small amounts of the oil at one time.

YANGU

Botanical Name: *Calodendrom capense*

Family: *Rutaceae*

The oil is obtained from the seeds.

History and Information

- Yangu is native to Africa, and is found in the forest off the coast, and in the mountains. The tree grows to a height of about 20–80 feet (6–24 meters), has dark-green aromatic leaves and a canopy of large pink or purple flowers that develop into brown fruit capsules with black seeds inside. The slow-growing tree takes more than twelve years to bloom. Yangu is also known as cape chestnut.

- The native people of Africa believe the seeds have magical properties.

- The bark is used in skin ointments and skin care formulations; the seeds are made into oil. The oil is bitter and not edible.

Practical Uses

Skin care

Hair care

Documented Properties

Antioxidant

CHAPTER 3

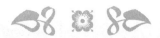

Essential Oils

Essential oils are the precious essences extracted from herbs, flowers, and trees. These wonderful, pure, and fragrant oils contain a natural living substance known as the "essence," which is the concentrated power and vital life force of the plant.

The following essential oils are covered in this chapter:

Ajowan
Allspice Berry
  (Pimento Berry)
Allspice Leaf (Pimento
  Leaf)
Almond (Bitter)
Ambrette Seed
Amyris
Angelica Root
Angelica Seed
Anise
Anise (Star)
Arina
Asafoetida
Balm of Gilead
Basil (Sweet)
Bay (Sweet)
Bay (West Indian)
Benzoin
Bergamot
Birch (Sweet)
Birch (White)
Black Cumin
Blue Mountain Sage
Bluegrass (African)
Bois de Rose
  (Rosewood)

Boldo
Buchu
Cabreuva
Cade
Cajeput
Calamint (Catnip)
Calamus (Sweet Flag)
Camphor
Camphor (Borneol)
Camphor Bush
Cananga
Cape Chamomile
Cape May
Cape Snowbush (Wild
  Rosemary)
Cape Verbena (Lippia
  or Zinziba)
Caraway
Cardamom
Carnation (Clove Pink)
Carrot Seed
Cascarilla Bark
Cassia
Cassia Bark
Cassie
Cedarwood
Cedarwood (Atlas)

Cedarwood
  (Himalayan or
  Deodar)
Cedarwood (Lebanon)
Celery
Chamomile (German)
Chamomile
  (Moroccan)
Chamomile (Roman)
Champaca Flower
Champaca Leaf
Chervil
Cinnamon Bark
Cinnamon Leaf
Citronella
Clary Sage
Clementine
Clove Bud
Clove Leaf
Clove Stem
Coffee
Combava
Copaiba
Coriander
Cornmint
Costus
Cubeb

Cumin
Cyperus (Cypriol)
Cypress
Cypress (Blue)
Cypress (Emerald)
Cypress (Jade)
Davana
Desert Rosewood
Dill Seed
Dill Weed
Dragon's Blood
  (Sangre de Grado)
Elecampane
Elemi
Eucalyptus
Eucalyptus Blue
  Mallee
Eucalyptus Citriodora
Eucalyptus Dives
Eucalyptus
  Macarthurii
Eucalyptus Radiata
Eucalyptus
  Sideroxylon
Eucalyptus Smithii
Eucalytpus Staigeriana
Fennel

Fenugreek Seed
Feverfew
Fir (Douglas)
Fir (Grand)
Fir Needles
Fir (Silver)
Fir Balsam Needles
Fir Balsam Resin
Fokienia (Bois de
    Siam)
Frankincense
    (Olibanum)
Galangal
Galbanum
Gardenia
Garlic
Geranium
Ginger
Ginger Lily
Gingergrass
Goldenrod
Grapefruit
Grapefruit (Pink)
Grapefruit (Red)
Guaiacwood
Gurjun Balsam
Helichrysum (Ever-
    lasting or Immortelle)
Helichrysum (African)
Heliotrope
Honeysuckle
Hops
Hyssop
Hyssop Decumbens
Jasmine
Juniper Berries
Kanuka
Katafray
Kava-Kava
Khella (Ammi Visnaga)
Kunzea
Labdanum (Cistus or
    Rock Rose)

Lantana
Larch
Lavandin
Lavender
Lavender (Spike)
Ledum
    Groenlandicum
Lemon
Lemon Verbena
Lemongrass
Lilac
Lime
Lime (Key)
Linaloe
Linden Blossom
Litsea Cubeba
Lovage
Magnolia (Bark)
Magnolia (Flowers)
Mandarin
Manuka (New
    Zealand Tea Tree)
Marjoram (Spanish)
Marjoram (Sweet)
Massoia Bark
Mastic
Melissa (Lemon Balm)
Mimosa
Monarda
Mugwort (Armoise)
Mullein
Mustard (Black)
Myrrh
Myrtle
Myrtle (Anise)
Myrtle (Lemon)
Neroli
Nerolina
Niaouli
Nutmeg
Onion
Opopanax
Orange (Bitter)

Orange (Blood)
Orange (Sweet)
Oregano
Orris Root
Osmanthus
Palmarosa
Parsley
Patchouli
Pennyroyal
Pepper (Black)
Pepper (Red)
    (Cayenne Pepper)
Peppermint
Perilla
Peru Balsam
Petitgrain
Pine
Rambiazana
    (Rambiaze)
Ravensara Anisata
    (Havozo Bark)
Ravensara Aromatica
Red Berry (Pepper
    Tree)
Rhododendron
Rose
Rosalina (Lavender
    Tea Tree)
Rosemary
Rue
Saffron
Sage
Sage (Spanish)
Sandalwood
Sandalwood
    (Australian)
Santolina (Lavender
    Cotton)
Sassafras
Savory
Schisandra
Spearmint
Spikenard

Spruce (Black)
Spruce (Sitka)
Spruce (White)
Spruce-Hemlock
St. John's Wort
Styrax (American)
Styrax (Asian)
Tagetes
Tana
Tangelo
Tangerine
Tarragon (Estragon)
Tansy
Tea Tree
Tea Tree (Black)
Tea Tree (Lemon)
Tea Tree (Lemon-
    Scented)
Tea Tree (Prickly
    Leaf)
Temple Orange
Terebinth
Thuja (Cedar Leaf)
Thyme
Tobacco Leaf
Tolu Balsam
Tonka Bean (Tonquin
    Bean)
Tuberose
Turmeric
Valerian
Vanilla
Vetiver
Vitex (Berry)
Vitex (Leaf)
Violet
Wintergreen
Wormwood
Yarrow
Ylang-Ylang
Yuzu
Zanthoxylum
Zedoary

AJOWAN

Botanical Name: *Trachyspermum ammi, Trachyspermum copticum*

Family: *Apiaceae*

The essential oil is obtained from the seeds.

History and Information

- Ajowan is native to Asia. The plant grows to a height of about 2 feet (.5 meter).
- The herb is utilized in Ayurvedic medicine in India to treat cholera and other intestinal problems.
- The seeds are used in curry powder as a seasoning for food.

Practical Uses

Heating; improves circulation

Promotes a restful sleep

Soothes sore and tight muscles

Documented Properties

Antibacterial, antifungal, antiseptic (strong), antiviral, aphrodisiac, carminative, parasiticide, tonic

Aromatherapy Methods of Use

Application, massage, mist spray

Caution: Ajowan oil is moderately toxic. Use only small amounts. People with dry or sensitive skin may require additional carrier oil when applying the essential oil topically.

ALLSPICE BERRY (Pimento Berry)
ALLSPICE LEAF (Pimento Leaf)

Botanical Name: *Pimenta dioica, Pimenta officinalis*

Family: *Myrtaceae*

Allspice berry essential oil and CO_2 extract are obtained from the unripe berries.

Allspice leaf essential oil is obtained from the twigs and leaves.

History and Information

- Allspice is an evergreen tree native to the West Indies, and Central and South America. The tree grows to a height of about 30–70 feet (9–21 meters), has light-green leathery leaves and small white flowers followed by green berries that turn brown when mature. The aromatic berries become black after being dried. The male and female flowers are on different trees.
- The berries have been used for digestive problems, muscle and joint pains, and congestion of mucous membranes. The warming effect is beneficial for chills and colds.
- In Latin America, before the fifteenth century, allspice was used as a seasoning and to embalm the dead.
- In Guatemala, crushed allspice berries are applied to painful muscles and joints.
- Allspice leaf oil is similar in composition to clove leaf oil, both containing high amounts of eugenol.

Practical Uses

Warming; improves circulation

Improves digestion

Purifying; helps in the reduction of cellulite

Calms the nerves, removes stress; promotes a restful sleep

Vapors open the sinus and breathing passages

Mood uplifting

Loosens tight muscles, lessens pain

Documented Properties

Analgesic, antidepressant, antioxidant, antiseptic, aphrodisiac, astringent, carminative, digestive, rubefacient, stomachic, tonic, tranquilizer

Aromatherapy Methods of Use

Application, aroma lamp, diffusor, inhaler, lightbulb ring, massage, mist spray, steam inhalation

Caution: People with dry or sensitive skin may require additional carrier oil when applying allspice essential oil topically. The berry oil is milder to the skin than the leaf oil.

ALMOND *(Bitter)*

Botanical Name: *Prunus amygdalus, Prunus dulcis*

Family: *Rosaceae*

The essential oil is obtained from the pulp of the nuts.

History and Information

- Bitter almond is native to Asia and belongs to the rose family. The tree grows to a height of about 35 feet (10.5 meters) and has white to pink flowers. There are approximately fifty species of the wild almond trees, most producing a bitter kernel.

- In China, bitter almond is used mainly for chest congestion.

- The essential oil is produced by distillation of the remains of the pulp from which almond oil has been previously expressed. Bitter almond is taken for coughs, added to flavor foods, and used as an ingredient in cosmetic skin preparations.

Documented Properties

Antispasmodic, antitussive, laxative, narcotic, tranquilizer

Aromatherapy Methods of Use

Fragrancing

Caution: Bitter almond contains prussic acid, which is converted in the body into a cyanide compound. The oil is toxic unless the prussic acid is extracted in the production process. The ingestion of approximately forty-five to fifty nuts at one time could prove to be fatal to an adult, while only twenty at one time could be fatal to a child.

AMBRETTE SEED

Botanical Name: *Abelmoschus moschatus, Hibiscus abelmoschus*

Family: *Malvaceae*

The essential oil and CO_2 extract are obtained from the seeds.

History and Information

- Ambrette is an evergreen shrub native to Asia. The bushy plant grows to a height of about 5 feet (1.5 meters) and has large yellow and purple flowers. The fruit is an oblong seedpod that splits at the tip when it matures. The seeds smell like musk.

- In China, ambrette seeds have been used as a remedy for headaches; the root for fever and coughs; and the flowers for the skin.

- In Latin America, the seeds are chewed to ease the stomach, calm the nerves, and for diuretic purposes. A seed tea is taken for muscle and joint aches, breathing congestion, and to expel intestinal parasites. A poultice from the seeds is placed topically on snakebites and a seed infusion is taken internally at the same time.

- In the Middle East, the seeds are used to flavor foods and coffee.

- The oil is an ingredient in cosmetics, perfumery, food flavorings, soft drinks, and alcoholic beverages.

Practical Uses

Calming, reduces stress, relieves nervous tension

Mood uplifting

Lessens aches and pains

Healing and moisturizing to the skin

A fixative to hold the scent of a fragrance

Documented Properties

Analgesic, antispasmodic, aphrodisiac, carminative, diuretic, nervine, sedative, stimulant, stomachic

Aromatherapy Methods of Use

Application, aroma lamp, bath, inhaler, lightbulb ring, massage, mist spray

Caution: Ambrette seed oil is phototoxic. Avoid exposure to direct sunlight for several hours after applying the essential oil on the skin.

AMMI VISNAGA

See Khella

AMYRIS

Botanical Name: *Amyris balsamifera, Schimmelia oleifera*

Family: *Rutaceae*

The essential oil is obtained from the wood chips.

History and Information

- Amyris is an evergreen tree native to the West Indies and Central America. The tree grows to about 60 feet (18 meters) high and has clusters of white flowers that develop into an edible black-bluish fruit.

- Amyris is also known as West Indian sandalwood. It is commonly used as a fixative in perfumery and to adulterate true sandalwood oil.

- The wood burns like a candle and is called candle-wood.

Practical Uses

Cooling

Calming, reduces stress and tension, releases anxiety, promotes a peaceful state

Helps to deepen the breathing

Reviving; improves mental clarity

Loosens tight muscles

A fixative to hold the scent of a fragrance

Documented Properties

Antiphlogistic, antiseptic, antispasmodic, aphrodisiac, balsamic, expectorant, fixative, hypotensive, lymphatic decongestant, sedative, tonic (heart)

Aromatherapy Methods of Use

Application, aroma lamp, bath, fragrancing, inhaler, lightbulb ring, massage, mist spray, steam inhalation, steam room and sauna

ANGELICA ROOT

ANGELICA SEED

Botanical Name: *Angelica archangelica, Angelica officinalis*

Family: *Apiaceae*

Angelica root essential oil and CO_2 extract are obtained from the roots.

Angelica seed essential oil is obtained from the seeds.

History and Information

- Angelica is native to Europe. The plant grows to about 6 feet (2 meters) in height and has clusters of yellow-green flowers.

- Paracelsus, the Swiss physician, used angelica during an epidemic in the sixteenth century.

- During the plague of 1665, the stems were chewed to prevent infection. The seeds and roots were burned to disinfect the air. The roots were also dried, powdered, and mixed with vinegar to disinfect linen and clothing when washing.

- The American Indians took angelica as an expectorant for respiratory congestion and tuberculosis, a tonic to recover from illness, and to expel worms.

- In Europe, the plant has been used as a remedy for coughs, colds, breathing congestion, stomach upsets, aching joints, urinary tract complaints, as a blood purifier, and to improve circulation.

- In England, angelica was incorporated into rituals and worn for protection against evil spirits and spells.

- In Asia, angelica is a highly regarded herb that is mainly taken as a remedy for females who have menopause or menstrual problems.

- In Chinese medicine, angelica is used to correct menstrual irregularities, promote female fertility, and as a tonic for the liver.

- Both the seeds and roots yield an essential oil. The seeds produce a greater oil content, and the root oil has a stronger odor. Angelica oil is highly valued as a fragrance in perfumes and is used as a flavoring ingredient in foods, soft drinks, and liqueurs.

- All parts of the plant are edible: the shoots are added to a salad, the stalks are eaten like celery or candied as a confectionery, the roots are steamed as vegetables, and the seeds are used to flavor baked goods.

Practical Uses

Cooling

Improves digestion, soothes the intestines, relieves nausea

Calming, reduces stress

Encourages dreaming; helpful for meditation

Vapors open the sinus and breathing passages; deepens the breathing

Improves mental clarity and alertness

Relieves aches, pains, and menstrual discomfort

Documented Properties

Analgesic, antibacterial, antifungal, anti-inflammatory, antirheumatic, antiseptic, antispasmodic, antiviral, aperitive, aphrodisiac, carminative, cephalic, depurative, diaphoretic, digestive, diuretic, emmenagogue, estrogenic, expectorant, febrifuge, healing (skin), hepatic, nervine, revitalizing, stimulant (uterine; nerves), stomachic, sudorific, tonic

Aromatherapy Methods of Use

Application, aroma lamp, bath, diffusor, inhaler, lightbulb ring, massage, mist spray, steam inhalation, steam room and sauna

Caution: Use small amounts. Angelica root oil is phototoxic. Avoid exposure to direct sunlight for several hours after applying the essential oil on the skin.

ANISE

Botanical Name: *Anisum officinalis, Anisum officinarum, Pimpinella anisum*

Family: *Apiaceae*

The essential oil is obtained from the plant.

History and Information

- Anise is native to the Mediterranean area. The plant reaches a height of about 2 feet (.5 meter) and has small white flowers, followed by seeds.

- During biblical times, anise was highly valued and used by the Romans to pay their taxes. When the Romans discovered the seeds of anise helped digestion, they added it to special cakes served after their large banquets.

- The Egyptians grew large amounts of anise for cooking, teas, and medicines.

- Hippocrates used the herb to clear mucous from the respiratory system.

- Theophrastus, the father of botany, wrote that anise, kept near the bed at night, promoted sweet dreams.

- Pliny, the Roman herbalist, recommended chewing anise as a breath freshener and digestive aid. Today, the seeds are chewed in India for those same reasons.

- In 1305, King Edward I declared anise a taxable commodity. The resulting taxes supplied funds to repair the London Bridge.

- The Aztec Indians chewed anise seeds to relieve flatulence.

- In the sixteenth century, Europeans discovered that mice were attracted to anise and used it as bait in mousetraps.

- The American Indians made a tea from the leaves and flowers for a cough remedy.

- The seeds are taken to facilitate childbirth, increase the flow of milk in nursing mothers, improve digestion, and as an aphrodisiac.

- The seeds yield 2 to 3 percent essential oil, which

is widely used in beverages, baked goods, foods, confectionery (licorice), cough drops, and liqueurs. Powdered anise seed is used to flavor horse and cattle feed.

Practical Uses

Improves digestion, soothes the intestines, relieves flatulence and aerophagy

Calming, relaxing; promotes a restful sleep

Vapors help open the sinus and breathing passages

Mood uplifting

Lessens pain and helps relieve menstrual discomfort

Increases lactation

Documented Properties

Abortifacient, analgesic, antiemetic, antiseptic, antispasmodic, aperitive, aphrodisiac, calmative, cardiac, carminative, digestive, disinfectant, diuretic (mild), estrogenic, expectorant, galactagogue, hepatic, insecticide, laxative, parasiticide, pectoral, stimulant (circulatory and digestive systems; respiratory tract), stomachic, tonic, warming

Aromatherapy Methods of Use

Application, aroma lamp, bath, inhaler, lightbulb ring, massage, mist spray, steam inhalation, steam room and sauna

Caution: People with dry or sensitive skin may require additional carrier oil when applying the essential oil topically. Anise tends to slow down reflexes. Avoid driving or doing anything that requires full attention after using the oil. Use small amounts.

ANISE *(Star)*

Botanical Name: *Illicium verum*

Family: *Illiciaceae*

The essential oil is obtained from the dried seeds.

History and Information

- Anise star is an evergreen tree native to Asia. The tree grows to a height of about 35 feet (10.5 meters), has shiny green leaves and small yellow flowers that develop into large star-shaped fruits with brown seeds. The fruits can be eaten fresh or dried; however, the leaves are poisonous.

- The use of star anise dates back centuries in Chinese medicine.

- Star anise was used as a folk remedy to move the bowels, freshen the breath, for muscle and joint aches, spasms, to help sleep, and for toothaches.

- In Asia, the seeds are chewed after meals to promote good digestion and sweeten the breath. The seeds and pods are added to make foods tastier.

- In Japan, the bark is an ingredient in cough medicines and cough drops, and burned as incense.

- Star anise is used as a flavoring agent in foods, confectionery, alcoholic drinks, and tobacco. The essential oil is added to toothpastes, soaps, skin creams, detergents, and perfumes.

Practical Uses

Improves digestion, soothes the intestines, relieves flatulence and aerophagy

Calming, relaxing; promotes a restful sleep

Vapors help open the sinus and breathing passages

Mood uplifting

Lessens pain and helps relieve menstrual discomfort

Increases lactation

Documented Properties

Analgesic, antiseptic, antispasmodic, aperitive, aphrodisiac, calmative, cardiac, carminative, digestive, disinfectant, diuretic (mild), estrogenic, expectorant, galactagogue, insecticide, stimulant (circulatory and digestive systems; respiratory tract), stomachic, tonic, warming

Aromatherapy Methods of Use

Application, aroma lamp, bath, inhaler, lightbulb ring, massage, mist spray, steam inhalation, steam room and sauna

Caution: People with dry or sensitive skin may require additional carrier oil when applying the essential oil topically. Star anise tends to slow down reflexes. Avoid driving or doing anything that requires full attention after using the oil. Use small amounts.

ARINA

Botanical Name: *Psiadia altissima*

Family Name: *Asteraceae*

The essential oil is obtained from the leaves.

History and Information

- Arina is native to Africa. The shrub grows on rocky lands. It has narrow pointy leaves and yellow flowers.

- The plant has been used for neurological problems and muscular atrophy caused by polio, to heal skin problems, and help muscle and joint discomfort.

Practical Uses

Warming; increases circulation

Calming, relaxing to the mind, reduces stress; promotes a restful sleep

Encourages dreaming

Opens the breathing

Loosens tight muscles

Documented Properties

Antimicrobial, antiseptic, tonic

Aromatherapy Methods of Use

Application, aroma lamp, bath, diffusor, inhaler, lightbulb ring, massage, mist spray, steam inhalation, steam room and sauna

ASAFOETIDA

Botanical Name: *Ferula assafoetida*

Family: *Apiaceae*

The essential oil is obtained from the roots.

History and Information

- Asafoetida is native to Asia. The plant grows to a height of about 8 feet (2.5 meters) and has large yellow-green flower heads.

- The ancient Egyptians and Greeks used the herb as a medicine and a spice.

- Chinese medicine used the plant as a nerve stimulant, laxative, and for chest ailments.

- In Ayurvedic medicine, asafoetida is mainly used to calm nervous disorders.

- The oil is used in perfumery as a fixative.

- Asafoetida has an intense onion-garlic odor and bitter taste. Some of its common names are devil's gum and devil's dung.

Documented Properties

Anticoagulant, antispasmodic, carminative, expectorant, hemostatic, hypotensor

Comments: Asafoeida oil has an odor that is disagreeable to most people. It is added to certain foods as a flavoring ingredient by the food industry, but it is not used in aromatherapy.

BALM OF GILEAD

Botanical Name: *Populus balsamifera, Populus candicans, Populus deltoides, Populus gileadensis, Populus tacamahaca*

Family: *Salicaceae*

The essential oil is obtained from the buds.

History and Information

- Balm of Gilead is native to the Northern Hemisphere. The tree grows to a height of about 30–100 feet (9–30.5 meters). The male and female flowers grow on separate trees.

- Early American settlers made a salve from the buds to heal skin sores. The leaves were used as a compress for headaches and earaches. The blossoms were steeped in water and taken to purify the blood, and the root bark was chewed for sore throats.

- In folk medicine, the bark and leaves were used for

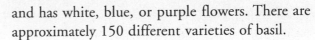

minor aches and pains, coughs, colds, bruises, and pimples.

- The leaf buds have been used to reduce inflammations, relieve congestion, increase circulation, soothe sore throats and coughs, for muscle and joint pains, and skin problems.

- The major use of balm of Gilead has been in cough remedies.

- Balm of Gilead contains salicin, which is an aspirin-like substance.

Practical Uses

Helps breathing congestion

Loosens tight muscles, reduces pain

Healing to the skin

A fixative to hold the scent of a fragrance

Documented Properties

Analgesic, antifungal, anti-inflammatory, antirheumatic, antiscorbutic, antiseptic, diuretic, expectorant, febrifuge, stimulant, tonic, vulnerary

Aromatherapy Methods of Use

Application, massage

Comments: The oil of balm of Gilead is usually extracted by solvents.

BASIL *(Sweet)*

Botanical Name: *Ocimum basilicum*

Family: *Lamiaceae*

The essential oil is obtained from the whole plant.

The CO_2 extract is obtained from the leaves.

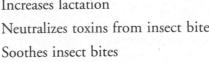

History and Information

- Sweet basil is native to Africa and Asia. The bushy plant grows to a height of about 2 feet (.5 meter)

and has white, blue, or purple flowers. There are approximately 150 different varieties of basil.

- Wreaths of basil have been found in the burial chambers of the ancient Egyptian pyramids.

- Kings were anointed with basil oil during ancient times.

- In Italy, basil symbolizes love. Traditionally, women put a pot of basil outside their window when they are ready for romance.

- Basil has been taken to increase the flow of milk in nursing mothers and to help ease nervous conditions.

- The herb is especially known in Asia for its ability to draw out the venomous poisons of snake or insect bites when applied directly on the skin.

- In South America and Africa, basil is taken for intestinal parasites.

- In China, the herb is used as a remedy for stomach problems.

- In India, the Hindus consider basil the most sacred of all plants. They plant the herb around their temples, graves, and homes. In Ayurvedic medicine, the plant is used for snakebites, skin problems, and as a tonic.

- In Arabic countries, a tea made from basil is used for menstrual cramps.

Practical Uses

Cooling

Improves digestion

Purifying; helps in the reduction of cellulite

Calming, reduces stress; promotes a restful sleep

Encourages dreaming; helpful for meditation

Mood uplifting; improves mental clarity and memory, sharpens the senses

Lessens pain

Increases lactation

Neutralizes toxins from insect bites

Soothes insect bites

Documented Properties

Abortifacient, analgesic, antibacterial, antidepressant, antiseptic, antispasmodic, antistress, antivenomous, aperitive, aphrodisiac, blood purifier, carminative, cephalic, diaphoretic, digestive, emmenagogue, estrogenic, expectorant, febrifuge, galactagogue, insect repellent, insecticide, laxative, nervine, refreshing, restorative, sedative, stimulant (adrenal glands; facilitates childbirth), stomachic, sudorific, tonic (nerves), uplifting, vermifuge

Aromatherapy Methods of Use

Application, aroma lamp, diffusor, inhaler, lightbulb ring, massage, mist spray

Caution: People with dry or sensitive skin may require additional carrier oil when applying basil essential oil topically. Use small amounts.

BAY *(Sweet)*

Botanical Name: *Laurus nobilis*

Family: *Lauraceae*

The essential oil is obtained from the leaves.

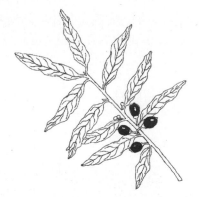

History and Information

- Sweet bay is an evergreen tree native to the Mediterranean area, Europe, and the United States. The tree grows to a height of about 10–60 feet (3–18 meters), has dark-green waxy aromatic leaves and small yellow flowers that develop into small purple or black berries.

- In the early Greek and Roman times, bay was the symbol of glory and reward. The greatest honor was bestowed on those fortunate enough to be crowned with the bay laurel wreath. The recipients of the crownings were kings, priests, prophets, poets, scholars, victorious athletes, and soldiers. The Roman generals crowned themselves with bay leaves when they returned home victorious from battle. The soldiers added the leaves to their baths to soothe fatigue and injuries.

- The Romans and Greeks valued bay for its memory-improvement property and used the leaves to flavor and preserve food.

- Dioscorides, the Greek physician, used the leaves for insect stings, inflammation, and bladder problems. Galen, the Greek physician, used bay leaves and berries for a variety of ailments, particularly for painful joints and promoting menstruation.

- In the Middle Ages, herbalists used bay to promote menstruation and induce abortions.

- During outbreaks of the plague in Rome, people were advised to live in the vicinity of bay trees.

- During Elizabethan times the leaves were strewn on the floors of homes to freshen stale air.

- In Greece, a leaf tea is taken as a contraceptive. A tea made from the dried berries is consumed to stimulate the appetite and aid digestion.

- A few drops of the leaf juice in water are used to promote the onset of menstruation and as a circulatory stimulant. The berries, mixed into foods, are eaten during childbirth to quicken delivery.

- Sweet bay oil is also known as laurel leaf oil.

Practical Uses

Warming; improves circulation, promotes perspiration

Digestive stimulant

Purifying; helps in the reduction of cellulite

Calming, reduces stress

Vapors open the sinus and breathing passages

Improves mental clarity and alertness, sharpens the senses

Relieves aching limbs and muscles, lessens pain; good for sprains

Disinfectant

Repels insects

Documented Properties

Abortifacient, analgesic, antibacterial, anticoagulant, antifungal, antineuralgic, antioxidant, antipruritic, antirheumatic, antiseptic, antispasmodic, aperient, aperitif, astringent, carminative, cholagogue, diaphoretic, digestive, diuretic, emetic, emmenagogue, expectorant, febrifuge, hepatic, hypotensor, insect repellent, laxative, nervine, sedative, stimulant (digestion), stomachic, tonic

Aromatherapy Methods of Use

Application, aroma lamp, diffusor, inhaler, lightbulb ring, massage, mist spray, steam inhalation

Caution: People with dry or sensitive skin may require additional carrier oil when applying bay essential oil topically. Use small amounts.

BAY *(West Indian)*

Botanical Name: *Myrcia acris, Pimenta acris, Pimenta racemosa*

Family: *Myrtaceae*

The essential oil is obtained from the leaves.

History and Information

- West Indian bay is a tropical evergreen tree native to the West Indies. The tree grows to a height of about 30–50 feet (9–15 meters), has aromatic leathery leaves and clusters of white or pink flowers that develop into black oval berries. Bay is also known as bay rum tree, wild cinnamon, and bayberry.

- During Victorian times, men used bay rum as a hair dressing. Over the years, bay has been used as a remedy for hair loss and to fragrance colognes and aftershave lotions.

- West Indian bay oil is also known as myrica oil or bay rum oil. It is an ingredient in foods and soft drinks.

Practical Uses

Warming; improves circulation, promotes perspiration

Digestive stimulant

Purifying; helps in the reduction of cellulite

Calming, reduces stress

Vapors open the sinus and breathing passages

Improves mental clarity and alertness, sharpens the senses

Relieves aching limbs and muscles, lessens pain; good for sprains

Disinfectant

Repels insects

Documented Properties

Analgesic, anticonvulsive, antifungal, antineuralgic, antirheumatic, antiseptic, antiviral, astringent, expectorant, hypertensor, parasiticide, stimulant, tonic

Aromatherapy Methods of Use

Application, aroma lamp, diffusor, inhaler, lightbulb ring, massage, mist spray, steam inhalation

Caution: People with dry or sensitive skin may require additional carrier oil when applying bay essential oil topically. Use small amounts.

BENZOIN

Botanical Name: *Styrax benzoin, Styrax tonkinensis*

Family: *Styracaceae*

The resin and essential oil are obtained from the bark.

History and Information

- Benzoin is native to Asia. The tree grows to a maximum height of 115 feet (35 meters) and has fragrant white flowers. The trunk secretes an aromatic resin when injured. The tree is also known as benjamin tree.

- The incense of benzoin has been used for thousands of years in temples during religious ceremonies.

- In France, the resin was burned and inhaled for respiratory problems.

- In southern Asia, benzoin was traditionally used for its healing qualities to mend the wound made by circumcision.

- Benzoin is a common ingredient in skin protective products and cosmetic preparations. It is also used as a preservative in ointments for extending their shelf-life, and as a fixative in soaps, perfumes, and creams. The food industry uses benzoin to flavor foods and beverages.

- The resin is also known as gum benjamin.

Practical Uses

Warming; improves circulation

Purifying; helps in the reduction of cellulite

Calming, reduces stress; promotes a restful sleep

Encourages dreaming; helpful for meditation

Improves the breathing and is especially helpful when rubbed on the chest

Mood uplifting

Reduces inflammation, relaxes tight muscles

Healing to the skin

Acts as a preservative in cosmetics

A fixative to hold the scent of a fragrance

Documented Properties

Anesthetic, antibacterial, antidepressant, anti-inflammatory, antimutagenic, antioxidant, antipruritic, antiseptic, antispasmodic, antistress, antitussive, antiviral, aphrodisiac, astringent, carminative, cephalic, cicatrizant, cordial, deodorant, disinfectant, diuretic, drying, euphoriant, expectorant, fixative, healing (skin), insecticide, laxative, pectoral, preservative, regulator, rejuvenator, sedative, soothing, stimulant (circulatory system), tonic, uplifting, vermifuge, vulnerary

Aromatherapy Methods of Use

Application, massage, mist spray

Caution: People with dry or sensitive skin may require additional carrier oil when applying benzoin resin or essential oil topically. Use small amounts.

BERGAMOT

Botanical Name: *Citrus bergamia*

Family: *Rutaceae*

The essential oil is obtained from the peels of the fruit.

History and Information

- Bergamot is an evergreen citrus tree native to Asia. The tree grows to a height of about 15 feet (4.5 meters) and bears nonedible green to yellow fruit. Bergamot was first discovered growing in Calabria, Italy, in the seventeenth century. The essence was initially sold in the city of Bergamo in the Lombardy region of Italy.

- In Italian folk medicine, the oil was used as a remedy for worms and fevers.

- Bergamot is renowned for its fragrant scent and is widely used in perfumery. The oil is produced from the rind of a fruit similar to the bitter orange. The bergamot fruit should not be confused with an herb in the mint family, monarda, which is also known as bergamot.

Practical Uses

Cooling

Purifying; helps in the reduction of cellulite

Balancing; calming, relieves anxiety, nervous tension and stress; promotes a restful sleep

Mood uplifting, refreshing; improves mental clarity, alertness, sharpens the senses

Disinfectant

Documented Properties

Analgesic, anthelmintic, antidepressant, antiseptic, antispasmodic, antistress, antitoxic, aperitive, calmative, carminative, cicatrizant, cordial, deodorant, digestive, expectorant, febrifuge, insecticide, laxative, parasiticide, refreshing, rubefacient, sedative, stomachic, tonic, uplifting, vermifuge, vulnerary

Aromatherapy Methods of Use

Application, aroma lamp, bath, diffusor, inhaler, lightbulb ring, massage, mist spray

Caution: People with dry or sensitive skin may require additional carrier oil when using the essential oil topically. Bergamot is phototoxic. Avoid exposure to direct sunlight for several hours after applying the oil on the skin.

BIRCH *(Sweet)*

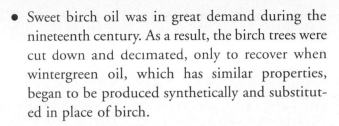

Botanical Name:
Betula lenta

Family: *Betulaceae*

The essential oil is obtained from the bark.

History and Information

- Sweet birch is native to North America. The tree grows to a height of about 50–80 feet (15–24 meters), has a black bark, leaves that smell of wintergreen, and yellow-green cones. The female cones produce seeds. The tree is also known as black birch.

- The American Indians used the birch leaves and dried bark as a tea to relieve headaches, muscle and joint aches, painful menstruation, abdominal cramps, colds, congestion, fevers, and digestive upsets. The leaves and branches were used in sweat lodge cleansing ceremonies. The essential oil, distilled from the bark, was used for gout, bladder infection, neuralgia, inflammation, muscle and joint aches, and pain. The tree sap was used as a syrup.

- Sweet birch oil was in great demand during the nineteenth century. As a result, the birch trees were cut down and decimated, only to recover when wintergreen oil, which has similar properties, began to be produced synthetically and substituted in place of birch.

- The Russian people have used birch leaves in steam baths throughout history. The tree sap is sold commercially as a tonic and is said to help skin, urinary, and muscle and joint problems.

- The sap is collected in the spring before the leaves appear and is made into a syrup, beer, wine, and liquor. The sap is used for good health, as a blood cleanser, and general tonic.

- Birch bark is used in medicated soaps for skin infections and blemishes; the branches for birch beer; and the wood to make canoes.

- In colder climates, a tea made from the young leaves or buds was brewed and taken to detox the body during the spring season. The young leaves are eaten in salads.

- The sweet birch tree and wintergreen plant produce an essential oil that is closely identical in smell and chemical composition, but sweet birch yields a greater amount of oil.

Practical Uses

Warming; improves circulation

Purifying; helps in the reduction of cellulite

Calming, relaxes the nerves, reduces tension and stress; promotes a restful sleep

Mood uplifting

Relieves achy, tense, and sore muscles, reduces inflammation, lessens pain, especially in the joints

Documented Properties

Analgesic, anthelmintic, anti-inflammatory, antirheumatic, antiseptic, antitoxic, astringent, deputative, detersive, disinfectant, diuretic, febrifuge, insect repellent, insecticide, laxative, rubefacient, stimulant (circulatory system), tonic

Aromatherapy Methods of Use

Application, aroma lamp, diffusor, inhaler, lightbulb ring, massage, mist spray, steam inhalation

Caution: Sweet birch is hardly produced anymore and is commonly falsified with the synthetic chemical, methyl salicylate. Due to the toxicity of the "true" oil, use small amounts. People with dry or sensitive skin may require additional carrier oil when applying the essential oil topically.

BIRCH (White)

Botanical Name: *Betula alba*

Family: *Betulaceae*

The essential oil is obtained from the buds and bark.

History and Information

- White birch is native to the Northern Hemisphere. The tree grows to a height of about 60 feet (18 meters).

- Early American settlers used the sap to prevent and treat scurvy and as a laxative and diuretic.

- The American Indians used the bark and leaves to cleanse and disinfect skin conditions.

- White birch oil has a smoky odor, unlike sweet birch oil. Birch tar is obtained from the bark. The oil extracted from the buds is referred to as birch bud oil and used primarily in shampoos and hair tonics.

Practical Uses

Purifying; helps in the reduction of cellulite

Relieves achy, tense, and sore muscles, reduces inflammation, lessens pain, especially in the joints

Documented Properties

Anti-inflammatory, antiseptic, cholagogue, diaphoretic, diuretic, febrifuge, tonic

Aromatherapy Methods of Use

Application, massage

BLACK CUMIN

Botanical Name: *Nigella sativa*

Family: *Ranunculaceae*

The essential oil is obtained from the seeds.

History and Information

See Black Cumin in Chapter 2, page 15.

Practical Uses

Warming

Helps to breathe easier

Loosens tight muscles

Documented Properties

Analgesic, antibacterial, antifungal, antioxidant, cholagogue

Aromatherapy Methods of Use

Application, inhaler, massage, mist spray

BLUE MOUNTAIN SAGE

Botanical Name: *Salvia stenophylla*

Family Name: *Lamiaceae*

The essential oil is obtained from the stems and leaves.

History and Information

- Blue mountain sage is native to Africa. The plant has aromatic narrow leaves and small blue flowers.

- The leaves are made into a tea and taken for digestive disturbances, coughs, colds, and chest congestion. It is also applied topically on scrapes, sores, and bites.

- The dried leaves are burned to repel insects.

Practical Uses

Cooling

Helps to breathe easier

Refreshing, energizing; improves mental clarity

Relaxes tight muscles

Documented Properties

Antibacterial, anti-inflammatory, healing (skin)

Aromatherapy Methods of Use

Application, aroma lamp, bath, diffusor, inhaler, light-bulb ring, massage, mist spray, steam inhalation, steam room and sauna

BLUEGRASS (African)

Botanical Name: *Cymbopogon validus*

Family: *Poaceae*

The essential oil is obtained from the whole plant.

History and Information

- African bluegrass is native to South Africa. The aromatic grass is grey-green with a lemony scent.

Practical Uses

Calming, reduces stress, relieves tension

Vapors open the sinus and breathing passages; deepens the breathing

Mood uplifting; improves mental clarity

Soothes insect bites

Documented Properties

Antifungal, antiseptic, astringent

Aromatherapy Methods of Use

Application, aroma lamp, bath, diffusor, inhaler, light-bulb ring, massage, mist spray, steam inhalation, steam room and sauna

BOIS DE ROSE (Rosewood)

Botanical Name: *Aniba rosaeodora*

Family: *Lauraceae*

The essential oil is obtained from the bark.

History and Information

- Bois de rose is native to the tropical parts of America, the West Indies, and India. The evergreen tree grows to a height of about 80 feet (24 meters), has leathery leaves and red flowers. Bois de rose is part of a species of forty evergreen trees.

- Amazonian natives have used the bark for its remarkable property to rejuvenate the skin.

Practical Uses

Calming, relieves nervousness and stress

Mood uplifting

Lessens pain

Regenerates and moisturizes the skin

Documented Properties

Analgesic, antibacterial, anticonvulsive, antidepressant, antifungal, antiseptic (throat), antiviral, aphrodisiac, calmative, cephalic, deodorant, emollient (skin), euphoriant, insecticide, parasiticide, regenerator (skin tissue), stimulant (immune system), tonic, uplifting

Aromatherapy Methods of Use

Application, aroma lamp, bath, diffusor, inhaler, light-bulb ring, massage, mist spray

BOLDO

Botanical Name: *Peumus boldus*

Family: *Monimiaceae*

The essential oil is obtained from the leaves.

History and Information

- Boldo is an evergreen tree native to South America. The aromatic tree grows to a height of about 20 feet (6 meters), has dark-green leaves and little white flowers that bear small edible fruit.

- Boldo is used medicinally and in the perfume industry worldwide.

Documented Properties

Cholagogue, digestive, diuretic, sedative, stimulant (liver, bladder)

Caution: Even in small amounts, boldo can have a very forceful effect on the body, causing convulsions. The essential oil should be avoided.

BUCHU

Botanical Name: *Agathosma betulina, Barosma betulina*

Family: *Rutaceae*

The essential oil is obtained from the dried leaves.

History and Information

- Buchu is native to Africa. The shrub grows to a height of about 3 feet (1 meter), has large light-green oval leaves, and white or pink flowers, followed by black seeds.

- Buchu is used as a remedy for urinary tract problems.

- The leaves yield approximately 2 percent essential oil and are mainly used as a flavoring for foods.

Documented Properties

Antirheumatic, antiseptic (urinary), antispasmodic, aperitive, carminative, digestive, diuretic, laxative, tonic (kidneys)

Caution: Buchu oil is not recommended for use in aromatherapy.

CABREUVA

Botanical Name: *Myrocarpus fastigiatus*

Family: *Fabaceae*

The essential oil is obtained from the wood chips.

History and Information

- Cabreuva is native to South America; it is found abundantly in forests off the coast of South America. The tree grows to a height of about 50 feet (15 meters).

- Cabreuva wood is heavy, hard, and durable. It is valued in the production of furniture. The oil is used in fragrances.

Practical Uses

Warming

Calming, reduces stress and tension

Helps to breathe easier

Mood uplifting, aphrodisiac, euphoric; improves mental clarity and alertness

Loosens tight muscles, reduces pain

Documented Properties

Anti-inflammatory, antiseptic, aphrodisiac, balsamic, cicatrizant, expectorant, fixative

Aromatherapy Methods of Use

Application, aroma lamp, bath, diffusor, lightbulb ring, inhaler, massage, mist spray, steam inhalation, steam room and sauna

CADE

Botanical Name: *Juniperus oxycedrus*

Family: *Cupressaceae*

The essential oil is obtained from the wood chips and branches.

History and Information

- Cade is an evergreen shrub native to the Asian and Mediterranean regions. The shrub grows to a height of about 15–35 feet (4.5–10.5 meters) with needlelike leaves and brownish-red cones. Cade is also known as prickly juniper or prickly cedar.

- Through the years, cade oil has been used for snakebites, leprosy, to soothe toothaches, kill lice and their eggs, and heal skin conditions, particularly psoriasis.

- Cade is used in perfumery, especially in men's fragrances, and as a food flavoring for a smoky taste. Veterinary practitioners use the oil for parasitic skin problems.

Practical Uses

Relieves aches and pains

Skin care

Documented Properties

Analgesic, antipruritic, antiseptic, disinfectant, parasiticide (skin), vermifuge

Aromatherapy Methods of Use

Application, aroma lamp, lightbulb ring, massage, mist spray

CAJEPUT

Botanical Name: *Melaleuca cajuputi, Melaleuca leucadendron, Melaleuca minor*

Family: *Myrtaceae*

The essential oil is obtained from the leaves and buds.

History and Information

- Cajeput is an evergreen tree native to Australia and Asia. The tree grows to a height of about 50–100 feet (15–30.5 meters), has a papery bark and narrow elliptical leaves. It is cultivated in many areas as an ornamental tree for its outstanding white, pink, or purple flowers. Cajeput belongs to a family of over 150 trees. The tree is also known as white tea tree, swamp tea tree, and paperbark tree.

- In Malaysia and Java, cajeput oil was a traditional remedy for cholera and muscle and joint pains. In Malaysia, the tree is called cajuputi, which means white wood.

- In Africa and Asia, the oil is used as an insecticide and parasiticide.

- Cajeput has been used for painful muscles and joints, muscular tension, sprains, and bruises.

Practical Uses

Slightly warming; improves circulation

Calming, reduces stress; promotes a restful sleep

Vapors open the sinus and breathing passages; deepens the breathing

Relieves aches and pains

Disinfectant

Repels insects

Documented Properties

Analgesic, anthelmintic, antibacterial, antidote, anti-inflammatory, antineuralgic, antipruritic, antirheumatic, antiseptic, antispasmodic, balsamic, calmative, carminative, cicatrizant, counterirritant, decongestant, diaphoretic, emollient (skin), estrogenic, expectorant, febrifuge, germicide, healing, insecticide, parasiticide, pectoral, stimulant (circulatory system), sudorific, tonic, vermifuge

Aromatherapy Methods of Use

Application, aroma lamp, bath, diffusor, inhaler, lightbulb ring, massage, mist spray, steam inhalation, steam room and sauna

CALAMINT *(Catnip)*

Botanical Name: *Calamintha clinopodium, Calamintha grandiflora, Calamintha officinalis, Nepeta cataria, Satureja calamintha*

Family: *Lamiaceae*

The essential oil is obtained from the flowering tops.

History and Information

- Calamint is a bushy plant native to Europe and Asia. The aromatic plant grows to a height of about 3 feet (1 meter), has a flowering spike with small pink flowers, and mint-scented leaves.

- Culpeper, the herbalist, found calamint useful for shortness of breath, cramps, and intestinal worms.

- In folk medicine, an herbal tea was brewed for colds, frazzled nerves, stomach upsets, diarrhea, fever, and to regulate the menstrual flow.

- In Europe, a leaf infusion was used for coughs and as a poultice for skin injuries.

- The leaves are chewed for toothache, made into a poultice to reduce swellings, and brewed into a tea to calm the nerves.

- Felines are attracted to, and become playful in, the presence of calamint.

Practical Uses

Calming

Mood uplifting; improves mental clarity and alertness

Lessens pain

Documented Properties

Analgesic, antirheumatic, antispasmodic, aperitive, astringent, carminative, diaphoretic, digestive, emmenagogue, expectorant, febrifuge, hypnotic, nervine, pectoral, sedative, stomachic, sudorific, tonic

Aromatherapy Methods of Use

Application, aroma lamp, bath, diffusor, inhaler, lightbulb ring, massage, mist spray, steam inhalation, steam room and sauna

CALAMUS *(Sweet Flag)*

Botanical Name: *Acorus calamus, Calamus aromaticus*

Family: *Araceae*

The essential oil and CO_2 extract are obtained from the roots.

History and Information

- Calamus is native to Europe, Asia, and North America. The plant grows to a height of about 2–6 feet (.5–2 meters), has swordlike leaves and yellow-green flowers.

- The herb has been used for 4,000 years.

- Ancient Egyptians used calamus as an aphrodisiac.

- Native Americans made a remedy from the plant for fevers, digestion, and colic.

- In Asia, the root is taken for its aphrodisiac effect.

- The Chinese use calamus to treat deafness, dizziness, and epileptic seizures.

- The Turkish people use the roots to treat infections. The candied roots are eaten as a preventative against disease and for coughs.

- In Europe, it is used as a digestive aid and for intestinal upsets.

- In India, the powdered herb serves as an insecticide.

- Calamus yields approximately 2 percent essential oil, which is used in cosmetics, shampoos, perfumes, and as an ingredient in foods and liqueurs. Chewing gum and breath fresheners are produced from the roots.

Documented Properties

Analgesic, antibacterial, anticonvulsive, anti-inflammatory, antirheumatic, antiseptic, antispasmodic, aperitive, aphrodisiac, carminative, diaphoretic, digestive, expectorant, febrifuge, hypotensor, insect repellent, refreshing, restorative (brain; nervous system), sedative, stimulant (salivary glands), stomachic, tonic, vermifuge

Caution: The calamus that grows in India contains a high content of the component asarone, which is potentially toxic and carcinogenic. Plants grown in Russia contain only a small percentage of asarone, while the North American variety has none.

CAMPHOR

Botanical Name: *Cinnamomum camphora, Laurus camphora*

Family: *Lauraceae*

The essential oil is obtained from the wood.

History and Information

- Camphor is a semi-evergreen tree native to Asia. The tree grows to a height of about 40–100 feet (12–30.5 meters), has red leaves that turn shiny green, and clusters of yellow flowers. Camphor is related to the cinnamon and cassia trees.

- Camphor has been used in Chinese medicine for 2,000 years.
- The price of camphor was once higher than the price of gold.
- Ayurvedic medicine uses the plant for headaches, infections, and snake and insect bites.
- The scent of camphor repels insects and was used in clothes and linen closets.

Practical Uses

Vapors open the sinus and breathing passages

Mood uplifting

Documented Properties

Analgesic, anthelmintic, antibacterial, antidepressant, anti-inflammatory, antirheumatic, antiseptic, antispasmodic, antiviral, cardiac, carminative, counterirritant, diaphoretic, diuretic, expectorant, febrifuge, hypertensive, insect repellent, insecticide, laxative, rubefacient, sedative, stimulant (central nervous system; adrenal glands; respiratory system), sudorific, tonic, vasoconstrictor, vermifuge, vulnerary

Caution: Camphor is an adrenal stimulant and can be harmful. The oil should be avoided by people prone to epileptic seizures. Do not use on children. If used on adults, use only very small amounts.

CAMPHOR *(Borneol)*

Botanical Name: *Dryobalanops aromatica, Dryobalanops camphora*

Family: *Dipterocarpaceae*

The essential oil is obtained from the wood.

History and Information

- Borneol camphor is a tall evergreen tree native to Asia. The tree grows to about 50–160 feet (15–49 meters) high, has leathery leaves and small white flowers.
- Camphor has been highly regarded in Asian countries for over 2,000 years. It was used as a remedy against plagues.

Practical Uses

Vapors open the sinus and breathing passages

Mood uplifting

Adrenal stimulant

Documented Properties

Analgesic, antidepressant, anti-inflammatory, antiseptic, antispasmodic, antiviral, carminative, diuretic, rubefacient, stimulant (adrenal glands), tonic

Caution: Borneol camphor should only be used in small amounts since it can cause an overstimulation of the adrenal glands. Exercise caution when using this essential oil.

CAMPHOR BUSH

Botanical Name: *Tarchonanthus camphoratus, Tarchonanthus minor*

Family: *Asteraceae*

The essential oil is obtained from the fresh leaves and flowers.

History and Information

- Camphor bush is an evergreen shrub native to Africa that can survive harsh environments from moist to arid locations, including strong winds and blowing sea mists. The shrub grows to a height of about 6–30 feet (2–9 meters), has an aromatic bark, narrow, leathery grey-green leaves, and white scented flowers that develop into fragrant fruits covered with fluffy cottonlike hairs. The male and female flowers are on separate shrubs. The shrub is also known as African wild sage, white cotton, camphor tree, and mikalambati.
- In Africa, a tea is made from the leaves for stomach problems, breathing congestion, coughs, colds, flu, headaches, muscle and joint aches, and toothaches. The crushed leaves are applied to the skin to heal cuts and wounds. The cottonlike seeds are stuffed into pillows to improve sleep.
- A poultice of the leaves is applied to the chest to relieve chest inflammations and breathing problems.

- The leaves are placed in bedding to promote a good night's sleep and used as an insect repellent.
- Animals have been observed brushing their body against the shrub in order to take on the scent to repel biting insects.
- The essential oil is also known as leleshwa.

Practical Uses

Calming

Reduces pain

Insect repellent

Healing to the skin

Acts as a preservative in formulations

Documented Properties

Antibacterial, antifungal, antiseptic, antiviral

Aromatherapy Methods of Use

Application, bath, inhaler, massage, mist spray

CANANGA

Botanical Name: *Cananga odorata*

Family: *Annonaceae*

The essential oil is obtained from flowers.

History and Information

- Cananga is an evergreen tree native to Asia. The tree grows to a height of about 100 feet (30.5 meters), has glossy leaves and large, fragrant, yellow flowers.
- In the nineteenth century, cananga was an ingredient in a European hair oil.

Practical Uses

Calming, reduces stress; promotes a restful sleep

Mood uplifting, euphoric

Lessens pain, relaxes the muscles

Documented Properties

Antidepressant, antiseptic, aphrodisiac, emollient,

euphoriant, fixative, hypotensor, nervine, relaxant, sedative, tonic

Aromatherapy Methods of Use

Application, aroma lamp, bath, diffusor, inhaler, light-bulb ring, massage, mist spray

CAPE CHAMOMILE

Botanical Name: *Eriocephalus punctulatus*

Family: *Asteraceae*

The essential oil is obtained from the stems, flowers, and leaves.

History and Information

- Cape chamomile is native to South Africa. The shrub is aromatic and has long and narrow needle-like leaves. It is also known as kapok bush.
- In South Africa, the leaves are used to lessen swellings.
- The plant was burned to fumigate and purify an area to remove negative spirits after a person died.

Practical Uses

Warming

Calming, reduces stress and anxiety; promotes a peaceful state

Mood uplifting, euphoric, aphrodisiac; encourages communication

Loosens tight muscles

Documented Properties

Analgesic, anticonvulsive, antidepressant, anti-inflammatory, antiseptic, antispasmodic, cholagogue, diuretic, emmenagogue, febrifuge, hepatic, nervine, sedative, stimulant (uterine), stomachic, sudorific, tonic, vasoconstrictor, vermifuge

Aromatherapy Methods of Use

Application, aroma lamp, bath, diffusor, inhaler, lightbulb ring, massage, mist spray, steam inhalation, steam room and sauna

CAPE MAY

Botanical Name: *Coleonema album*

Family: *Rutaceae*

The essential oil is obtained from the stems and leaves.

History and Information

- Cape May is an evergreen shrub native to South Africa. The shrub grows to a height of about 6 feet (2 meters), has small aromatic green pointed needlelike leaves and many small white flowers followed by brown fruit. The plant is also known as white confetti bush.

- Cape May has been used to reduce body aches and joint problems, to repel insects, and as a deodorant.

Practical Uses

Cooling

Helps to breathe easier

Mood uplifting

Documented Properties

Antiseptic, diuretic, febrifuge, insecticide, sedative

Aromatherapy Methods of Use

Application, aroma lamp, bath, diffusor, inhaler, lightbulb ring, massage, mist spray, steam inhalation, steam room and sauna

CAPE SNOWBUSH
(Wild Rosemary)

Botanical Name: *Eriocephalus africanus*

Family: *Asteraceae*

The essential oil is obtained from the leaves and stems.

History and Information

- Cape snowbush is native to South Africa. The plant grows to a height of about 3 feet (1 meter), has small aromatic greyish-green leaves, and pur-

ple centered white flowers followed by white hairy seeds.

- In Africa, a tea is made for coughs, colds, stomach problems, menstrual cramps, and can be used as a diuretic.

Practical Uses

Helps to breathe easier; deepens the breathing

Mood uplifting; improves mental clarity

Documented Properties

Antidepressant, antiseptic, antispasmodic, balsamic, carminative, cephalic, decongestive, digestive, diuretic, sedative, stomachic, styptic, sudorific, tonic, vulnerary

Aromatherapy Methods of Use

Application, aroma lamp, bath, diffusor, inhaler, lightbulb ring, massage, mist spray, steam inhalation, steam room and sauna

CAPE VERBENA
(Lippia or Zinziba)

Botanical Name: *Lippia javanica*

Family: *Verbenaceae*

The essential oil is obtained from the leaves and twigs.

History and Information

- Cape verbena is native to South Africa. The woody aromatic shrub grows to a height of about 3–7 feet (1–2 meters), has strongly lemon-scented leaves and small yellow-white flowers that develop into small fruit. The shrub is also known as fever tree, wild tea, and lemon bush.

- The natives of South Africa make a tea beverage from the leaves for colds, coughs, fever, breathing congestion, headaches, and nervousness. A poultice is applied on rashes and insect bites. The leaves, mixed with a vegetal oil, are rubbed into the muscles to relieve soreness. The oil has been diluted in water and used as a gargle for sore throats, the vapors have been inhaled for coughs and colds, and it is applied externally for insect bites and used as an insect repellent.

Practical Uses

Helps to breathe easier; deepens the breathing

Calming, reduces stress, relieves tension, promotes a peaceful state, and a restful sleep

Helpful for meditation

Mood uplifting, euphoric; slightly energizing, improves mental clarity

Loosens tight muscles

Documented Properties

Analgesic, antidepressant, antipruritic, antiseptic, disinfectant, emollient, expectorant, febrifuge, hemostatic, insecticide, uplifting

Aromatherapy Methods of Use

Application, aroma lamp, bath, inhaler, lightbulb ring, massage, mist spray, steam inhalation, steam room and sauna

CARAWAY

Botanical Name:
Apium carvi, Carum carvi

Family: *Apiaceae*

The essential oil and CO_2 extract are obtained from the seeds.

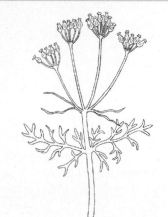

History and Information

- Caraway is native to Europe and Asia. The plant grows to a height of about 2 feet (.5 meter), has carrotlike leaves and small white or pink flowers with seed capsules that bursts open when mature, and a fleshy root that looks like a carrot.

- Caraway seeds have been in use for 5,000 years. In the Ebers Papyrus in 1550 B.C., the ancient Egyptians recommended caraway for digestive upsets.

- Dioscorides, the Greek physician, suggested eating the seeds to aid digestion.

- Caraway is used to promote menstruation, lactation in nursing mothers, and for menstrual cramps. A cream made from the herb was used by European women to remove wrinkles and beautify their skin.

- Caraway was once an essential ingredient in love potions.

- Country people fed their animals caraway to keep them from straying.

- The seeds yield 3 to 5 percent essential oil, which is used to flavor two digestive aid liqueurs: Scandinavian Aquavit and German Kümmel. Caraway seeds are often used in breads, pastries, and sauces to aid the digestive process and relieve flatulence.

Practical Uses

Improves digestion, soothes the intestines, relieves flatulence

Relieves pain, and menstrual discomfort

Documented Properties

Abortifacient, antibacterial, antiseptic, antispasmodic, aperitive, astringent, cardiac, carminative, depurative, digestive, disinfectant, diuretic, emmenagogue, expectorant (mild), galactagogue, parasiticide, regenerator (tissue), stimulant (circulation; digestive and glandular systems), stomachic, tonic (nerves and digestive organs), vermifuge

Aromatherapy Methods of Use

Application, aroma lamp, bath, diffusor, inhaler, lightbulb ring, massage, mist spray

CARDAMOM

Botanical Name: *Elettaria cardamomum*

Family: *Zingiberaceae*

The essential oil and CO_2 extract are obtained from the seeds.

History and Information

- Cardamom is native to Asia. The plant grows to a height of about 10 feet (3 meters) and has small yellow flowers. The fruit holds eighteen seeds.

- Cardamom was first brought to the West by soldiers of Alexander the Great upon returning from India.

- The earliest reports of Ayurvedic medicine mentioned cardamom for its use in urinary problems and reducing body fat. Cardamom has also been a remedy for hemorrhoids, nausea, headaches, and fever.

- The Romans ate the seeds to aid digestion.

- In India, the seeds are chewed as a breath freshener.

- Chinese medicine considers cardamom invaluable for intestinal problems. It is also used for pulmonary conditions and fevers.

- Cardamom is the most popular spice in the Arab countries. A coffee made from the seeds is consumed regularly by the people of Saudi Arabia. In Scandinavian countries, the seeds are used in pastries.

- Approximately 80 percent of the world's supply of cardamom is produced in India. The fruits and seeds yield approximately 4 to 7 percent essential oil.

Practical Uses

Warming; improves circulation

Improves digestion, soothes the intestines, relieves flatulence

Mood uplifting; energizing, improves mental clarity, improves physical strength, increases sexual strength

Relieves pain, menstrual pains and cramps

Documented Properties

Antiseptic, antispasmodic, aperitif, aperitive, aphrodisiac, calmative, carminative, cephalic, digestive, diuretic, expectorant, refreshing, stimulant (circulation; digestion), stomachic, tonic, uplifting

Aromatherapy Methods of Use

Application, aroma lamp, bath, diffusor, inhaler, lightbulb ring, massage, mist spray

CARNATION *(Clove Pink)*

Botanical Name: *Dianthus caryophyllus*

Family: *Caryophyllaceae*

The absolute/essential oil is obtained from the flowers.

History and Information

- The carnation plant originated in Europe. The bushy plant reaches a height of about 2 feet (.5 meter). The white, yellow, orange, pink, red, or purple flowers emit a fragrance that intensifies towards the evening.

- Carnations were the most popular flower used in garlands, chaplets, and coronets at coronation ceremonies; thus, its name was derived from the word "coronation."

- The oil is extracted from the double-flowered variety of clove pink, which has a spicy fragrance.

Practical Uses

Mood uplifting

Fragrancing

Documented Properties

Antidepressant, antistress, calmative, sedative

Aromatherapy Methods of Use

Application, aroma lamp, fragrancing, inhaler, lightbulb ring, massage, mist spray

CARROT SEED

Botanical Name: *Daucus carota*

Family: *Apiaceae*

The essential oil and CO_2 extract are obtained from the seeds.

History and Information

See Carrot Root in Chapter 2, page 21

Practical Uses

Warming

Calming, relieves tension

Opens the breathing

Mood uplifting; energizing, improves mental clarity

Loosens tight muscles

Documented Properties

Anthelmintic, antilithic, antioxidant, antipruritic, antisclerotic, aperitive, astringent, carminative, diuretic, emmenagogue, galactagogue, hemostatic, hepatic, laxative, parasiticide, rejuvenator (skin cells), stimulant (uterine), tonic, vasodilator, vermifuge, vulnerary

Aromatherapy Methods of Use

Application, aroma lamp, bath, diffusor, inhaler, lightbulb ring, massage, mist spray

CASCARILLA BARK

Botanical Name: *Croton eleuteria*

Family: *Euphorbiaceae*

The essential oil is obtained from the bark.

History and Information

• Cascarilla is native to the West Indies and Central America. The tree grows to a height of about 40 feet (12 meters), has an aromatic bark, and small white, pink, or red fragrant flowers that develop into a seed capsule.

• In Latin America, a stimulating drink is brewed from the leaves and bark. The tea is also taken to reduce fevers. It is sold commercially as a substitute for quinine.

• In China, the bark is used for malaria, pain, and nausea.

• The bark emits an aromatic scent when burned. Cascarilla is used extensively in cigarettes for the aroma when smoked. The oil is an ingredient to flavor foods and beverages and to fragrance soaps, detergents, cosmetics, and perfumes. The yield of essential oil is approximately 2 percent. An oil is also made from the seeds, but it is dangerous due to the strong purgative effect.

Practical Uses

Warming

Calming, reduces stress, relieves tension

Helps to deepen the breathing

Mood uplifting, euphoric

Documented Properties

Antiseptic, astringent, carminative, digestive, expectorant, stomachic, tonic

Aromatherapy Methods of Use

Application, bath, massage, mist spray

CASSIA

CASSIA BARK

Botanical Name: *Cinnamomum aromaticum, Cinnamomum cassia, Laurus cassia*

Family: *Lauraceae*

The essential oil is obtained from the young leaves and twigs.

The essential oil and CO_2 extract are obtained from the bark.

History and Information

- Cassia is an evergreen tree native to Asia. The tree grows to a height of about 40–80 feet (12–24 meters), has small green flowers and a thin peeling bark.

- Cassia was considered one of the most important herbs used in the Greek and Roman pharmacopoeia. Cassia leaves were also mentioned as a spice in a first century Roman cookbook.

- Its name was derived from the Greek word kassia, which means "to strip off the bark." This refers to the way the essential oil is obtained by stripping the bark and boiling it. The bark yields approximately 2 percent of essential oil. Cassia has a stronger aroma than cinnamon, is cheaper in price, and is sometimes referred to as "poor man's cinnamon."

Practical Uses

Heating; improves circulation

Helps in the reduction of cellulite

Mood uplifting; reviving, helps to relieve a fatigued state

Lessens pain, increases mobility in the joints

Disinfectant

Repels insects

Documented Properties

Analgesic, anesthetic, antibacterial, antiemetic, antifertility, antifungal, anti-inflammatory, antimutagenic, antioxidant, antipyretic, antiseptic, antitumor, antiviral, aphrodisiac, astringent, cardiotonic, carminative, diaphoretic, digestive, diuretic, emmenagogue, expectorant, febrifuge, hepatic, hypotensor, immunostimulant, laxative, parasiticide, purgative, sedative, stimulant (increases contractions during childbirth; circulatory system), tonic, vasodilator

Aromatherapy Methods of Use

Aroma lamp, diffusor, lightbulb ring, mist spray

Caution: Cassia and cassia bark essential oils are heating and can cause skin irritation. Avoid use on the skin.

CASSIE

Botanical Name: *Acacia farnesiana, Cassia ancienne*
Family: *Mimosaceae*
The absolute/essential oil is obtained from the flowers.

History and Information

- Cassie is native to the West Indies and tropical America. The bush grows to a height of about 5–25 feet (1.5–7.5 meters), has leathery leaflets and tiny, sweet, fragrant yellow flowers that develop into kidney-shaped seeds in a pod.

- In Central America, a drink from the infused flowers is taken for stomach troubles, headaches, and to calm the nerves.

- In India, cassie is made into a perfume.

- In China, the flowers are used for muscle and joint pains and chest ailments.

- The oil is added to fragrances and expensive perfumes and used as a food flavoring ingredient.

Practical Uses

Mood uplifting

Documented Properties

Antirheumatic, antiseptic, antispasmodic, aphrodisiac, balsamic, insecticide

Aromatherapy Methods of Use

Fragrancing

CEDARWOOD

Botanical Name: *Juniperus virginiana*
Family: *Cupressaceae*
The essential oil is obtained from the sawdust and wood chips.

History and Information

- Cedarwood is an evergreen tree native to North America. The tree grows to a height of over 100 feet (30.5 meters).

- The American Indians burned the twigs and inhaled the smoke to relieve head colds and chest congestion. The fumes were also used to promote childbirth delivery.

- Pencils are made from the wood of the tree.

- The wood repels moths and other insects and is made into furniture to store clothing.

Practical Uses

Calming, relieves anxiety and nervous tension; promotes a restful sleep

Encourages dreaming; helpful for meditation

Vapors open the sinus and breathing passages; eases chest congestion when rubbed on the chest

Lessens pain

Repels insects

Documented Properties

Abortifacient, antipruritic, antiseptic, antispasmodic, astringent, balsamic, diuretic, emmenagogue, emollient, expectorant, healing (skin), insect repellent, sedative, stimulant (circulatory system)

Aromatherapy Methods of Use

Application, aroma lamp, bath, inhaler, lightbulb ring, massage, mist spray, steam inhalation, steam room and sauna

Caution: Due to the toxicity of the essential oil, use small amounts.

CEDARWOOD *(Atlas)*
CEDARWOOD *(Himalayan or Deodar)*
CEDARWOOD *(Lebanon)*

Botanical Name: *Cedrus atlantica* (Cedarwood atlas), *Cedrus deodara* (Himalayan cedarwood, Deodar cedarwood), *Cedrus libani* (Cedar-of-Lebanon, Lebanon cedarwood)

Family: *Pinaceae*

The essential oil is obtained from the wood.

History and Information

- Cedarwood atlas is an evergreen tree native to Africa. The tree grows to a height of about 130–140 feet (39.5–42.5 meters), has bluish-green needlelike leaves and cones. If undisturbed, the tree can reach an age of 1,000 to 2,000 years.

- Himalayan/Deodar cedarwood is an evergreen tree native to the Himalayas. The tree reaches 150 feet (46 meters), has dark-blue-green needlelike leaves, yellow male cones, and green female seed cones.

- Lebanon cedarwood is an evergreen tree native to Lebanon. The tree grows to more than 100–150 feet (46 meters), has grey-green needlelike leaves and cones.

- A grove of cedars from which King Solomon built his temple still exists today on Mount Lebanon. The first cedar planted in Great Britain, in 1646, is still living today.

- The wood was thought to be indestructible and, therefore, was used in the building palaces, mummy cases, and furniture.

- Cedarwood was highly prized and valued by the Egyptians for its use in cosmetics. It was also burned in the temples of Egypt and Greece.

- In the Middle East, the branches of cedar lebanon are burned and the smoke inhaled for breathing problems.

- The oil is used extensively in hair and skin care products. In France, it is added to shampoos and lotions to protect the hair and prevent hair loss.

Practical Uses

Cooling

Calming, relieves anxiety and nervous tension; promotes a restful sleep

Encourages dreaming; helpful for meditation

Vapors open the sinus and breathing passages; eases chest congestion when rubbed on the chest

Improves mental clarity

Loosens tight muscles, lessens pain,

Repels insects

A fixative to hold the scent of a fragrance

Documented Properties

Antibacterial, antidepressant, antifungal, antiputrid, antiseptic, aphrodisiac, astringent, detoxifier (cellulite), diuretic, expectorant, fixative, insect repellent, regenerator (skin), sedative, stimulant (circulatory system), tonic

Aromatherapy Methods of Use

Application, aroma lamp, bath, inhaler, lightbulb ring, massage, mist spray, steam inhalation, steam room and sauna

CELERY

Botanical Name: *Apium graveolens*

Family: *Apiaceae*

The essential oil and CO_2 extract are obtained from the seeds.

History and Information

- Celery is native to the Mediterranean area. The biennial plant grows to a height of about 1–2 feet (.5 meter) and has green-white flowers that develop into seeds.

- The Romans and Greeks grew celery for medicinal purposes. The Greeks also made a celery wine, which was given to victorious athletes.

- Ayurvedic physicians in India have used celery seeds since ancient times for water retention, joint problems, and indigestion.

- In Latin America, the root is made into a tea and taken several times a day to dry up breast milk. The tea is also consumed to help the nervous system, relieve joint and muscle aches, urinary problems, to regulate menstruation, and improve digestion.

- In Europe, the seeds are a common medicinal treatment for gout, as well as muscle and joint pains.

- Celery stimulates childbirth labor and is said to lower blood pressure.

- The seeds yield approximately 2 percent essential oil. Celery oil is an ingredient in foods, liqueurs, perfumes, and soaps.

Practical Uses

Cooling

Purifying; helps in the reduction of cellulite

Calming, relaxing; promotes a restful sleep

Documented Properties

Abortifacient, analgesic, antiarthritic, anticonvulsive, antigalactogogue, antilithic, antioxidant, antiphlogistic, antirheumatic, antiscorbutic, antispasmodic, aperitive, aphrodisiac, carminative, cholagogue, depurative, diaphoretic, digestive, diuretic, emmenagogue, hepatic, hypotensor, nervine, sedative, stimulant (uterine contractions), stomachic, tonic, vulnerary

Aromatherapy Methods of Use

Application, aroma lamp, bath, inhaler, lightbulb ring, massage, mist spray

Caution: Celery tends to slow down reflexes. Avoid driving or doing anything that requires full attention after using the essential oil. Due to celery's detoxifying effect, use in small amounts.

CHAMOMILE *(German)*
CHAMOMILE *(Roman)*

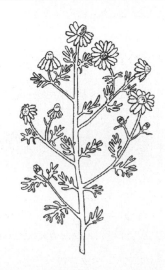

Botanical Name:
Matricaria chamomilla,
Matricaria recutita
(German chamomile);
Anthemis nobilis,
Chamaemelum nobile
(Roman chamomile)

Family: *Asteraceae*

The essential oil is
obtained from the
flowers and leaves.

German chamomile
CO_2 extract is obtained
from the flowers.

History and Information

- German chamomile is native to Europe and Asia. The plant grows to a height of about 3 feet (1 meter) and has small daisylike yellow flowerheads with white petals.

- Roman chamomile is native to Europe and Asia. The plant grows to a height of about 1 foot (.5 meter) and has flowers that are similar in appearance to daisies.

- The Greek physicians, Dioscorides and Galen, used chamomile for female ailments and fevers. In southern Europe, chamomile is still used for childbearing and female problems.

- The Egyptian sages dedicated the plant to the sun for its ability to reduce fevers. The flowers were powdered and used to relieve pain.

- In Latin America, the flowers from Roman chamomile are taken as a nerve tonic, to aid digestion, for muscle and joint aches, and menstrual problems.

- A tea made from the flowers of German chamomile is used for menstrual conditions, stomach upsets, breathing difficulties, and nervous problems.

- Chamomile is one of the most popular herbal teas in the Western world.

- Chamomile contains a component called azulene, which is formed after the essential oil is distilled. The German variety yields a greater amount. Azulene has been found to be an excellent anti-inflammatory agent.

- Roman chamomile is used in cosmetics, perfumes, creams, lotions, soaps, detergents, soft drinks, alcoholic beverages, and liquers.

Practical Uses

Improves digestion, soothes the intestines

Calming; promotes a restful sleep

Mood uplifting

Lessens pain, relieves menstrual discomfort, soothes inflammation

Healing to the skin

Soothes insect bites

Documented Properties

Analgesic, antianemic, antibacterial, anticonvulsive, antidepressant, antiemetic, antifungal, anti-inflammatory, antineuralgic, antipruritic, antirheumatic, antiseptic, antispasmodic, antistress, antitoxic, aperitive, calmative, carminative, cholagogue, cicatrizant, diaphoretic, digestive, diuretic, emmenagogue, emollient, febrifuge, healing, hepatic, hypotensor, laxative, nervine, regenerator (skin), sedative, stimulant (digestive system; spleen, uterine), stomachic, sudorific, tonic, vermifuge, vulnerary

Aromatherapy Methods of Use

Application, aroma lamp, bath, diffusor, inhaler, light-bulb ring, massage, mist spray

CHAMOMILE *(Moroccan)*

Botanical Name: *Anthemis mixta, Ormenis mixta, Ormenis multicaulis*

Family: *Asteraceae*

The essential oil is obtained from the flowering tops.

History and Information

- Moroccan chamomile is native to Africa and the Mediterranean area. The plant grows to a height of about 2 feet (.5 meter) and has yellow flowers.

Practical Uses

Calming

Documented Properties

Anti-inflammatory, antiseptic, antispasmodic, calmative, cholagogue, emmenagogue, hepatic, parasiticide, sedative, tonic

Aromatherapy Methods of Use

Application, aroma lamp, bath, diffusor, inhaler, light-bulb ring, massage, mist spray

CHAMPACA FLOWER
CHAMPACA LEAF

Botanical Name: *Michelia alba, Michelia champaca*

Family: *Magnoliaceae*

The champaca flower essential oil is obtained from the flowers.

The champaca leaf essential oil is obtained from the leaves.

History and Information

- Champaca is an evergreen tree native to Asia. The tree grows to a height of about 65 feet (6–20 meters), has long glossy green leaves and small, fragrant white, yellow, or orange flowers that develop into yellow-green fruits.

- The tree is planted in India around temples to supply flowers for religious ceremonies. It is held in reverence and considered sacred by the Hindus.

- In India, the bark of the tree is used as a remedy to reduce fever, and the roots are used for skin disorders.

- The flowers have been used for inflamed eyes and urinary tract problems.

- The essential oil from the flowers is added to perfumes, cosmetics, and after-bath and hair care products.

Practical Uses for the Flower Oil

Warming

Calming, reduces stress, promotes a peaceful state

Helps to breathe easier

Mood uplifting, euphoric

A fixative to hold the scent of a fragrance

Practical Uses for the Leaf Oil

Warming

Calming, reduces stress

Helps to breathe easier

Euphoric; improves mental clarity

Documented Properties

Aphrodisiac, emollient, febrifuge

Aromatherapy Methods of Uses

Application, aroma lamp, bath, fragrancing, inhaler, lightbulb ring, massage, mist spray

CHERVIL

Botanical Name: *Anthriscus cerefolium*

Family: *Apiaceae*

The essential oil is obtained from the seeds or fruits.

History and Information

- Chervil is native to Europe. The plant reaches a height of about 1–2 feet (.5 meter), has bright-green leaves and small clusters of white flowers.

- Pliny, the Roman herbalist, recommended chervil for hiccoughs.

- The Greeks and Romans made a poultice with chervil leaves to heal wounds.

- Chervil is used in Europe to lower blood pressure.

Documented Properties

Antigalactagogue, anti-inflammatory, antilithic, antiseptic, aperitive, carminative, cholagogue, cicatrizant, depurative, diaphoretic, digestive, diuretic, expectorant, hepatic, laxative, stimulant, stomachic, tonic

Caution: Chervil oil is said to be toxic and is not used in aromatherapy.

CINNAMON BARK
CINNAMON LEAF

Botanical Name: *Cinnamomum verum, Cinnamomum zeylanicum, Laurus cinnamomum*

Family: *Lauraceae*

Cinnamon bark essential oil and CO_2 extract are obtained from the bark.

Cinnamon leaf essential oil is obtained from the leaves.

History and Information

- Cinnamon is an evergreen tree native to Asia, and prefers moist soils. The tree grows to a height of about 30–50 feet (9–15 meters), has leathery green leaves and small white to yellowish flowers that develop into blue to black berries.

- Cinnamon is one of the oldest spices mentioned in the Old Testament. Chinese herbalists wrote about cinnamon as early as 2700 B.C., and used it for fever, diarrhea, and menstrual problems.

- The cinnamon tree has been cultivated in Ceylon since 1200 A.D.

- The Egyptians used cinnamon in their embalming procedures.

- In ancient Greece and Rome, only royalty could afford cinnamon. The Greek and Roman pharmacopoeia recognized cinnamon as one of the most important herbs for its strong antiseptic properties.

- Cinnamon was one of the most sought-after spices during the explorations of the fifteenth and sixteenth centuries. At one time the spice was more valuable than gold. Cinnamon was one of the most expensive gifts among royalty and the privileged upper class in Europe.

- In Europe, cinnamon was a component of remedies recommended for coughs, colds, headaches, chest pain, and digestion problems.

- The spice has been taken to help with appetite, digestive problems, and applied topically to get rid of lice.

- In Chinese medicine, many herbal remedies require the inclusion of cinnamon. Some of the uses include a tonic for depression, a calmative, and a strengthener for the heart.

- In recent years, research has shown cinnamon to be effective in lowering blood sugar levels.

- Studies by Japanese researchers have shown that cinnamon kills fungi, bacteria, and other microorganisms, including the bacteria responsible for botulism poisoning and staph infections.

- The bark yields 0.5 to 1.5 percent essential oil, which becomes darker when it is exposed to air.

- The unripe berry buds are dried and used for flavoring.

- Cinnamon is the second most popular spice used by the Western world. It is only superceded by black pepper.

Practical Uses

Heating; improves circulation

Improves digestion

Purifying; helps in the reduction of cellulite

Reduces stress

Mood uplifting; reviving, helps to relieve a fatigued state

Loosens tight muscles, lessens pain

Disinfectant

Repels insects

Documented Properties

Analgesic, anesthetic, anthelmintic, antibacterial, anticonvulsant, antidepressant, antidiabetic, antidiarrhea, antidote, antiemetic, anti-inflammatory, antioxidant, antiputrid, antirheumatic, antiseptic (strong), antispasmodic, antitussive, antiviral, aperitif, aphrodisiac, astringent (mild), cardiac, carminative, digestive, emmenagogue, emollient, estrogenic, expectorant, febrifuge, hemostatic, hepatic, insecticide, parasiticide, stimulant (circulatory, glandular, nervous, and respiratory systems; production of secretions: saliva, tears, and mucous; uterine contractions), stomachic, tonic, vermifuge

Aromatherapy Methods of Use for Cinnamon Bark

Aroma lamp, diffusor, inhaler, lightbulb ring, mist spray

Aromatherapy Method of Use for Cinnamon Leaf

Application, aroma lamp, diffusor, inhaler, lightbulb ring, massage, mist spray

Caution: People with dry or sensitive skin may require additional carrier oil when applying cinnamon essential oil topically. Use small amounts.

CITRONELLA

Botanical Name: *Andropogon nardus, Cymbopogon nardus*

Family: *Poaceae*

The essential oil is obtained from the grass.

History and Information

- Citronella is an aromatic tall grass native to Asia.
- Citronella is also known as mana grass and is widely used in soaps, perfumery, sanitary products, and insect repellents.
- Since the oil is inexpensive, it is used to adulterate other essential oils such as rose oil.

Practical Uses

Cooling

Calming, reduces stress

Mood uplifting; mental stimulant, improves mental clarity and alertness

Repels insects

Documented Properties

Antibacterial, antidepressant, antifungal, anti-inflammatory, antiseptic, antispasmodic, deodorant, deodorizer, diaphoretic, disinfectant, diuretic, emmenagogue, febrifuge, insect repellent, insecticide, parasiticide, stimulant (digestion), stomachic, tonic, uplifting, vermifuge

Aromatherapy Methods of Use

Application, aroma lamp, diffusor, inhaler, lightbulb ring, massage, mist spray

Caution: People with dry or sensitive skin may require additional carrier oil when using the essential oil topically. Citronella is phototoxic. Avoid exposure to direct sunlight for several hours after applying the oil on the skin.

CLARY SAGE

Botanical Name: *Salvia sclarea*

Family: *Lamiaceae*

The essential oil is obtained from the flowering tops.

History and Information

- Clary sage is native to Europe. The plant grows to a height of about 3 feet (1 meter) and has flowers that are pink, white, or blue, depending on the variety.
- In the 1500s, clary sage was cultivated in Europe mainly for brewing ales and adding to wine to make it more intoxicating.
- Clary sage is known to contain a hormone similar to estrogen, which is useful in helping women with sexual problems, menstrual discomfort, and premenstrual tension.

Practical Uses

Improves digestion

Calming, reduces stress, relieves tension; promotes a restful sleep

Mood uplifting, aphrodisiac; increases sexual strength

Relieves menstrual pain and cramps; regulates the female reproductive system

Documented Properties

Analgesic, anticonvulsive, antidepressant, anti-inflammatory, antiseptic, antispasmodic, antistress, antisudorific, aphrodisiac, astringent, balsamic, calmative, carminative, deodorant, digestive, emmenagogue, emollient, estrogenic, euphoriant, fixative, healing (skin), hypotensor, nervine, refreshing, relaxant (strong), regenerator (skin cells), sedative, stimulant (uterine contractions), stomachic, tonic, tonifying, uplifting, warming

Aromatherapy Methods of Use

Application, aroma lamp, bath, inhaler, lightbulb ring, massage, mist spray

Caution: Due to the relaxing effect of the essential oil, clary sage should not be used before driving or doing anything that requires full attention. Clary sage can dull the senses. Use small amounts.

CLEMENTINE

See Mandarin

CLOVE BUD
CLOVE LEAF
CLOVE STEM

Botanical Name: *Caryophyllus aromaticus, Eugenia aromatica, Eugenia caryophyllata, Eugenia caryophyllus, Syzygium aromaticum*

Family: *Myrtaceae*

Clove bud essential oil is obtained from the buds.

Clove leaf essential oil is obtained from the leaves.

Clove stem essential oil is obtained from the stems.

The CO_2 extract is obtained from the buds.

History and Information

- Clove is a tropical evergreen tree native to Asia. The tree grows to a height of about 40 feet (12 meters), has dark-green leaves and bright-pink buds that develop into yellow flowers followed by purple berries.

- In ancient Persia, clove was used in love potions.

- In Chinese medicine, clove is known for its antibacterial and antifungal properties.

- Ayurvedic healers in India have used clove to treat fevers, respiratory ailments, and digestive problems.

- The people of the Molucca Islands were devastated by previously unknown epidemics after the Dutch destroyed all the clove trees.

- In Africa, the bark, leaf, and roots have been used to increase lactation in nursing mothers.

- A folk remedy for the relief of headaches consisted of clove and apple-cider vinegar.

- Folk healers, pharmacists, and dentists have recommended cloves or clove oil to relieve toothaches.

- Clove oil was used to disinfect large public places like theaters.

- In Latin America, a tea made from the leaves and buds is consumed for breathing congestion.

- The buds yield 16 percent essential oil, the stems 4 to 6 percent, and the leaves 2 percent. The oils are used in perfumes, soaps, toothpastes, and mouthwashes. It is reported that Indonesian people consume almost 65 percent of the world's supply of cloves to make their own cigarettes by mixing it with tobacco.

Practical Uses

Heating

Improves digestion, relieves flatulence

Vapors open the sinus and breathing passages

Mood uplifting; aphrodisiac; reviving, mental stimulant, improves mental clarity and memory

Reduces pain by numbing the area

Disinfectant

Repels insects

Documented Properties

Abortifacient, analgesic, anesthetic (local), anthelmintic, antibacterial, antidepressant, antiemetic, antifungal, antineuralgic, antioxidant, antirheumatic, antiseptic (strong), antispasmodic, antistress, antiviral, aperitif, aphrodisiac, carminative, caustic, cicatrizant, counterirritant, disinfectant, emmenagogue, expectorant, insect repellent, insecticide, parasiticide, stimulant (vitality), stomachic, tonic, vermifuge

Aromatherapy Methods of Use

Application, aroma lamp, diffusor, inhaler, lightbulb ring, massage, mist spray

Caution: People with dry or sensitive skin may require additional carrier oil when applying clove essential oil topically. Use small amounts. The oil from clove bud is the only clove oil suitable for use in aromatherapy, since it is less irritating than the leaf and stem oils.

COFFEE

Botanical Name: *Coffea arabica*

Family: *Rubiaceae*

The essential oil is obtained from the beans.

History and Information

See Coffee in Chapter 2, page 26.

Practical Uses

Warming

Increases appetite

Mood uplifting; energizing, stimulating, improves mental clarity

Documented Properties

Diuretic, stimulant

Aromatherapy Methods of Use

Application, aroma lamp, bath, lightbulb ring, massage, mist spray

Caution: Coffee oil is an adrenal gland and nervous system stimulant. In large amounts, it can be deleterious to a person's health.

COMBAVA

Botanical Name: *Citrus hystrix*

Family: *Rutaceae*

The essential oil is obtained from the leaves and twigs.

History and Information

- Combava is native to Asia and thrives in tropical locations. The shrub has aromatic green leaves and white flowers, followed by edible citrus fruits that have a rough texture and a small amount of juice.

- The leaves have been used for fevers and colds, and as a purgative to cleanse the liver. The fruits and peels are used for fragrances, food flavoring, personal care products, and cleaners.

Practical Uses

Cooling

Calms the nerves, relieves anxiety, tension and mental stress; promotes a restful sleep

Helpful for meditation

Mood uplifting; improves mental clarity and alertness

Soothes inflamed and irritated skin tissue

Documented Properties

Antidepressant, antiseptic, antispasmodic, antistress, astringent, calmative, deodorant, digestive, fixative, nervine, parasiticide, refreshing, sedative, stimulant (digestive system), stomachic, tonic, uplifting

Aromatherapy Methods of Use

Application, aroma lamp, bath, diffusor, inhaler, lightbulb ring, massage, mist spray

COPAIBA

Botanical Name: *Copaifera officinalis*

Family: *Fabaceae*

The resin and essential oil are obtained from the tree trunk.

History and Information

- Copaiba is an evergreen tree native to tropical America and Africa. The tree grows to a height of about 60–100 feet (18–30.5 meters) and has small yellow flowers that turn from brown to red fruits. Copaiba is part of a species of about forty evergreen trees.

- The resin is extracted by drilling holes in the tree trunk; one tree can yield up to twelve gallons.

- In Brazil, copaiba sap is made into an ointment to heal the skin. The oil is recommended as an anti-inflammatory, for stomach disorders, and is used for hair care and to eliminate dandruff.

Practical Uses

Warming; improves circulation

Soothes the intestines

Calming, reduces stress, promotes a peaceful state of mind, and a restful sleep

Helpful for meditation

Opens the breathing passages for deeper breathing

Mood uplifting; improves mental clarity and alertness

Healing and moisturizing to the skin

A fixative to hold the scent of a fragrance

Documented Properties

Anthelmintic, antibacterial, anti-inflammatory, anti-ulcer, balsamic, decongestant, disinfectant, diuretic, expectorant, stimulant

Aromatherapy Methods of Use

Application, aroma lamp, bath, inhaler, lightbulb ring, massage, mist spray, steam inhalation, steam room and sauna

CORIANDER

Botanical Name: *Coriandrum sativum*

Family: *Apiaceae*

The essential oil is obtained from the seeds of the ripe fruits and the leaves.

The CO_2 extract is obtained from the seeds.

History and Information

- Coriander is native to the Mediterranean area. The plant grows to a height of about 3 feet (1 meter) and has small white flowers that develop into green seeds. Coriander is also known as cilantro and Chinese parsley.

- The use of coriander dates back to 5000 B.C.

- The Chinese used coriander in the third century B.C. They believed the seeds contained the power of immortality.

- In Ayurvedic medicine, coriander was used to relieve constipation and help sleep.

- Greek and Roman physicians, including Hippocrates, made medicines with coriander. It was also highly prized as a spice and used as an ingredient in Roman vinegar to preserve meat and flavor bread.

- The Egyptians added coriander seeds to wine to increase intoxication.

- In the Middle East and Europe, coriander has been valued as a love potion and aphrodisiac.

- To ease the pain and facilitate childbirth, a preparation of coriander seeds was placed on a woman's thighs while she was in labor.

- In European cultures, a tea or soup made from the leaves and mixed with barley water is taken to help a person regain strength while recovering from an illness.

- In China, coriander seeds are used to break up phlegm, stop bleeding, and for hemorrhoids. The herb is taken for indigestion, nausea, and constipation.

- Coriander was listed in the United States Pharmacopoeia from 1820 to 1980.

- The seeds yield 0.5 to 1 percent essential oil. The oil is used as an ingredient in perfumes, candy, chocolate, baked goods, brewing, many liqueurs, and to flavor beer.

Practical Uses

Improves digestion, relieves flatulence, aerophagy and nausea; strengthens and tones the stomach

Reviving, energizing, helps to relieve a fatigued state, improves mental clarity and memory

Relieves pain

Documented Properties

Abortifacient, analgesic, anesthetic, antibacterial, anti-inflammatory, antimutagenic, antioxidant, antirheumatic, antispasmodic, antitumor, aperitif, aperitive, aphrodisiac, calmative, cardiotonic, carminative, deodorant, depurative, detoxifier, diaphoretic, digestive, diuretic, emmenagogue, febrifuge, hepatic, nervine, refreshing, regenerator, revitalizing, stimulant (circulatory system), stomachic, tonic, uplifting, warming

Aromatherapy Methods of Use

Application, aroma lamp, bath, diffusor, inhaler, lightbulb ring, massage, mist spray

Caution: Use small amounts.

CORNMINT

Botanical Name: *Mentha arvensis*

Family: *Lamiaceae*

The essential oil is obtained from the leaves.

History and Information

- Cornmint is native to North America and Asia. The plant grows to a height of about 1–3 feet (.5–1 meter), has aromatic leaves and small clusters of white or purplish flowers.

- The leaves yield an essential oil that is comprised of approximately 85 percent menthol. The oil is dementholized because the high menthol content causes it to solidify at room temperature. A large portion of the world's supply of menthol is derived from the cornmint plant.

Practical Uses

Cooling

Improves digestion, relieves flatulence

Vapors open the sinus and breathing passages; deepens the breathing

Mood uplifting especially to people who have a slow metabolism; refreshing, reviving, energizing, improves mental clarity and alertness, sharpens the senses

Lessens pain

Repels insects

Documented Properties

Antibacterial, antiseptic, antispasmodic, carminative, digestive, expectorant, refreshing, refrigerant, stimulant, stomachic

Aromatherapy Methods of Use

Aroma lamp, diffusor, fragrancing, inhaler, lightbulb ring, mist spray, steam inhalation, sauna and steam room

Comments: For applications other than fragrancing, it is best to use peppermint or spearmint oil, since cornmint is a fractionated oil.

Caution: People with dry or sensitive skin may require additional carrier oil when applying cornmint essential oil topically. Use small amounts. Avoid using before bedtime since the oil can overstimulate the nervous system.

COSTUS

Botanical Name: *Saussurea costus, Saussurea lappa*

Family: *Asteraceae*

The essential oil is obtained from the roots.

History and Information

- Costus is native to India. The plant grows to a height of about 8 feet (6–2.5 meters).

- Costus root has been used for centuries in Asia as a remedy for cholera, typhoid, and infections.

- In Ayurvedic medicine, costus is used to help muscle and joint pains, breathing congestion, coughs, digestive problems, reduce headaches, sleeping sickness, purify the blood, and heal the skin.

- The oil is used to scent perfumes and as a food flavoring.

Practical Uses

Cooling

Calming; promotes a restful sleep

Improves alertness

Documented Properties

Analgesic, anthelmintic, antibacterial, anti-inflammatory, antioxidant, antiseptic, antispasmodic, antistress, antiulcer, antiviral, aphrodisiac, astringent, cardiotonic, carminative, contraceptive, depurative, digestive, diuretic, emmenagogue, expectorant, febrifuge, hypotensor, stimulant, stomachic, tonic, vasodilator

Aromatherapy Methods of Use

Application, aroma lamp, fragrancing, lightbulb ring, massage, mist spray

CUBEB

Botanical Name: *Cubeba officinalis, Piper cubeba*

Family: *Piperaceae*

The essential oil is obtained from the berries.

History and Information

- Cubeb is an evergreen shrub native to Indonesia. The climbing woody shrub grows to a height of about 20 feet (6 meters) and has clusters of flowers that develop into small berries resembling peppers.

- In the nineteenth century, the dried berries were rolled up into cigarettes and smoked to relieve breathing problems and chest congestion.

- Cubeb has been used as a spice in Europe as early as the eleventh century.

- The oil has been used as a urinary antiseptic and as an ingredient in cosmetics.

- In Asia, the berries are eaten to promote good digestion and balance blood sugar.

Practical Uses

Improves circulation

Improves digestion

Vapors open the sinus and breathing passages; deepens the breathing

Relieves aches, pains, and inflammation

Documented Properties

Antibacterial, anti-inflammatory, antiseptic (strong; urinary), antispasmodic, antiviral, carminative, diuretic, expectorant, stimulant (circulatory system), stomachic, tonic

Aromatherapy Methods of Use

Application, aroma lamp, bath, diffusor, inhaler, lightbulb ring, massage, mist spray, steam inhalation, steam room and sauna

CUMIN

Botanical Name:
*Cuminum cyminum,
Cuminum odorum*

Family: *Apiaceae*

The essential oil is obtained from the seeds and fruit.

The CO_2 extract is obtained from the seeds.

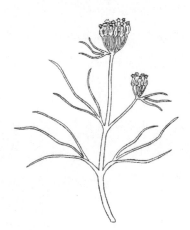

History and Information

- Cumin is native to the Mediterranean area. The plant grows to a height of about 1 foot (.5 meter), has threadlike leaves, small white or pink flowers, and aromatic seeds.

- Cumin was mentioned as a medicinal herb in the Papyrus Ebers in 1550 B.C. Dioscorides, the Greek physician, praised the herb in the first century. In ancient Rome, cumin was added to foods as a substitute for pepper.

- Cumin has been an ingredient in perfumes, love potions, and baths for its aphrodisiac effect.

- In Latin America, a tea made from the leaves was taken to help increase the flow of breast milk. The seeds are eaten to regulate menstruation, rid the body of excess water, and improve digestion.

- In Ayurvedic medicine, cumin is used to aid digestion and strengthen convalescing patients.

- In the Middle East, cumin seeds are recommended to ease discomfort after childbirth.
- In Africa, the seeds are taken for colds and digestive problems.
- Cumin is an important spice in Arab, European, and Vietnamese cuisines. It is also used as an ingredient in Indian curry.
- Natural health researchers has shown cumin to be effective in lowering blood sugar levels.
- The seeds yield 2 to 4 percent essential oil.

Practical Uses

Warming; improves circulation

Improves digestion, relieves flatulence

Purifying; helps in the reduction of cellulite

Calming, reduces stress

Helpful for meditation

Mood uplifting, euphoric; reviving, helps to relieve fatigue

Relieves pain

Documented Properties

Abortifacient, analgesic, anesthetic, anthelmintic, antibacterial, antidiabetic, antidysentery, anti-inflammatory, antimicrobial, antimutagenic, antioxidant, antiseptic, antispasmodic, antitoxic, antitumor, aperitive, aphrodisiac, astringent, cardiac, carminative, decongestant, depurative, diaphoretic, digestive, disinfectant, diuretic, emmenagogue, estrogenic, galactagogue, larvicide, nervine, parasiticide, revitalizing, sedative, stimulant (circulatory, digestive, and nervous systems), tonic

Aromatherapy Methods of Use

Application, aroma lamp, diffusor, inhaler, lightbulb ring, massage, mist spray

Caution: People with dry or sensitive skin may require additional carrier oil when using the essential oil topically. Use small amounts. Cumin is phototoxic. Avoid exposure to direct sunlight for several hours after applying the oil on the skin.

CYPERUS *(Cypriol)*

Botanical Name: *Cyperus scariosus*

Family: *Cyperaceae*

The essential oil is obtained from the flowers.

History and Information

- Cyperus is a sedge native to the Mediterranean region and Africa, and is found in damp locations. The plant is a grasslike rhizomatous herb with flowers and brown tubers. Cyperus is part of a species of six hundred plants growing in the tropics and subtropics.
- The plant was used by the Egyptians around 1550 B.C. to make a paper known as papyrus. The Egyptians also used the plant for fragrancing and making cloth.

Practical Uses

Warming; improves circulation

Calming, promotes a peaceful state of mind and a restful sleep

Documented Properties

Decongestant, hepatic, insect repellent, tonic (digestive system)

Aromatherapy Methods of Use

Application, aroma lamp, bath, inhaler, lightbulb ring, massage, mist spray

CYPRESS

Botanical Name: *Cupressus sempervirens*

Family: *Cupressaceae*

The essential oil is obtained from the leaves and twigs.

History and Information

- Cypress is an evergreen tree native to Asia and the Mediterranean area. The tree grows to a height of about 80–160 feet (24–48 meters), has dark-green leaves and cones. Some cypress trees are believed to be older than 3,000 years.

- Early physicians recommended that patients with lung ailments go to the island of Crete, which had dense forests of cypress trees.

- From early times, cypress trees were associated with the transition of the soul crossing over from this life to the afterlife. Ancient cultures burned cypress branches at funerals, and the Egyptians made coffins from the wood. Cypress trees were planted around burial sites.

- Cypress contains a hormone that normalizes the female sex hormones and can be helpful during menopause.

Practical Uses

Purifying; helps in the reduction of cellulite

Balancing to the nervous system; calming, relieves nervous tension and stress; promotes a restful sleep

Helps the breathing

Mood uplifting; refreshing, improves mental clarity and alertness

Contracts weak connective tissue, relieves muscle tension

Lessens perspiration

Regulates the female reproductive and hormonal systems

Documented Properties

Antirheumatic, antiseptic, antispasmodic, antisudorific, antitussive, astringent, calmative, cicatrizant, deodorant, deodorizer, diuretic, febrifuge, hemostatic, hepatic, insect repellent, insecticide, refreshing, restorative (nervous system), sedative, tonic, vasoconstrictor, warming

Aromatherapy Methods of Use

Application, aroma lamp, bath, diffusor, inhaler, lightbulb ring, massage, mist spray, steam inhalation, steam room and sauna

CYPRESS (Blue)
CYPRESS (Emerald)
CYPRESS (Jade)

Botanical Name: *Callitris columellaris* (Emerald cypress), *Callitris glaucophylla* (Jade cypress), *Callitris intratropica* (Blue cypress)

Family: *Cupressaceae*

Blue cypress essential oil is obtained from the wood.

Emerald cypress essential oil is obtained from the wood.

Jade cypress essential oil is obtained from the twigs and wood.

History and Information

- Blue cypress is native to Australia. The tree grows to a height of about 80 feet (24 meters) and has dark-green leaves. The genus has nineteen species.

- The blue cypress tree was used by the native Australian Tiwi people for muscle and joint aches, abdominal discomfort, bruises, wounds, insect bites, and as an insect repellent.

- Emerald cypress is an evergreen tree native to Australia. The tree grows in dry inland areas to a height of about 100 feet (30.5 meters), has dark-grey bark, dark-green leaves, and small seed cones. The tree is also known as Bribie Island pine and sand cypress pine.

- Jade cypress is an evergreen tree native to Australia; it is often found in dry inland areas, as well as near the coasts. The tree grows to a height of about 85–100 feet (26–30.5 meters) and has grey-green needlelike leaves with silver-grey cones containing small seeds inside. The tree is also known as white cypress pine.

Practical Uses

Cooling

Increases circulation

Purifying; helps in the reduction of cellulite

Mood uplifting; refreshing, energizing, improves mental clarity and alertness

Contracts weak connective tissue

Documented Properties

Analgesic, antibacterial, anti-inflammatory, antiviral

Aromatherapy Methods of Use

Application, aroma lamp, bath, diffusor, inhaler, lightbulb ring, massage, mist spray

DAVANA

Botanical Name: *Artemisia pallens*

Family: *Asteraceae*

The essential oil is obtained from the stems, leaves, and flowers.

History and Information

- Davana is native to India. The plant grows to a height of about 1 foot (.5 meter).

- The oil is used to flavor foods, and in perfumery.

Practical Uses

Relaxing

Mood uplifting, euphoric, aphrodisiac; improves mental awareness

Perfumery

Aromatherapy Methods of Use

Application, aroma lamp, bath, diffusor, fragrancing, inhaler, lightbulb ring, massage, mist spray

DESERT ROSEWOOD

Botanical Name: *Eremophila mitchellii*

Family: *Myoporaceae*

The essential oil is obtained from the bark and wood.

History and Information

- Desert rosewood is an evergreen shrub native to Australia. The shrub grows to a height of about

8–20 feet (2.5–6 meters), has glossy dark-green broomlike leaves and white or mauve bell-shaped fragrant flowers followed by fleshy fruits. The tree flowers most of the year. It is also known as false sandalwood, buddhawood, and budtha.

- The wood yields 3 percent essential oil.

Practical Uses

Calming, relaxes muscles; strengthens the nervous system

Helps to focus

A fixative to hold the scent of a fragrance

Documented Properties

Analgesic

Aromatherapy Methods of Use

Application, bath, inhaler, massage, mist spray

DILL SEED
DILL WEED

Botanical Name:
*Anethum graveolens,
Fructus anethi,
Peucedanum graveolens*

Family: *Apiaceae*

Dill seed essential oil and CO_2 extract are obtained from the seeds.

Dill weed essential oil is obtained from the whole plant.

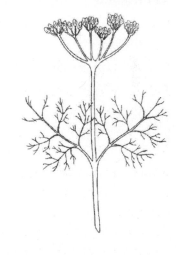

History and Information

- Dill is native to the Mediterranean countries and Russia. The plant grows to a height of about 3 feet (1 meter) and has small yellow flowers.

- Dill was mentioned in the Papyrus Ebers in 1550 B.C. as a medicinal herb.

- Writings found in Egyptian tombs show evidence that dill was used to help digestion.

- The Greek physician, Dioscorides, prescribed dill so frequently that it became known as the "herb of Dioscorides." Some of his recommended uses were for hiccups, flatulence, to increase lactation in nursing mothers, and stimulate urination.

- In medieval times, wounded knights placed dill seeds on their open cuts to speed the healing.

- Emperor Charlemagne insisted on having dill at his banquets as a remedy for hiccups and flatulence from indigestion.

- Dill has been used over the centuries as an ingredient in exotic love potions and aphrodisiacs.

- The leaves and seeds have been used to increase lactation when taken daily by nursing mothers. Before they started nursing, mothers also rubbed their chests with dill seeds that were soaked in water.

- Since early times, dill has had a reputation of helping crying babies fall asleep.

- In Latin America, a tea is made from the dill plant to increase breast milk, improve digestion, and help relieve water retention.

- India's Ayurvedic and Unani practitioners use dill for indigestion, fever, and ulcers.

- Dill has been used to sweeten the breath.

- The seeds yield 2 to 4 percent essential oil.

Practical Uses

Improves digestion, soothes and freshens the intestines, relieves flatulence and fermentation

Calming, relaxing; promotes a restful sleep

Relieves pain and menstrual discomfort

Repels insects

Documented Properties

Antibacterial, antimutagenic, antioxidant, antiseptic, antispasmodic, antitumor, aperitive, calmative, carminative (prevents flatulence and fermentation and stops hiccoughs), detersive, diaphoretic, digestive, disinfectant, diuretic, emmenagogue, emollient, estrogenic, galactagogue, laxative, parasiticide, resolvent, sedative, seductive, stomachic, vasodilator

Aromatherapy Methods of Use

Application, aroma lamp, bath, diffusor, inhaler, lightbulb ring, massage, mist spray

Caution: Dill tends to slow down reflexes. Avoid driving or doing anything that requires full attention after using the essential oil.

DRAGON'S BLOOD
(Sangre de Grado)

Botanical Name: *Croton lechieri*

Family: *Euphorbiaceae*

The resin is obtained from the inner bark.

History and Information

- Dragon's blood is native to South and Central America. The tree grows to a height of about 30–60 feet (9–18 meters), has green leaves and greenish-white flowers.

- The dark-red resin exudes out when the trunk is cut.

- The red sap is used by the indigenious people of the rainforest for its ability to stop bleeding, help quicken the healing and regeneration of the skin, and restore health and vitality to the tissues of the body. It is said to be one of the strongest antioxidants.

Practical Uses

Healing to the skin; stops bleeding

Documented Properties

Antibacterial, anti-inflammatory, antioxidant, antiseptic, antiviral, astringent, hemostatic, tonic, vulnerary

Aromatherapy Methods of Use

Application

ELECAMPANE

Botanical Name: *Aster officinalis, Helenium grandiflorum, Inula helenium*

Family: *Asteraceae*

The essential oil is obtained from the roots.

History and Information

- Elecampane is native to Europe and Asia. The plant grows to a height of about 4–8 feet (1.2–2.5 meters) and has large yellow daisylike flowers.

- Throughout history, the roots were eaten to relieve indigestion, asthma, and coughs.

- The ancient Greeks and Romans used elecampane as a remedy for colds, an expectorant, and to promote sweating. The Romans also ate the plant as a vegetable.

- The American Indians used the plant for bronchial and other lung ailments.

- In the nineteenth century, the roots were boiled in sugar water to make asthma lozenges, cough drops, and candy.

Practical Uses

Helps the breathing

Mood uplifting

Documented Properties

Analgesic, anthelmintic, antibacterial, antifungal, anti-inflammatory, antiseptic, antispasmodic, antitussive, astringent, carminative, cholagogue, diaphoretic, digestive, diuretic, emmenagogue, expectorant, parasiticide, relaxant, sedative, stimulant, stomachic, sudorific, tonic, vermifuge, warming

Aromatherapy Methods of Use

Application, aroma lamp, inhaler, lightbulb ring, massage, mist spray, steam inhalation, steam room and sauna

Caution: People with dry or sensitive skin may require additional carrier oil when applying elecampane essential oil topically. Use small amounts.

ELEMI

Botanical Name: *Canarium commune, Canarium luzonicum*

Family: *Burseraceae*

The resin and essential oil are obtained from the wood.

History and Information

- Elemi is an evergreen tree native to Asia. The tree grows to a height of about 80–100 feet (24.5–30.5 meters) and has small, yellow-white, fragrant flowers that develop into purple-black fruits the size of plums with nuts inside. The nuts are called kenari nut, pili nut, Philippine nut, and java almond; they taste similar to an almond and serve as an important food source to millions of people. The tropical tree thrives in low elevations and warm climates and can bear up to seventy pounds of nuts annually per tree. There are about seventy-five different varieties of pili nuts.

- The ancient Egyptians used elemi resin in the embalming process.

- In Europe, during the eighteenth and nineteenth centuries, the aromatic resin of elemi was applied as an ointment to speed the healing of wounds.

- In Asia, the tree bark is used to treat malaria, and the lemon-scented resin is burned as incense.

- The nuts are said to act as a purgative, while the roasted nuts are easily digestible. Infants are fed an emulsion of the powdered roasted nuts mixed with water as a substitute for milk.

- Pili nut oil is a vegetal oil, extracted from the nuts, and has a high oil content of about 72 percent. The nuts do not store well and go rancid quickly.

- Elemi resin/oil is used for incense and as a perfume fixative to fragrance soaps, detergents, and cosmetics, as well as to flavor foods and beverages.

Practical Uses

Warming; improves circulation

Calming, relaxing, reduces stress; promotes a restful sleep

Helpful for meditation

Opens the breathing passages for deeper breathing; breaks up mucous (mild effect)

Mood uplifting; encourages communication of inner feelings

Heals skin tissue

A fixative to hold the scent of a fragrance

Documented Properties

Analgesic, antibacterial, antifungal, antiseptic, antiviral, balsamic, cicatrizant, expectorant, nervine, stimulant (immune system), stomachic, tonic, vulnerary

Aromatherapy Methods of Use

Application, aroma lamp, bath, inhaler, lightbulb ring, massage, mist spray, steam inhalation, steam room and sauna

Caution: Elemi tends to slow down reflexes. Avoid driving or doing anything that requires full attention after using the essential oil.

EUCALYPTUS
EUCALYPTUS BLUE MALLEE
EUCALYPTUS DIVES
EUCALYPTUS MACARTHURII
EUCALYPTUS RADIATA
EUCALYPTUS SIDEROXYLON
EUCALYPTUS SMITHII

Botanical Name:
Eucalyptus dives,
Eucalyptus globulus
(Eucalyptus),
Eucalyptus
macarthurii,
Eucalyptus
polybractea
(Eucalyptus
Blue Mallee),

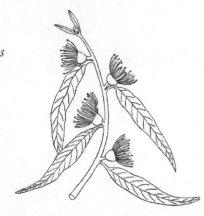

Eucalyptus radiata, Eucalyptus sideroxylon, Eucalyptus smithii

Family: *Myrtaceae*

The essential oil is obtained from the leaves and twigs.

History and Information

- Eucalyptus is native to Australia. The forests of Australia are made up of over 90 percent eucalyptus trees. There are approximately seven hundred different species of eucalyptus.

- Eucalyptus dives grows to about 60 feet (18 meters) high, has glossy dark-green leaves with a peppermint aroma and small white flowers. The tree is also known as broad-leafed peppermint.

- Eucalyptus globulus is one of the tallest trees, reaching as high as 480 feet (146 meters). The trees grow up to 100 feet (30.5 meters) tall in ten years. The bark is grey, the fragrant green leaves are long and leathery, the flowers are white, and the fruit is contained in a capsule. The tree is also known as the blue gum, fever tree, and gum tree, and its roots are said to store a large quantity of water in order to survive the dry seasons. People have been known to dig up a root and gather the water during times of drought. The roots release a poisonous chemical that kills nearby plants.

- Eucalyptus macarthurii grows to a height of about 125 feet (38 meters), has a rough bark and dull green leaves. The tree is also known as camden woollybutt.

- Eucalyptus polybractea reaches a height of about 30 feet (9 meters), has bluish-grey leaves and profuse white flowers.

- Eucalyptus radiata grows to a height of about 150–170 feet (46–52 meters), and has a dark bark, narrow green aromatic leaves, and cream-colored flowers. The tree is also known as narrow-leaved peppermint. The essential oil is high in cineole and used for medicinal purposes.

- Eucalyptus sideroxylon reaches a height of about 100 feet (30.5 meters), has a black bark, strongly aromatic grey-green leaves, and clusters of narrow white, pink, or red flowers. The tree is also known as red ironbark and mugga. The essential oil contains 70 percent cineole.

- Eucalyptus smithii grows to about 100 feet (30.5 meters) tall, has green leaves and small white flowers followed by seed capsules. The tree favors streams and wet areas. It is also known as gully gum, gully peppermint, and blackbutt peppermint. The essential oil is high in cineole and used for medicinal purposes.

- The aboriginal people in Australia used eucalyptus as a remedy for colds, sore throats, breathing difficulties, congestion relief, infections, and pain.

- Eucalyptus has a long tradition of uses in medicine and is known to be an excellent antiseptic for purifying the environment. It became known as catheter oil when British hospitals, in the nineteenth century, used it to sterilize urinary catheters.

- Historically, to improve their health, people who were ill were relocated to areas where the trees grew. In the latter part of the nineteenth century, eucalyptus oil was regarded as a cure-all.

- Eucalyptus has been used over the years to clear congestion from the head and breathing passages.

- Koala bears feed exclusively on the leaves of the tree.

- The essential oil of Eucalyptus dives contains between 45 to 50 percent pipertone. Pipertone is used in the industry for the production of synthetic thymol and menthol.

- The eucalyptus leaves yield approximately 2 to 3 percent essential oil.

- Pharmacopoeias require a minimum content of 70 percent of the component cineole to be present in the oil in order for the essential oil to be considered for medicinal purposes. Cineole is the active therapeutic agent of eucalyptus. If the oil has a lower content of the component, additional cineole is taken from another oil and combined.

- Most of the essential oil is produced for medicinal and industrial purposes; a smaller amount is used for perfumery. Industrial applications include disinfectants, deodorizers, and air fresheners. The oil is also used in: soaps, gargles, deodorants, inhalants, cough lozenges, spot and stain removers, antiseptics, and germicides.

Practical Uses

Cooling

Stimulating to the nervous system

Vapors open the sinus and breathing passages; deepens the breathing; improves circulation

Refreshing, reviving, energizing, improves mental clarity and alertness

Relieves pain, aching and sore muscles

Disinfectant

Repels insects

Documented Properties

Analgesic, anthelmintic, antibacterial, antidiabetic, antidote, antifungal, anti-inflammatory, antineuralgic, antipruritic, antiputrid, antirheumatic, antiseptic (strong), antispasmodic, antivenomous, antiviral (respiratory tract), astringent, balsamic, cephalic, cicatrizant, cooling, decongestant, deodorant, deodorizer, depurative, diaphoretic, disinfectant, diuretic, expectorant, febrifuge, germicide, hemostatic, insect repellent, insecticide, invigorating, parasiticide, pectoral, purifying, regenerator (skin tissue), rubefacient, stimulant (circulatory system), tonic, uplifting, vermifuge, vulnerary

Aromatherapy Methods of Use

Application, aroma lamp, bath, diffusor, inhaler, light-bulb ring, massage, mist spray, steam inhalation, steam room and sauna

Caution: Use small amounts of the globulus variety. Eucalyptus radiata is considered to be gentler than Eucalyptus globulus.

EUCALYPTUS CITRIODORA
EUCALYPTUS STAIGERIANA

Botanical Name: *Eucalyptus citriodora, Eucalyptus staigeriana*

Family: *Myrtaceae*

The essential oil is obtained from the leaves and twigs.

History and Information

- Eucalyptus citriodora is an evergreen tree native to Australia. The tree grows to a height of about 90–120 feet (27.5–36.5 meters), has a smooth white bark, narrow pointed leathery leaves, and white flowers that develop into brown fruits. Every part of the tree has a strong lemony scent. It is also known as lemon-scented gum or spotted gum tree.

- Eucalyptus staigeriana is native to Australia. The tree reaches a height of about 60 feet (18 meters), has oblong lemon-scented leaves containing a high amount of citral and white flowers. The tree is also referred to as lemon-scented ironbark and is grown for ornamental purposes. The leaves yield about 3 percent essential oil, which is used in perfumery.

- Eucalyptus citriodora is grown for ornamental purposes and is easily cultivated.

- Eucalyptus citriodora contains 65 to 85 percent of citronella, giving it its lemony scent. The richest source of the component is in the leaves.

- The essential oil yield is about 2 percent and is used in perfumery.

Practical Uses

Calming

Mood uplifting; reviving, helps to relieve a fatigued state

Documented Properties

Antibacterial, antidepressant, antifungal, anti-inflammatory, antirheumatic, antiseptic, antiviral, calmative, expectorant, febrifuge, insect repellent, pectoral, sedative, tonic, vulnerary

Aromatherapy Methods of Use

Application, aroma lamp, diffusor, inhaler, lightbulb ring, massage, mist spray

FENNEL

Botanical Name:
*Anethum foeniculum,
Foeniculum officinale,
Foeniculum vulgare*

Family: *Apiaceae*

The essential oil and CO_2 extract are obtained from the seeds.

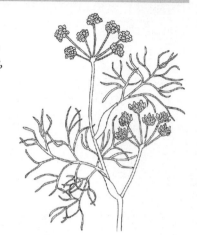

History and Information

- Fennel is native to Europe and Asia. The plant grows to a height of about 3–7 feet (1–2 meters), has green feathery leaves and clusters of small yellow flowers.

- The Romans and Greeks used the herb to lose weight. The Greeks also consumed fennel for courage and to prolong life. The Greek physicians, Hippocrates and Dioscorides, recommended fennel for nursing mothers to increase their lactation. Dioscorides also used fennel to suppress hunger, decrease fluid retention, and relieve inflammations related to the urinary system.

- Pliny, the Roman herbalist, recommended eating fennel to strengthen the eyesight. In later years, other herbalists corroborated with Pliny's findings and prescribed extracts of the root to treat cataracts and the whole plant as a remedy for poor vision.

- The Hindus and Chinese used fennel as an antivenomous agent against snake and scorpion bites.

- Emperor Charlemagne ordered the herb grown in all of his imperial gardens.

- The household of King Edward I of England consumed more than eight pounds of fennel a month.

- In China, the seeds are powdered and used as a poultice for snakebites.

- Fennel is said to stimulate the estrogen level, which is useful in helping women with sexual problems. It is also helpful for women who experience menstrual discomforts and premenstrual tension.

- Fennel is used for digestive problems and to soothe coughs.

- Farmers have reported that adding fennel to the feed of nursing animals increases their lactation.

- The seeds yield 4 to 5 percent essential oil. Fennel oil is used as an ingredient in perfumes, soaps, cough syrups, licorice candy, sour pickles, and liqueurs. It has also been used as an ingredient in antiwrinkle creams for the skin.

Practical Uses

Warming; improves circulation

Improves digestion, soothes and purifies the intestines, relieves flatulence and aerophagy

Purifying; helps in the reduction of cellulite

Reduces stress; promotes a restful sleep

Helps the breathing

Relieves pain and menstrual discomfort

Increases lactation

Disinfectant

Repels insects

Documented Properties

Antibacterial, antidote, antiemetic, antifungal, antiphlogistic, antiseptic, antispasmodic, antitoxic, aperitif, appetite, astringent, calmative, carminative, decongestant, depurative, detoxifier, diaphoretic, digestive, diuretic, emmenagogue, estrogenic, expectorant, galactagogue, hepatic, insect repellent, insec-

ticide, laxative, parasiticide, regulator (female reproductive system), resolvent, revitalizing, stimulant (uterine contractions, estrogen levels), stomachic, tonic, vermifuge

Aromatherapy Methods of Use

Application, aroma lamp, bath, inhaler, lightbulb ring, massage, mist spray, steam inhalation, steam room and sauna

Caution: People with dry or sensitive skin may require additional carrier oil when applying the essential oil topically. Fennel tends to slow down reflexes. Avoid driving or doing anything that requires full attention after using the oil. Use small amounts. Fennel should be avoided by people prone to epileptic seizures.

FENUGREEK SEED

Botanical Name: *Trigonella foenum-graecum*
Family: *Fabaceae*
The essential oil is obtained from the seeds.

History and Information

See Fenugreek Seed in Chapter 2 on page 30.

Practical Uses

Warming

Improves digestion, soothes the intestines

Calming, reduces stress, relieves tension

Helps to breathe easier

Helps premenstrual stress

Loosens tight muscles

Documented Properties

See Fenugreek Seed in Chapter 2 on page 30.

Aromatherapy Methods of Use

Application, bath, inhaler, massage, mist spray

FEVERFEW

Botanical Name: *Tanacetum parthenium*

Family Name: *Asteraceae*

The CO_2 extract is obtained from the flowers and leaves.

History and Information

- Feverfew is native to Europe. The bushy plant grows to about 3 feet (1 meter) high, has green leaves and small daisylike flowers with white rays and a yellow center. Feverfew is in the daisy family.

- Dioscorides, the Greek physician, used feverfew for inflammations.

- The Roman women used the herb to induce delayed menstruation and to help in difficult childbirths.

- Culpeper, the British physician, recommended feverfew for women to strengthen the reproductive system.

- In Europe, the herb is used for headaches, digestive upsets, toothaches, and menstrual problems.

- Feverfew is taken as a remedy for headaches and joint problems. Externally, the plant is used for insect bites.

Practical Uses

Calming, relaxing, reduces stress and tension; promotes a restful sleep

Mood uplifting; helps to focus

Loosens tight muscles

Documented Properties

Abortifacient, anti-inflammatory, antiseptic, antispasmodic, carminative, depurative, emmenagogue, febrifuge, laxative, sedative (mild), stomachic, vermifuge

Aromatherapy Methods of Use

Application, massage

FIR BALSAM NEEDLES
FIR NEEDLES

Botanical Name: *Abies alba* (Silver fir), *Abies balsamea* (Fir balsam needles), *Abies grandis* (Grand fir), *Pseudotsuga menziesii* (Douglas fir)

Family: *Pinaceae*

The essential oil is obtained from the needles.

History and Information

- Fir is an evergreen tree native to North America and Europe. The trees range in height from 40–80 feet (12–24 meters) for the fir balsam and 100–300 feet (30.5–91.5 meters) for the fir needle. The leaves are needlelike, and the wood is soft and odorless. Fir trees are popularly used as a Christmas tree because their needles remain on the branches long after the tree has been cut. There are approximately forty species of the fir tree. The life span of the needles on the tree is up to ten years.

- The American Indians used every part of the tree for a different remedy. The inner bark was prepared into a tea to alleviate chest pains, the twigs were used as a laxative, the powdered roots were placed in the mouth to soothe sores, and the needles were used in sweat baths. Balsam needles and resin were inhaled in the sauna to help relieve colds and coughs. The resin was also applied to the skin to heal burns, sores, cuts, wounds, inflammation, and relieve congestion and itching.

- The resin has been used as a source of turpentine, an adhesive for microscope slides and optical lenses, and an ingredient in hemorrhoid ointments. Dentists use the balsam to seal root canals.

Practical Uses

Purifying; removes lymphatic deposits from the body, helps in the reduction of cellulite

Calming

Vapors open the sinus and breathing passages; deepens the breathing

Mood uplifting: refreshing, reviving, improves mental clarity; encourages communication

Lessens pain

Documented Properties

Analgesic, antiseptic, antitussive, astringent, cicatrizant, diuretic, expectorant, purgative, sedative, stimulant (respiratory system), tonic, vulnerary

Aromatherapy Methods of Use

Application, aroma lamp, bath, diffusor, inhaler, lightbulb ring, massage, mist spray, steam inhalation, steam room and sauna

FIR BALSAM RESIN

Botanical Name: *Abies balsamea, Abies balsamifera, Pinus balsaamea*

Family: *Pinaceae*

The resin is obtained from the inner bark.

History and Information

See Fir Balsam Needles

Practical Uses

Warming; improves circulation

Purifying; helps in the reduction of cellulite

Calming; promotes a restful sleep

Mood uplifting

Reduces and soothes swollen tissue

Soothes insect bites

Documented Properties

Antiscorbutic, antiseptic, expectorant, pectoral, sedative, tonic, vulnerary, warming

Aromatherapy Methods of Use

Application, massage

FOKIENIA (Bois de Siam)

Botanical Name: *Fokienia hodginsii*

Family: *Cupressaceae*

The essential oil is obtained from the wood.

History and Information

- Fokienia is an evergreen conifer tree native to Asia. The tree grows to a height of about 40–50 feet (12–15 meters), has aromatic peeling bark, green leaves, and spherical cones. Fokienia is related to the cypress tree family.

- The Vietnamese believe the tree brings eternal life.

- In Asian countries, the wood from the fokienia tree is used to make coffins and is called coffin wood.

- An essential oil extracted from the roots is used in fragrancing and is called pemou oil.

Practical Uses

Helps to breathe easier

Calming, reduces stress

Mood uplifting; improves mental clarity

Helps to relieve pain

Aromatherapy Methods of Use

Application, massage

FRANKINCENSE (Olibanum)

Botanical Name: *Boswellia carteri, Boswellia sacra, Boswellia thurifera*

Family: *Burseraceae*

The resin, essential oil, and CO_2 extract are obtained from the bark resin.

History and Information

- Frankincense is native to the Mediterranean area; it is found in hot, dry locations. The small tree grows to a height of about 20 feet (6 meters), has glossy leaves and white flowers. When the bark is damaged, a resin exudes from the injured area.

- Nearly 5,000 years ago, the ancient Egyptians burned the incense of frankincense in the temples during religious ceremonies and later used the gum as a facial mask to rejuvenate their skin.

- The ancients used frankincense to improve circulation, relieve congestion of the breathing passages, ease muscle and joint aches, regulate menstruation, and reduce inflammations.

- Traditionally, frankincense was used to fumigate sickrooms. The Chinese used the gum in the treatment of leprosy and tuberculosis.

- The yield of essential oil is approximately 5 percent. The oil is used as an ingredient in Oriental perfumes, soaps, and cosmetics. The incense is still burned in many churches.

Practical Uses

Calming, relaxing; promotes a restful sleep

Helpful for meditation

Vapors open the sinus and breathing passages

Mood uplifting, brings out feelings

Reduces inflammation

Soothes and heals inflamed skin; bruises, burns

Documented Properties

Abortifacient, analgesic, antibacterial, antidepressant, anti-inflammatory, antioxidant, antiseptic, antispasmodic, antitussive, astringent, balsamic, carminative, cephalic, cicatrizant, cytophylactic, digestive, diuretic, emmenagogue, emollient, expectorant, fixative, nervine, pectoral, purgative, rejuvenator (skin), revitalizing, sedative, stimulant (cells, immune system), tonic, tonifying (skin), uplifting, vulnerary, warming

Aromatherapy Methods of Use

Application, aroma lamp, bath, diffusor, inhaler, lightbulb ring, massage, mist spray, steam inhalation, steam room and sauna

GALANGAL

Botanical Name: *Alpinia galanga, Alpinia officinarum, Languas officinarum*

Family: *Zingiberaceae*

The essential oil is obtained from the rhizomes.

History and Information

- Galangal is native to Asia. The plant grows to a height of about 5 feet (1.5 meters), has green sword-shaped leaves, white flowers, and an aromatic rhizome.

- During the Middle Ages, galangal was used as an aphrodisiac.

- In folk medicine, galangal was used for coughs, fevers, inflammation, stomach upsets, and aches and pains.

- A leaf tea is made to help with muscle and joint pains, and to stimulate the metabolism. Galangal is also used as a remedy for cholera, congestion, digestion, and skin problems.

- In Asian cooking, the rhizome is substituted for ginger while the shoots and flowers are eaten fresh in a salad or cooked.

Practical Uses

Improves digestion

Reduces stress

Mood uplifting

Relieves aches and pains

General stimulant

Disinfectant

Documented Properties

Analgesic, anti-inflammatory, antiseptic, antispasmodic, antitussive, aphrodisiac, balsamic, carminative, cicatrizant, digestive, diuretic, emmenagogue, expectorant, hypotensive, pectoral, restorative, stimulant, stomachic, tonic

Aromatherapy Methods of Use

Application, aroma lamp, diffusor, inhaler, lightbulb ring, massage, mist spray

Comments: Since galangal oil is relatively expensive, ginger oil can be used as a substitute instead.

GALBANUM

Botanical Name: *Ferula galbaniflua, Ferula gumosa, Ferula rubricaulis*

Family: *Apiaceae*

The resin and essential oil are obtained from the bark.

The CO_2 extract is obtained from the resin.

History and Information

- Galbanum is native to the Mediterranean region. The thin and resinous plant grows to a height of about 3 feet (1 meter), has long, greyish-green, hairy leaves and umbels of very small yellow flowers that bear seeds.

- Galbanum is mentioned in the Bible as one of the ingredients in the holy ointment. It was also used by the Greeks, Hippocrates, and Pliny, the Roman herbalist.

Practical Uses

Calming, reduces stress

Mood uplifting

Relieves pain and inflammation

Documented Properties

Analgesic, anti-inflammatory, antiseptic, antispasmodic, aphrodisiac, balsamic, carminative, cicatrizant, digestive, diuretic, emmenagogue, expectorant, hypotensive, nervine, resolvent, restorative, stimulant, tonic, vulnerary

Aromatherapy Methods of Use

Application, aroma lamp, bath, inhaler, lightbulb ring, massage, mist spray

GARDENIA

Botanical Name: *Gardenia grandiflora*

Family: *Rubiaceae*

The absolute/essential oil is obtained from the flowers.

History and Information

- Gardenia is an evergreen bush native to Asia. The shrub grows to a height of about 7–10 feet (2–3 meters), and has fragrant waxy-white flowers that develop into orange fruits.

- In China, the flowers are added to scent tea, and the roots and leaves are used to reduce fevers and cleanse the body.

- In Africa, the fruits are used as a spice in cooking.

- In Thailand, a yellow food coloring is made from the fruits.

Practical Uses

Mood uplifting

Fragrancing

Documented Properties

Alterative, analgesic, anthelmintic, antibacterial, anticonvulsive, antidepressant, anti-inflammatory, antiseptic, aphrodisiac, calmative, choleretic, febrifuge, hemostatic, hepatic, hypnotic, hypotensor, sedative, stomachic, uplifting

Aromatherapy Methods of Use

Application, aroma lamp, bath, fragrancing, lightbulb ring, massage, mist spray

GARLIC

Botanical Name: *Allium sativum*

Family: *Liliaceae*

The essential oil and CO_2 extract are obtained from the bulbs.

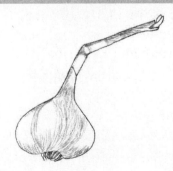

History and Information

- Garlic is native to Europe and Asia. The plant grows to a height of about 1–3 feet (.5–1 meter).

- The builders of the pyramids in Egypt were fed garlic daily to keep them healthy.

- Dioscorides, the Greek physician, used garlic for intestinal worms.

- Pliny, the Roman herbalist, listed garlic as a treatment for sixty-one different ailments.

- In the Middle Ages, garlic was used for leprosy.

- The American Indians applied garlic to draw out the poisons of insect stings and snakebites. As a treatment for intestinal worms, they steeped crushed bulbs in water and drank the tea on an empty stomach.

- In the eighteenth century, French priests ate garlic to successfully protect themselves against a highly contagious disease in London, while their English counterparts, who didn't eat garlic, succumbed to the disease.

- In World War I and World War II, European doctors dressed wounds with sterilized swabs containing garlic to prevent gangrene.

- The garlic bulb yields 1 percent essential oil.

Documented Properties

Analgesic, antibacterial, anticoagulant, antifungal, antilithic, antiputrid, antisclerotic, antiseptic, antispasmodic, antiviral, aperitive, calmative, carminative, cholagogue, cicatrizant, decongestant, diaphoretic, digestive, disinfectant, diuretic, expectorant, febrifuge, hypotensor, insecticide, laxative, parasiticide, resolvent, stomachic, stimulant, tonic (heart), tonifying (lymphatic system), vasodilator, vermifuge, warming

Comments: Garlic oil has a strong odor that is disagreeable to many people. It is added to foods as a flavoring ingredient by the food industry, but not used in aromatherapy.

Caution: Garlic oil is irritating to the skin.

GERANIUM

Botanical Name: *Pelargonium graveolens*

Family: *Geraniaceae*

The essential oil is obtained from the leaves, stems, and flowers.

History and Information

- Geranium is a small fragrant plant native to Africa. The plant grows to a height of about 3 feet (1 meter), has fragrant leaves and red, purple, or other colored flowers. There are over seven hundred different species of geranium.

- In ancient times, geranium was regarded as an exceptional healing agent for wounds and bone fractures.

- The American Indians drank a tea made from the powdered roots for dysentery, hemorrhaging, and ulcers. Poultices were made from the same preparation for hemorrhoids and arthritis.

- Early American women regularly drank a tea made from the roots, which was thought to prevent pregnancy.

Practical Uses

Cooling

Purifying; helps in the reduction of cellulite

Calming to the nervous system in small amounts and stimulating in large amounts; reduces tension

Mood uplifting; encourages communication

Lessens pain and inflammation

Stimulates the adrenal glands

Disinfectant

Repels insects

Soothes insect bites, lice, ticks

Documented Properties

Analgesic, antibacterial, anticoagulant, antidepressant, antidiabetic, antifungal, anti-inflammatory, antineuralgic, antiseptic, antispasmodic, antistress, astringent, cicatrizant, cytophylactic, deodorant, depurative, diuretic, healing, hemostatic, insect repellent, insecticide, parasiticide, protectant (cells), refreshing, regulator (glandular functions and hormones), rejuvenator (skin tissue), sedative (mild) (anxiety), stimulant (adrenal glands; circulatory and lymphatic systems), tonic, tonifying (skin), uplifting (menopause and premenstrual tension), vasoconstrictor, vermifuge, vulnerary

Aromatherapy Methods of Use

Application, aroma lamp, bath, diffusor, inhaler, light-bulb ring, massage, mist spray

GINGER

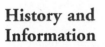

Botanical Name:
Amomum zingiber,
Zingiber officinale

Family: *Zingiberaceae*

The essential oil and CO_2 extract are obtained from the roots.

History and Information

- Ginger is native to Asia. The plant grows to a height of about 3 feet (1 meter) and has white or yellow flowers.

- The ancient people of India used ginger in cooking, to preserve food, and for digestive problems.

- Dioscorides, the Greek physician, recommended the root to aid digestion and as a poison antidote. The Romans and Greeks later also used ginger to improve digestion.

- In the sixteenth century, Henry VIII recommended ginger root as a remedy for the plague.

- In Oriental medicine, ginger root is incorporated in about half of the herbal formulations. In China, the herb has been used for thousands of years as a general tonic, a remedy for colds, coughs, flu, hangovers, digestive disorders, congestion, inflammatory conditions, pain relief, to promote perspiration, warm cold extremities, and strengthen the heart. Chinese sailors chewed ginger to prevent seasickness. Tibetans used ginger to stimulate the vital energies of one who was debilitated, lethargic, or recovering from an illness. In Japan, a massage with ginger oil is a traditional treatment for spinal and joint pains. The root is used to relieve morning nausea during pregnancy and alleviate motion dizziness during traveling.

- In Ayurvedic medicine, ginger was employed as a remedy for liver problems, intestinal gas, hemorrhoids, and anemia.

- Herbalists have recommended compresses of hot ginger to relieve gout, headaches, aches and pains, sinus congestion, and menstrual cramps, and a warm ginger footbath to invigorate the body.

- In Africa, ginger is used for headaches and parasites. It is said to be effective against intestinal worms.

- In Latin America, the herb is taken for nausea, morning sickness, dizziness, muscle and joint aches, chest congestion, to improve circulation, and relieve fatigue.

- Ginger is one of the most widely used herbal remedies for morning nausea during pregnancy. It is also taken for ulcers and to aid digestion.

- The crushed root is placed on inflamed gums and teeth to relieve discomfort and made into a compress for eye inflammations.

- The root yields 1 to 3 percent essential oil. Ginger is an ingredient in perfumery as well as an additive in foods, ginger ale, and ginger beer. It is significantly used as an antioxidant in food products.

Practical Uses

Warming; improves circulation

Improves digestion, soothes the intestines, relieves flatulence

Mood uplifting; improves mental clarity and memory

General stimulant to the entire body; relieves dizziness and nausea caused by traveling

Relieves aches and pains

Cleanses the bowels

Disinfectant

Documented Properties

Analgesic, antibacterial, anticoagulant, antiemetic, anti-inflammatory, antioxidant, antiscorbutic, antiseptic, antispasmodic, antitoxic, antitussive, aperitif, aperitive, aphrodisiac, astringent (stops bleeding), carminative, cephalic, diaphoretic, digestive (nausea), diuretic, emmenagogue, expectorant, febrifuge, laxative, rubefacient, stimulant (circulatory and nervous systems), stomachic, tonic, tonifying (digestive system), vermifuge

Aromatherapy Methods of Use

Application, aroma lamp, diffusor, inhaler, lightbulb ring, massage, mist spray

Caution: People with dry or sensitive skin may require additional carrier oil when applying ginger essential oil topically. Use small amounts.

GINGER LILY

Botanical Name: *Hedychium spicatum*

Family: *Zingiberaceae*

The essential oil and CO_2 extract are obtained from the rhizomes.

History and Information

- Ginger lily is native to India. The plant grows to a height of about 3 feet (1 meter) and has yellow flowers.

- In the Amazon region, the rhizomes are boiled and added to bathwater to soothe aches, discomforts, and inflammations.

- In Asia, ginger lily is an ingredient in chewing tobacco, incense, and perfumes.

Practical Uses

Calming, reduces stress, relieves tension

Helps to breathe easier; deepens the breathing

Mood uplifting, euphoric; mentally stimulating, energizing, improves mental clarity

Loosens tight muscles

Documented Properties

Analgesic, anti-inflammatory, antirheumatic, carminative, insecticide, stimulant, stomachic, tonic

Aromatherapy Methods of Use

Application, aroma lamp, inhaler, lightbulb ring, massage, mist spray, steam inhalation, steam room and sauna

GINGERGRASS

Botanical Name: *Cymbopogon martinii var. sofia*

Family: *Poaceae*

The essential oil is obtained from the plant.

History and Information

- Gingergrass is a grass native to Asia and thrives in moist soils. The plant is closely related to palmarosa.

Practical Uses

Warming; improves circulation

Calming, reduces stress

Vapors open the sinus and breathing passages

Mood uplifting, aphrodisiac, euphoric; improves mental clarity

Documented Properties

Antibacterial, antifungal, antiviral, tonic

Aromatherapy Methods of Use

Application, aroma lamp, diffusor, inhaler, lightbulb ring, massage, mist spray

Caution: People with dry or sensitive skin may require additional carrier oil when applying gingergrass essential oil topically. Use small amounts.

GOLDENROD

Botanical Name: *Solidago canadensis, Solidago odora*

Family: *Asteraceae*

The essential oil is obtained from the flowers.

History and Information

- Goldenrod is native to North America. The plant grows to a height of 3–7 feet (1–2 meters) and has thin leaves and yellow flowers.

- The American Indians made a lotion from the flowers for bee stings. The roots were taken for liver problems.

- Early American settlers used the flowers to help the gums and teeth.

- In Europe, the flowers are taken as a laxative and for sinus and joint problems. The seeds are used for diarrhea.

- The herb was made as a tea during the American revolt against the British tea tax. The tea was known as "patriot tea."

- In Chinese medicine, the herb is used for malaria, headaches, and sore throats.

- Herbalists use goldenrod leaves for wounds, abrasions, and insect bites.

Practical Uses

Warming; improves circulation

Calming, reduces stress

Helpful for meditation

Mood uplifting; improves mental clarity, encourages communication

Relieves pain

Documented Properties

Analgesic, astringent, carminative, diaphoretic, diuretic, hepatic, laxative, tonic

Aromatherapy Methods of Use

Application, aroma lamp, bath, diffusor, lightbulb ring, inhaler, massage, mist spray

GRAPEFRUIT
GRAPEFRUIT *(Pink)*
GRAPEFRUIT *(Red)*

Botanical Name:
Citrus paradisi

Family: *Rutaceae*

The essential oil is obtained from the peel of the fruit.

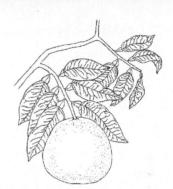

History and Information

- Grapefruit is an evergreen citrus tree that grows to a height of about 30–50 feet (9–15 meters) and has fragrant white flowers that develop into large yellow fruits.

- The earliest record of the grapefruit is in the West Indies in the early eighteenth century. Scientists believe that the tree developed as a mutation from the pomelo fruit. The first grapefruit trees in Florida were planted in about 1820.

- The peel contains a bitter component called naringin, which is used as a flavoring in chocolate and bitter tonic beverages. The seeds produce grapefruit seed oil, which is a dark, bitter oil. The seed oil can be used in salads and as a cooking oil after it is refined to extract the bitter taste.

- Pink and red grapefruit are high in vitamin A.

Practical Uses

Cooling

Purifying; reduces cellulite and obesity; balances the fluids in the body

Reduces stress

Mood uplifting; refreshing, reviving, improves mental clarity and awareness, sharpens the senses

Increases physical strength and energy

Documented Properties

Antibacterial, antidepressant, antiseptic, antistress, antitoxic, aperitif, aperitive, astringent, balancing (central nervous system), cephalic, cholagogue, depurative, detoxifier, digestive, disinfectant, diuretic, hemostatic, resolvent, restorative, reviving, stimulant (digestive and lymphatic systems, and neurotransmitters), tonic (liver), tonifying (skin)

Aromatherapy Methods of Use

Application, aroma lamp, bath, diffusor, inhaler, lightbulb ring, massage, mist spray

Caution: People with dry or sensitive skin may require additional carrier oil when using the essential oil topically. Use small amounts. Grapefruit is phototoxic. Avoid exposure to direct sunlight for several hours after applying the oil on the skin.

GUAIACWOOD

Botanical Name: *Bulnesia sarmienti, Guaiacum officinale*

Family: *Zygophyllaceae*

The resin/essential oil is obtained from the wood.

History and Information

- Guaiacwood is a slow-growing evergreen tree native to the Central and South America, and the West Indies. It is found in dry coastal areas. The tree reaches a height of about 30–40 feet (9–12 meters), has glossy oval green leathery leaves and clusters of small deep blue or purple flowers that develop into yellow-orange fruit containing a seed. Guaiacwood is also known as guaiacum, guayacan, pockwood, and lignum vitae, which means "wood of life." The wood of the tree has a rich supply of fats and resins that make it very hard and impervious to water. It is the heaviest of all woods and will sink in water.

- During the sixteenth century, guaiacwood was widely used in the treatment of syphilis.

- Guaiacwood is used in perfumery to smoothe out and balance strong or harsh aromas.

- The oil is also known as champaca wood, bulnesol, and essence bois de guaiac.

Practical Uses

Purifying to the tissues

Calming and relaxing, reduces stress and tension; promotes a restful sleep

Helpful for meditation

Mood uplifting; improves mental clarity

Reduces inflammation; loosens tight muscles

Soothes swollen and injured skin tissue

A fixative to hold the scent of a fragrance

Documented Properties

Anti-inflammatory, antirheumatic, antiseptic, aphrodisiac, astringent, balsamic, diaphoretic, diuretic, laxative, stimulant (genitourinary system), sudorific, tonifying (skin)

Aromatherapy Methods of Use

Application, aroma lamp, bath, lightbulb ring, massage, mist spray

Caution: Guaiacwood tends to slow down reflexes. Avoid driving or doing anything that requires full attention after using the resin or essential oil.

GURJUN BALSAM

Botanical Name: *Dipterocarpus gracilis, Dipterocarpus griffithi, Dipterocarpus jourdainii, Dipterocarpus palasus, Dipterocarpus turbinatus*

Family: *Dipterocarpaceae*

The resin/essential oil is obtained from the wood.

History and Information

- Gurjun balsam is native to Asia. The tree grows to a height of about 120 feet (36.5 meters) and has large pink flowers. The genus has seventy species of trees.

- The balsam has been used for skin ulcers, ringworm, and other skin problems.
- The vegetal oil extracted from the seeds of Dipterocarpus lamellantus is used in Chinese medicine for leprosy.
- The oil has industrial uses in varnishes, anti-corrosive coatings, and printing inks.

Practical Uses

Warming

Calming; promotes a restful sleep

A fixative to hold the scent of a fragrance

Documented Properties

Anti-inflammatory, antiseptic, disinfectant

Aromatherapy Methods of Use

Application, massage

HELICHRYSUM (*Everlasting* or *Immortelle*)

Botanical Name: *Helichrysum angustifolium, Helichrysum italicum*

Family: *Asteraceae*

The essential oil is obtained from the flowers.

History and Information

- Helichrysum is an evergreen plant native to the Mediterranean area and Asia. The plant grows to a height of about 2 feet (.5 meter) and has daisy-like yellow flowers. There are approximately five hundred species of helichrysum.
- The plant was used in Europe over the years to freshen the air, repel insects, and for medicinal purposes.

Practical Uses

Cooling

Relaxing, reduces stress

Vapors open the sinus and breathing passages

Mood uplifting, euphoric; reviving, strengthening, improves mental clarity and alertness

Relieves aches, pains and menstrual discomfort

Increases muscle endurance

Disinfectant

Documented Properties

Analgesic, antibacterial, anticoagulant, antidepressant, antifungal, anti-inflammatory, antiseptic, antispasmodic, antistress, antitussive, antiviral, astringent, blood purifier, cephalic, cholagogue, cicatrizant, cytophylactic, detoxifier, diuretic, emollient, expectorant, hepatic, nervine, regenerator (skin cells), sedative, stimulant (dreaming), tonic

Aromatherapy Methods of Use

Application, aroma lamp, bath, diffusor, lightbulb ring, inhaler, massage, mist spray, steam inhalation, steam room and sauna

HELICHRYSUM (*African*)

Botanical Name: *Helichrysum splendidum*

Family: *Asteraceae*

The essential oil is obtained from flowers.

History and Information

- African helichrysum is native to Africa. The shrub grows to a height of about 6 feet (2 meters), has aromatic silver-grey leaves and sweet-scented bright-yellow flowers.

Practical Uses

Relaxing, reduces stress

Vapors open the sinus and breathing passages

Mood uplifting; reviving, strengthening

Loosens tight muscles, relieves aches, pains, and menstrual discomfort

Documented Properties

Antifungal, antimicrobial, vulnerary (burns)

Aromatherapy Methods of Use

Application, aroma lamp, bath, diffusor, lightbulb ring, inhaler, massage, mist spray, steam inhalation, steam room and sauna

HELIOTROPE

Botanical Name: *Heliotropium arborescens*

Family: *Boraginaceae*

The essential oil is obtained from the flowers.

History and Information

- Heliotrope is an evergreen shrub native to South and Central America. The shrub grows to a height of about 3–6 feet (1–2 meters), has glossy narrow leaves, and many sweet-scented, lilac-colored blossoms that develop into small olivelike fruits. Heliotrope belongs to a species of two hundred fifty herbaceous plants.

- The Incas of Peru use the flowers to relieve fevers.

- The essential oil is added to fragrances in the perfume industry. The powder made from the flowers is used as an ingredient to scent various body and skin care products.

Practical Uses

Mood uplifting

Fragrancing

Aromatherapy Methods of Use

Fragrancing

HONEYSUCKLE

Botanical Name: *Lonicera fragrantissims, Lonicera japonica*

Family: *Caprifoliaceae*

The absolute/essential oil is obtained from the flowers.

History and Information

- Honeysuckle is an evergreen bush native to Asia. The bush grows to a height of about 10–20 feet (3–6 meters), has blue-green leaves and highly fragrant white, pink, or yellow tubular flowers. The small honeysuckle berries are poisonous to humans. The Lonicera japonica variety has white or purple flowers that develop into black fruit.

- Dioscorides, the Greek physician, recommended the seeds and flowers for the liver, spleen ailments, and breathing problems.

- The Algonquin Indians made a tea from the bark to relieve constipation.

- A flower decoction was made for colds, loss of the voice, and joint aches.

- In China, the honeysuckle flowers are used to relieve inflammation and the leaves are used for fevers and colds.

- In Japan, the flowers and leaves are brewed into a tea beverage.

- The oil is used in perfumery and to fragrance products.

Practical Uses

Improves circulation

Relieves inflammation of the breathing passages

Mood uplifting

Lessens pain, relieves inflammation

Inflamed skin

Fragrancing

Documented Properties

Alterative, antibacterial, anti-inflammatory, antimicrobial, antiseptic, antispasmodic, antiviral, diaphoretic, diuretic, expectorant, febrifuge, laxative, refrigerant, uplifting

Aromatherapy Methods of Use

Fragrancing

HOPS

Botanical Name:
Humulus lupulus

Family: *Moraceae*

The essential oil is obtained from the buds and flowers.

The CO_2 extract is obtained from the hop cones.

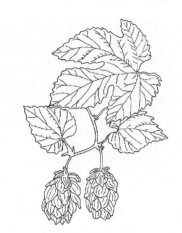

History and Information

- Hops is native to Europe and Asia. The climbing vine grows to about 19–25 feet (5.5–7.5 meters) and has pale-green, bell-shaped flowers. The male and female flowers grow on separate plants. Hops belong to the same family as marijuana.

- In ancient Rome and Greece, the young shoots of the plant were eaten as a vegetable in salads.

- During the ninth and tenth centuries, brewers in Germany and France widely used hops as a preservative in the beer they produced.

- Native Americans used hops to relieve pain and get a restful sleep.

- In Europe, hops were used to relax the body, relieve aching muscles and joints, lower fevers, help nervous conditions, digestion, alleviate menstrual cramps, intestinal parasites, and improve skin problems.

- In the seventeenth century, the herb was taken to relieve stress and tension, digestive upsets, menstrual pain, and headaches.

- Herbalists mixed hops into their herbal remedies to stimulate estrogen production, relieve pain, sleeplessness, muscle and joint aches, jaundice, and other conditions.

- The female flowers contain conelike catkins that ripen into small egg-shaped, fruiting cones. Brewers use the whole cones to give beer a bitter taste and calming effect.

Practical Uses

Calming; promotes a restful sleep

Mild pain reliever

Documented Properties

Analgesic, antibacterial, anticonvulsive, anti-inflammatory, antilithic, antipruritic, antispasmodic, aperitive, aphrodisiac (for women), astringent, blood purifier, calmative, carminative, digestive, diuretic, emmenagogue, emollient, estrogenic, febrifuge, galactagogue, hepatic, hypnotic, nervine, sedative, sudorific, tonic, tranquilizer, vermifuge

Aromatherapy Methods of Use

Application, massage, mist spray

Comments: The fresh hops fruits can cause hypersomnia, vomiting, profuse perspiration, overexcitement, and dermatitis.

Caution: Hops oil is moderately toxic. Use small amounts.

HYSSOP

HYSSOP DECUMBENS

Botanical Name: *Hyssopus officinalis* (Hyssop); *Hyssopus officinalis var. decumbens* (Hyssop decumbens)

Family: *Lamiaceae*

The essential oil is obtained from the leaves and flowering tops.

History and Information

- Hyssop is a semi-evergreen plant native to Europe and Asia. The bushy plant grows to a height of about 1–4 feet (.5–1 meter), has aromatic leaves and spikes of white, pink, blue, or dark-purple flowers.

- In ancient times, the herb was used to fragrantly scent and purify the air during religious services and celebrations. An ancient pharmacopoeia mentioned hyssop as the major ingredient in numerous preparations, elixirs, and syrups.

- Hyssop was prescribed by Hippocrates, Galen, and Dioscorides for its healing effects on the respiratory system.

- In the sixteenth and seventeen centuries, herbalists used the plant to soothe coughs and congestion.

- In folk medicine, hyssop was used for congestion of breathing passages, to improve blood circulation, help stomach problems, and for menstrual conditions.

- In England, hyssop was added to baths to relieve aching muscles and joints.

- In Latin America, the syrup of the flowering tops is consumed to break up chest congestion and soothe the stomach. The juice from the plant is taken to improve eyesight, expel parasites, and for toothaches.

- The strong fragrance of hyssop attracts bees and adds a sweet smell to the honey.

Practical Uses

Relaxing

Vapors open the sinus and breathing passages; deepens the breathing

Mood uplifting; reviving, improves mental clarity and alertness

Fragrancing

Documented Properties

Antibacterial, anti-inflammatory, antirheumatic, antiseptic, antispasmodic, antiviral, aperient, astringent, balsamic, cardiac, carminative, cephalic, cicatrizant, depurative, diaphoretic, digestive, diuretic, emmenagogue, emollient, expectorant, febrifuge, healing (skin), hypertensor, laxative (mild), nervine, parasiticide, pectoral, regulator (blood pressure), resolvent, stimulant (adrenal glands), stomachic, sudorific, tonic, vermifuge, vulnerary

Aromatherapy Methods of Use

Application, aroma lamp, bath, diffusor, inhaler, lightbulb ring, massage, mist spray, steam inhalation, steam room and sauna

Comments: Hyssop decumbens is gentler than the other hyssop variety.

Caution: Use small amounts. Hyssop oil should be avoided by people prone to epileptic seizures.

JASMINE

Botanical Name:
Jasminum officinale

Family: *Oleaceae*

The absolute/
essential oil is
obtained from the
flower petals.

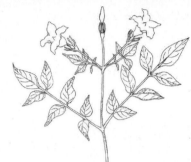

History and Information

- Jasmine is native to Asia and belongs to the olive family. The climbing plant grows to a height of about 30–40 feet (9–12 meters) and has fragrant white flowers.

- Persian women soaked jasmine flowers in sesame oil to massage into their body and hair.

- The Chinese so highly prize the fragrance of jasmine that they add the flowers to scent beverages, cosmetics, massage oils, and to freshen the air. Medicinally, the flowers are taken for liver problems and as a blood purifier. The root is used for insomnia, headaches, and other pains.

- Jasmine flowers are picked after the sun has set to capture their aromatic scent.

- Jasmine garlands are part of Buddhist ceremonies to symbolize respect.

Practical Uses

Mood uplifting, aphrodisiac

Fragrancing

Documented Properties

Analgesic, antidepressant, anti-inflammatory, antipruritic, antiseptic, antispasmodic, antistress, aphrodisiac, calmative, carminative, cicatrizant, decongestant, emollient, euphoriant, expectorant, galactagogue, moisturizer (skin), rejuvenator (skin), sedative, stimulant (uterine contractions), tonic (female reproductive system), uplifting

Aromatherapy Methods of Use

Application, aroma lamp, bath, fragrancing, lightbulb ring, massage, mist spray

JUNIPER BERRIES

Botanical Name:
Juniperus communis

Family: *Cupressaceae*

The essential oil and CO_2 extract are obtained from the ripe berries.

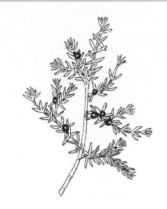

History and Information

- Juniper is an evergreen bush native to Europe, Asia, and the Northern Hemisphere. The bush is about 2–6 feet (.5–2 meters) in height and sometimes reaches as high as 25 feet (7.5 meters). The male trees have yellow cones and the female trees have bluish-green cones. The silvery-green leaves are needlelike. The green berries take three years to ripen to a blue color. The maximum life span of the bush is 2,000 years.

- The Romans used the berries as an antiseptic and to help with digestion, coughs, colds, urinary tract problems, tumors, and snakebites, as well as to flavor foods.

- In the Middle Ages, juniper was burned to protect people against the plague.

- The tree was a source of food for the American Indians. They ate the inner bark, drank a tea from the leaves, and ground up the berries to make cakes. The berries were combined with the twigs to make a tea high in vitamin C. For medicinal uses, a tea was brewed from the juniper twigs for stomachaches and colds. The berries were taken as a blood tonic, to aid digestion, lower fevers, for muscle and joint pains, and as a urinary tract cleanser. They were also applied topically to stop bleeding and heal wounds. During and after illnesses, the branches were burned to fumigate the living quarters, as well as during ceremonial rituals for good luck. The smoke was also inhaled to help respiratory problems. Every part of the tree was used as an antiseptic.

- In folk medicine, the berries were infused in water and used as an antidote for poisonous bites. In Europe, juniper was regarded as helpful for cholera, typhoid, and to expel worms.

- The berries are used to make gin. They are also roasted and used as a coffee substitute.

Practical Uses

Purifying; helps in the reduction of cellulite; cleansing to the intestines and the tissues in the body

Relaxing, reduces stress

Mood uplifting; refreshing, reviving, improves mental clarity and memory

Lessens pain, painful swellings, painful menstruation, fluid retention

Disinfectant

Repels insects

Soothes insect bites

Documented Properties

Abortifacient, analgesic, antifungal, anti-inflammatory, antilithic, antirheumatic, antiscorbutic, antiseptic, antispasmodic, antitoxic, aphrodisiac, astringent, blood purifier, carminative, cholagogue, cicatrizant, depurative, detoxifier, digestive, disinfectant, diuretic (strong), emmenagogue, expectorant, healing, hemostatic, insecticide, nervine, parasiticide, refreshing, rubefacient, sedative, stimulant (genitourinary tract), stomachic, sudorific, tonic, tonifying, vermifuge, vulnerary

Aromatherapy Methods of Use

Application, aroma lamp, bath, diffusor, inhaler, lightbulb ring, massage, mist spray

Caution: Because of juniper berry's strong stimulating effect on the kidneys, use small amounts. Avoid use on a person who has weak kidneys.

KANUKA

Botanical Name: *Kunzea ericoides, Leptospermum ericoides*

Family: *Myrtaceae*

The essential oil is obtained from the leaves and branches.

History and Information

- Kanuka is native to New Zealand. The tree grows to a height of about 30–60 feet (9–18 meters), has green needlelike leaves and a profuse number of small aromatic white flowers. The tree is also known as white tea tree and white manuka.

Practical Uses

Calming, reduces stress, relieves tension

Helps to breathe easier

Mood uplifting, aphrodisiac, euphoric; improves mental clarity

Loosens tight muscles, relieves aches and pains

Disinfectant

Healing to the skin

Documented Properties

Antibacterial, antiseptic

Aromatherapy Methods of Use

Application, aroma lamp, bath, lightbulb ring, massage, mist spray, steam inhalation, steam room and sauna

KATRAFAY

Botanical Name: *Cedrelopsis grevei*

Family: *Ptaeroxylaceae*

The essential oil is obtained from the bark and leaves.

History and Information

- Katrafay is native to Madagascar, and thrives in wet forests. The tree grows to a height of about 20 feet (6 meters), has a fragrant bark and small green flowers followed by a brown capsule. The tree is also known as white mahogany and bois de catafaye. There are eight species of trees in Madagascar.

- The bark has been used as a tonic and given as a tea to women after child delivery. It was also used to eliminate intestinal parasites, abdominal cramps, and fevers.

Practical Uses

Relaxing, reduces stress

Opens the breathing

Mood uplifting

Documented Properties

Analgesic, antibacterial, anti-inflammatory, anti-rheumatic

Aromatherapy Methods of Use

Application, aroma lamp, bath, inhaler, lightbulb ring, massage, mist spray

KAVA-KAVA

Botanical Name: *Piper methysticum*

Family: *Piperaceae*

The CO_2 extract is obtained from the rhizomes.

History and Information

- Kava-kava is an evergreen shrub native to Asia. The shrub grows to a height of about 10–20 feet (3–6 meters), and has heart-shaped leaves with a large rhizome underneath. The small male and female flowers are on separate plants. There are over twenty varieties of the plant.

- The herb has been cultivated in the Pacific Islands for thousands of years, where it is consumed as a beverage to calm nerves, open breathing passages, relieve muscle and joint aches, headaches, stomach cramps, and as a tonic.

Practical Uses

Relaxing; promotes a restful sleep

Reduces pain

Documented Properties

Analgesic, anesthetic, antianxiety, antibacterial, antidepressant, antifungal, anti-inflammatory, antiseptic, antispasmodic, aphrodisiac, diaphoretic, diuretic, hypnotic, nervine, relaxant, sedative, tonic, tranquilizer

Aromatherapy Methods of Use

Application, massage

Caution: Kava-kava tends to slow down reflexes. Avoid driving or doing anything that requires full attention after using the essential oil. Use small amounts.

KHELLA *(Ammi Visnaga)*

Botanical Name: *Ammi visnaga*

Family: *Apiaceae*

The essential oil is obtained from the seeds.

History and Information

- Khella is native to the Mediterranean region. The plant is also known as bishop's weed and greater ammi.

- The herb was used in ancient Egypt and mentioned in the Ebers Papyrus, written about 1550 B.C.

- The fruits have a long history of use. They have a relaxing effect on the muscles, especially on the breathing passages. The dried fruits were used for urinary conditions, pain relief, and as a diuretic.

- The seeds have been made into a tea and taken for a diuretic effect, spasms, menstrual conditions, and to ease breathing problems.

Practical Uses

Calming, reduces stress, relieves tension

Vapors open the sinus and breathing passages; deepens the breathing

Mood uplifting, euphoric; improves mental clarity

Loosens tight muscles

Documented Properties

Analgesic, antispasmodic, dilator, muscle relaxant

Aromatherapy Methods of Use

Application, aroma lamp, bath, diffusor, inhaler, lightbulb ring, massage, mist spray, steam inhalation, steam room and sauna

KUNZEA

Botanical Name: *Kunzea ambigua*

Family: *Myrtaceae*

The essential oil is obtained from the leaves, twigs, and small branches.

History and Information

- Kunzea is native to Australian costal areas. The aromatic shrub grows to a height of about 12 feet (3.5 meters), has narrow dark-green leaves and a profuse amount of small white flowers that develop into fluffy balls. The flowers can be pink in color when the plant is cultivated. The shrub is also known as white kunzea tree. The kunzea family consists of about thirty species of plants.

Practical Uses

Relaxing, eases nervous tension

Muscle and joint aches; reduces pain and swelling

Documented Properties

Analgesic

Aromatherapy Methods of Use

Application, aroma lamp, bath, inhaler, lightbulb ring, massage, mist spray

LABDANUM *(Cistus or Rock Rose)*

Botanical Name: *Cistus creticus, Cistus incanus, Cistus ladanifer*

Family: *Cistaceae*

The resin, absolute, and essential oil are obtained from the leaves.

History and Information

- Labdanum is a small evergreen bush native to the Mediterranean area and Middle East. The bush grows to a height of about 5–10 feet (1.5–3 meters), has dark-green leaves and large white flowers with yellow stamens in the center.

- Labdanum is used in expensive perfumes because of its excellent fixative qualities.

Practical Uses

Warming; increases circulation

Calming, reduces stress; promotes a restful sleep

Helpful for meditation

Mood uplifting, euphoric; brings out feelings, encourages communication

Loosens tight muscles

A fixative to hold the scent of a fragrance

Documented Properties

Antiarthritic, anticoagulant, antioxidant, antiseptic, antispasmodic, antitussive, astringent, balsamic, cardiotonic, cicatrizant, depurative, diuretic, drying, emmenagogue, expectorant, fixative, hemostatic, insecticide, sedative, tonic, vulnerary

Aromatherapy Methods of Use

Application, aroma lamp, inhaler, lightbulb ring, massage, mist spray

LANTANA

Botanical Name: *Lantana camara*

Family: *Verbenaceae*

The essential oil is obtained from the leaves.

History and Information

- Lantana is a vigorous growing evergreen shrub native to the United States that reaches a height of about 4–13 feet (1–4 meters). The flowers are orange and develop into black berries. The berries and dry leaves are poisonous.

- The flowers and roots have been taken to clear congestion from the breathing passages.

- In Latin America, a tea is made for muscle and joint pains, colds, fevers, and to soothe the stomach. For snakebites, the tea is taken while the leaves are placed on the bitten area. A tea from the flowers is made to relieve water retention and to help the urinary tract and regulate menstruation. The root tea is used for breathing problems.

- In Brazil, an infusion of the plant is dispersed in warm baths to help with muscle and joint aches, and regulate the menstrual cycle. A boiled leaf infusion is used to soothe itching.

- The lantana plant is highly toxic to grazing animals, causing death. Children have been poisoned by eating the green berries.

Practical Uses

Cooling

Calming, reduces stress; promotes a restful sleep

Mood uplifting

Documented Properties

Antiseptic, antispasmodic, antiviral, cicatrizant, emmenagogue, expectorant, febrifuge, hepatic

Aromatherapy Methods of Use

Application, aroma lamp, bath, inhaler, lightbulb ring, massage, mist spray

Caution: Lantana is moderately toxic. Use small amounts. The essential oil tends to slow down reflexes. Avoid driving or doing anything that requires full attention after using the oil.

LARCH

Botanical Name: *Larix europaea*

Family: *Pinaceae*

The essential oil is obtained from the needles.

History and Information

- Larch is a deciduous conifer native to the Northern Hemisphere. The tree is one of the fastest growing of all trees and reaches a height of about 65 feet (20 meters). It has soft needlelike leaves and bears a flower called the larch rose. The wood is strong and durable.

- Native Americans made a tea from the needles and bark for urinary tract infections, breathing congestion, coughs, and colds.

Practical Uses

Vapors open the sinus and breathing passages

Mood uplifting

Documented Properties

Analgesic, antidepressant, antiseptic, astringent, diuretic, hemostatic, laxative, vulnerary

Aromatherapy Methods of Use

Application, aroma lamp, bath, inhaler, lightbulb ring, massage, mist spray, steam inhalation, steam room and sauna

Caution: Use small amounts.

LAVANDIN

Botanical Name: *Lavandula fragrans, Lavandula hortensis, Lavandula hybrida*

Family: *Lamiaceae*

The essential oil is obtained from the flowers.

History and Information

- Lavandin is an evergreen plant native to the Mediterranean area. The plant grows to a height of about 3 feet (1 meter) and bears lilac-colored flowers.

- Lavandin is a hybrid plant of lavender. The hybridization occurs naturally by the work of bees. Compared to lavender, the lavandin plant has greater resistance to disease and can tolerate harsher weather conditions. It also produces a greater number of flowers and approximately four times the amount of oil, but of a lower grade. Lavandin oil is less expensive than lavender oil, but it is often sold falsely as lavender.

Practical Uses

Improves digestion; soothing to the intestines

Purifying; helps in the reduction of cellulite

Calming and strengthening to the nerves, relaxes the muscles; promotes a restful sleep

Calming in small amounts and stimulates the nervous system in large amounts

Vapors open the sinus and breathing passages

Mood uplifting, balances mood swings

Lessens aches and pains; gently reduces fluid retention

Disinfectant

Repels insects, kills parasites and lice

Healing to the skin: bruises, cuts, wounds, burns, sunburn, scars, sores, insect bites, and injuries

Documented Properties

Analgesic, anticonvulsive, antidepressant, antirheumatic, antiseptic, antitoxic, carminative, cholagogue, choleretic, cicatrizant, cordial, cytophylactic, deodorant, deodorizer, disinfectant, diuretic, emmenagogue, expectorant, hypotensor, insect repellent, nervine, parasiticide, sedative, stimulant (respiratory system), sudorific, tonic, vermifuge, vulnerary

Aromatherapy Methods of Use

Application, aroma lamp, bath, diffusor, inhaler, lightbulb ring, massage, mist spray, steam inhalation, steam room and sauna

LAVENDER

LAVENDER *(Spike)*

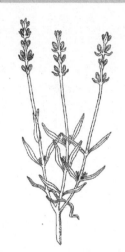

Botanical Name:
Lavandula angustifolia,
Lavandula officinalis,
Lavandula vera
(Lavender); *Lavandula*
latifolia, Lavandula
spica (Spike lavender)

Family: *Lamiaceae*

The essential oil and CO_2 extract are obtained from the flowers.

History and Information

- Lavender is an evergreen plant native to the Mediterranean area. The plant grows to a height of about 3 feet (1 meter) and has lilac-colored flowers.

- Spike lavender grows to about 3 feet (1 meter), has grey-green leave, and purple flowers. There are twenty-eight species of lavender.

- Lavender is regarded as one of the most useful and versatile essences for therapeutic purposes. Herbalists have used the essential oil for head pains, loss of consciousness, and cramps. Lavender's relaxing properties are used on lions and tigers in zoos to keep them calm. Lavender is also known to have a powerful antivenom property that starts neutral-

izing the poison of a snake or insect bite immediately after it is applied.

- Lavender is used to scent soaps, detergents, lotions, and perfumes.

Practical Uses

Improves digestion, soothing to the intestines

Purifying; helps in the reduction of cellulite

Calming and strengthening to the nerves, relaxes the muscles, lessens tension; promotes a restful sleep

Vapors open the sinus and breathing passages

Mood uplifting, balances mood swings

Lessens aches and pains; gently removes fluid retention

Disinfectant

Repels insects, kills parasites and lice

Healing to the skin: bruises, cuts, wounds, burns, sunburns, scars, sores, insect bites, and injuries

Documented Properties

Analgesic, antibacterial, anticonvulsive, antidepressant (premenstrual syndrome and menopause), antifungal, anti-inflammatory, antirheumatic, antiseptic, antispasmodic, antistress, antitoxic, antitussive, antivenomous, antiviral, aperitive, calmative, carminative, cephalic, cholagogue, cicatrizant, cordial, cytophylactic, decongestant, deodorant, detoxifier, diuretic, emmenagogue, healing (skin), hypotensor, insect repellent, nervine, parasiticide, regenerator (skin tissue), restorative, reviving, sedative (heart), stimulant (respiratory system), stomachic, sudorific, tonic, vermifuge, vulnerary

Aromatherapy Methods of Use

Application, aroma lamp, bath, diffusor, inhaler, lightbulb ring, massage, mist spray, steam inhalation, steam room and sauna

Comments: Spike lavender is more camphorous than the other lavender varieties.

Caution: Spike lavender should be avoided during pregnancy.

LEDUM GROENLANDICUM

Botanical Name: *Ledum groenlandicum*

Family: *Ericaceae*

The essential oil is obtained from the leaves.

History and Information

- Ledum groenlandicum is an evergreen shrub native to North America. The shrub grows to a height of about 3 feet (1 meter), has dark-green leathery leaves and clusters of white fragrant flowers.

- The native Canadian people brewed a tea from the leaves called labrador tea. The tea was used as an expectorant and for colds.

Practical Uses

Warming; improves circulation

Calming, reduces stress

Helpful for meditation

Improves mental clarity and alertness

Documented Properties

Analgesic, antibacterial, anti-inflammatory, antiseptic, antispasmodic, decongestant, diaphoretic, digestive, diuretic, emmenagogue, expectorant, febrifuge, hepatic, insecticide, stimulant, stomachic

Aromatherapy Methods of Use

Application, aroma lamp, bath, inhaler, lightbulb ring, massage, mist spray

Caution: Ledum tends to slow down reflexes. Avoid driving or doing anything that requires full attention after using the essential oil. Use small amounts.

LEMON

Botanical Name: *Citrus limon*

Family: *Rutaceae*

The essential oil is obtained from the peel of the fruit.

History and Information

- Lemon is an evergreen citrus tree native to Asia. The tree grows to a height of about 10–20 feet (2–6 meters) and has fragrant white flowers that develop into yellow fruits.

- The Greeks used lemon to perfume clothing.

- The demand for lemon fruit increased enormously in the 1800s after physicians discovered that the high content of vitamin C and other valuable nutrients it contained could help prevent and alleviate the illness of scurvy.

- Many health-conscious people start the day off by having a freshly squeezed lemon in a glass of warm pure water with honey. This daily drink is said to help cleanse the blood vessels, intestinal tract, liver, and other organs, and provide an important amount of vitamin C for the body.

Practical Uses

Cooling

Purifying; breaks down cellulite, cleanses the tissues

Calming, relaxing, reduces stress; promotes a restful sleep

Mood uplifting; refreshing, reviving, improves mental clarity, alertness, and memory; sharpens the senses

Disinfectant

Soothes insect bites

Documented Properties

Antianemic, antibacterial, antidepressant, antifungal, antilithic, antineuralgic, antioxidant, antipruritic, antirheumatic, antisclerotic, antiscorbutic, antiseptic

131

(strong), antispasmodic, antistress, antitoxic, antitussive, aperitive, astringent, blood purifier, calmative, carminative, cephalic, cicatrizant, coagulant, cooling, decongestant, depurative, detoxifier, diaphoretic, digestive, disinfectant, diuretic, emollient, febrifuge, hemostatic, hepatic, hypotensor, insect repellent, insecticide, invigorating (immune system), laxative, parasiticide, refreshing, rubefacient, sedative, stimulant (circulatory and lymphatic systems), stomachic, tonic, uplifting, vermifuge

Aromatherapy Methods of Use

Application, aroma lamp, bath, diffusor, inhaler, lightbulb ring, massage, mist spray

Caution: People with dry or sensitive skin may require additional carrier oil when using the essential oil topically. Use small amounts. Lemon is phototoxic. Avoid exposure to direct sunlight for several hours after applying the oil on the skin.

LEMON VERBENA

Botanical Name: *Aloysia citriodora, Aloysia triphylla, Lippia citriodora, Lippia triphylla, Verbena triphylla*

Family: *Verbenaceae*

The essential oil is obtained from the leaves and branches.

History and Information

- Lemon verbena is native to South America. The bush grows to a height of about 6–10 feet (2–3 meters), has strong, lemon-scented, green leaves and clusters of aromatic, small, white or purple flowers that have a tiny yellow dot in the center. When touched, the flower releases a refreshing fragrance.

- Lemon verbena was a folk remedy for fevers and spasms.

- In Latin America, a tea is made from the leaves and stems for sore throats, colds, fevers, diarrhea, digestive problems, breathing congestion, and to have a restful sleep.

- The leaves are used as a cardiotonic.

- The oil is an ingredient in perfumes and liqueurs. Lemon verbena oil is rare and expensive, and frequently adulterated with cheaper oils like citronella or lemongrass.

Practical Uses

Mood uplifting; reviving, improves mental clarity and alertness

Documented Properties

Antidepressant, antiseptic, antispasmodic, aphrodisiac, aperitive, calmative, carminative, cholagogue, cooling, detoxifier, digestive, diuretic, emollient, expectorant, febrifuge, galactagogue, hepatic, insect repellent, insecticide, nervine, pectoral, refreshing, sedative, stimulant (circulatory system), stomachic, sudorific, tonic (nerves), tonifying (skin), uplifting

Aromatherapy Methods of Use

Application, aroma lamp, inhaler, lightbulb ring, massage, mist spray

Caution: People with dry or sensitive skin may require additional carrier oil when using the essential oil topically. Use small amounts. Lemon verbena is phototoxic. Avoid exposure to direct sunlight for several hours after applying the oil on the skin.

LEMONGRASS

Botanical Name: *Cymbopogon citratus, Cymbopogon flexuosus*

Family: *Poaceae*

The essential oil is obtained from the whole plant.

History and Information

- Lemongrass is native to Asia, and thrives in warm and sunny locations. The grass grows to a height of about 2 feet (.5 meter), has swordlike leaves and an aromatic rhizome. Lemongrass is also known as fever grass, oil grass, and citronnelle.

- Dioscorides and Pliny the Elder reported on the use of aromatic grasses in the first century.

- The plant has been taken for water retention, muscle stiffness, nervous upsets, and infections.

- In the Amazon region, lemongrass is mainly used to help digestion, regulate menstrual cycles, and reduce fevers.

- In Latin America, a leaf tea is taken for the stomach, lung congestion, urinary spasms, muscle and joint aches, colds, fevers, flu, headaches, nervousness, and to lower blood pressure. The leaves are chewed to relieve toothaches. The sap from the plant is made into a compress for eye infections. The rhizome tea is used as a mouthwash to help the gums and teeth, and for colds, stomach, and intestinal discomfort.

- In Indonesia, the plant is taken for coughs, headaches, digestion, to promote sweating, and for urinary tract problems.

- In India, the oil is applied on the skin for ringworm. The leaves are used for fevers, as well as menstrual and digestion problems.

- In Thailand, lemongrass is a popular food flavoring ingredient.

- In Asia, a tea is made for menstrual conditions and to regulate blood sugar.

- Lemongrass is highly aromatic and widely cultivated in the Asian tropics for the essential oil. It is used in perfumery, to fragrance skin care products and soaps, and as a flavoring agent in cooking, soft drinks, candy, ice cream, and baked goods.

Practical Uses

Improves digestion

Balancing to the nervous system; calming, reduces stress; promotes a restful sleep

Vapors help open the sinus and breathing passages

Mood uplifting; reviving, improves alertness

Reduces inflammation and swollen tissues; contracts weak connective tissue, tones the skin

Increases lactation

Repels insects

Documented Properties

Abortifacient, analgesic, antibacterial, antidepressant, antidiabetic, antifungal, antioxidant, antiseptic, antispasmodic, aperitive, astringent, calmative, carminative, deodorant, deodorizer, depurative, diaphoretic, digestive, disinfectant, diuretic, emmenagogue, expectorant, febrifuge, galactagogue, hypotensor, insect repellent, insecticide, nervine, parasiticide, regulator (parasympathetic system), reviving, sedative, stimulant (circulatory system), stomachic, tonic, tonifying (skin)

Aromatherapy Methods of Use

Application, aroma lamp, diffusor, inhaler, lightbulb ring, massage, mist spray

Caution: People with dry or sensitive skin may require additional carrier oil when applying lemongrass essential oil topically. Use small amounts.

LILAC

Botanical Name: *Syringia vulgaris*

Family: *Oleaceae*

The absolute/essential oil is obtained from the flowers.

History and Information

- Lilac is a deciduous bush native to Europe. The bush grows to a height of about 6–20 feet (2–6 meters) and has clusters of fragrant lilac or white-colored flowers. Lilac belongs to the olive family.

Practical Uses

Mood uplifting

Fragrancing

Documented Properties

Antidepressant

Aromatherapy Methods of Use

Fragrancing

LIME

LIME *(Key)*

Botanical Name:
Citrus aurantiifolia,
Citrus limetta (Lime);
Citrus aurantiifolia
var. swingle (Key lime)

Family: *Rutaceae*

The essential oil is
obtained from the
peel of the fruit.

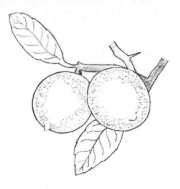

History and Information

- Lime is an evergreen citrus tree native to Asia. The tree grows to a height of about 10 feet (3 meters) and has fragrant white flowers that develop into green fruits with an acid pulp.

- Key lime is a small evergreen tree native to Asia. The tree grows to a height of about 20 feet (6 meters), has yellow-green to dark-green leaves and white fragrant flowers followed by green fruits.

- Lime fruit increased in popularity after physicians in the 1800s discovered that the high content of vitamin C helped prevent and cure scurvy. English sailors were called "limeys" because they added limes to their diet as a preventative.

Practical Uses

Cooling

Purifying; helps in the reduction of cellulite

Strengthens the nerves; used when there is weakness in the body

Reduces stress

Mood uplifting; refreshing, reviving, improves mental clarity and alertness, sharpens the senses

Disinfectant

Soothes insect bites

Documented Properties

Antibacterial, antidepressant, antilithic, antioxidant, antirheumatic, antisclerotic, antiscorbutic, antiseptic, antispasmodic, antitoxic, antiviral, aperitif, astringent, cooling, depurative, disinfectant, febrifuge, hemostatic, hepatic, insecticide, refreshing, restorative, stimulant (digestive and lymphatic systems), tonic (immune system), uplifting

Aromatherapy Methods of Use

Application, aroma lamp, bath, diffusor, inhaler, lightbulb ring, massage, mist spray

Caution: People with dry or sensitive skin may require additional carrier oil when using the essential oil topically. Use small amounts. Lime is phototoxic. Avoid exposure to direct sunlight for several hours after applying the oil on the skin.

LINALOE

Botanical Name: *Bursera glabrifolia*

Family: *Burseracea*

The essential oil is obtained from the wood, leaves, twigs, and seeds.

History and Information

- The linaloe is an evergreen tree native to South America. The tree produces small flowers. There are fifty species of linaloe.

- The oil is used in soaps and perfumes.

Practical Uses

Calming, reduces nervous tension and stress

Documented Properties

Antibacterial, anticonvulsant, anti-inflammatory, antiseptic, calmative, tonic

Aromatherapy Methods of Use

Application, aroma lamp, bath, diffusor, inhaler, lightbulb ring, massage, mist spray

LINDEN BLOSSOM

Botanical Name: *Tilia europaea, Tilia vulgaris*

Family: *Tiliaceae*

The absolute/essential oil is obtained from the flowers.

History and Information

- Linden is native to the Northern Hemisphere. The tree grows to a height of about 100–130 feet (30.5–36.5 meters) and has clusters of fragrant yellow-white flowers, followed by green fruits. Linden is also known as lime tree and basswood.

- In Europe, the leaves were brewed to make a tea for relaxation and sleep.

- The flowers have been taken for calming purposes, digestive problems, to ease breathing congestion, improve circulation, headaches, and increase sweating.

Practical Uses

Calming, reduces stress; promotes a restful sleep

Fragrancing

Documented Properties

Antidepressant, antineuralgic, antiseptic, antispasmodic, antistress, antitussive, astringent, calmative, carminative, cephalic, decongestant, detoxifier, diaphoretic, diuretic, emollient, hypotensor, nervine, sedative, stomachic, sudorific, tonic (nervous system)

Aromatherapy Methods of Use

Application, aroma lamp, bath, inhaler, lightbulb ring, massage, mist spray

Caution: Linden blossom oil should not be used over a prolonged period of time. Use in small amounts.

LITSEA CUBEBA

Botanical Name: *Litsea citrata, Litsea cubeba*

Family: *Lauraceae*

The essential oil is obtained from the fruit.

History and Information

- Litsea cubeba is an evergreen tree native to Asia. The tree grows to a height of about 30–40 feet (9–12 meters), has green leaves and small fragrant white or yellow flowers that develop into small red or black berries. Litsea cubeba is part of a family of sixty species of trees.

- In Chinese medicine, litsea cubeba is used for chest congestion.

- The fruits are edible and have been used for their medicinal value to improve nerve impulses, memory, and digestion.

- The seeds are applied to the scalp for ringworm.

- The properties of litsea cubeba are similar to those of lemongrass oil.

- The oil is mainly produced and extensively used in China. The herb is also known as may-chang.

- All parts of the tree contain essential oil.

Practical Uses

Cooling

Improves digestion

Calming, reduces stress; promotes a restful sleep

Mood uplifting, euphoric; reviving, improves mental clarity and alertness

Relieves pain

Documented Properties

Antibacterial, anticongestive, antidepressant, anti-inflammatory, antiseptic, antistress, aperitive, astringent, bronchodilator, calmative, carminative, deodorant, deodorizer, detoxifier, digestive, disinfectant, emollient, expectorant (bronchitis), galactagogue, healing (skin), insecticide, revitalizing, sedative, stimulant (digestion), stomachic, tonic, uplifting, vulnerary

Aromatherapy Methods of Use

Application, aroma lamp, diffusor, inhaler, lightbulb ring, massage, mist spray

Caution: People with dry or sensitive skin may require additional carrier oil when applying litsea cubeba essential oil topically. Use small amounts.

LOVAGE

Botanical Name: *Angelica levisticum, Levisticum officinale, Ligusticum levisticum*

Family: *Apiaceae*

The essential oil and CO_2 extract are obtained from the roots.

History and Information

- Lovage is native to Europe. The plant grows to a height of about 6 feet (2 meters), has large dark-green leaves, and small green flowers. Lovage is also known as love parsley

- Herbalists recommend various preparations of lovage roots to stimulate urine flow and menstruation.

- In Asian countries, the stems are eaten to strengthen the body's defenses against infection and for cholera disease.

- The plant and roots are eaten fresh in salads; the seeds flavor baked goods and cooked dishes.

- The root yields approximately 1 percent essential oil and is used extensively in perfumery and as a food flavoring ingredient.

Practical Uses

Purifying; helps in the reduction of cellulite

Calming, reduces stress

Helps to breathe easier

Mood uplifting, aphrodisiac, euphoric; improves mental clarity and alertness

Documented Properties

Antibacterial, antifungal, antiseptic, antispasmodic, aphrodisiac, carminative, deodorizer, depurative, detoxifier, diaphoretic, digestive, diuretic, emmenagogue, expectorant, febrifuge, laxative, parasiticide, revitalizing, stimulant (digestive system and kidneys), stomachic, warming

Aromatherapy Methods of Use

Application, aroma lamp, bath, inhaler, lightbulb ring, massage, mist spray

Caution: Lovage is phototoxic. Avoid exposure to direct sunlight for several hours after applying the essential oil on the skin.

MAGNOLIA *(Bark)*

Botanical Name: *Magnolia officinalis*

Family: *Magnoliaceae*

The essential oil is obtained from the bark.

History and Information

- Magnolia is a deciduous tree native to Asia. The tree grows to a height of about 65 feet (20 meters), has light-green leaves and large fragrant white flowers that develop into fruits with seeds. This species of magnolia now only survives as a cultivated tree. The trees became extinct in the wild due to the stripping of the bark for use in medicinal remedies.

- The dried tree bark was used in folk medicine to induce sweating and as a bitter tonic.

- In Chinese medicine, the bark has been used since the first century for anxiety, stress, and nervous related digestive conditions.

Documented Properties

Antioxidant, antiseptic, antispasmodic, calmative (neuromuscular blocking effect; relaxation of the skeletal muscles), diuretic, expectorant, hypotensor, stimulant (uterine contractions), stomachic, tonic

Caution: Large amounts of the bark can cause respiratory paralysis. The essential oil is not recommended for use in aromatherapy.

MAGNOLIA (Flowers)

Botanical Name: *Magnolia grandiflora, Magnolia liliiflora*

Family: *Magnoliaceae*

The absolute/essential oil is obtained from the flowers.

History and Information

- Magnolia is an evergreen tree native to North America and thrives in moist locations. The tree grows to a height of about 60–80 feet (18–24 meters), has glossy, dark-green, leathery leaves and fragrant, twelve-inch, lemon-scented, white flowers that develop into red or purple fruits with seeds. Magnolia liliiflora grows to a height of about 10 feet (3 meters), has green leaves and purple flowers. The tree is also known as lily-tree, laurel magnolia, hindi-andachampa, and him champa.

- The bark was used for malaria and muscle and joint aches.

- Magnolia is named after Pierre Magnol, a French horticulturist. Prior to receiving the name magnolia the tree was known as laurel-tulip tree.

- In Latin America, a tea from the bark is taken as a stimulant and tonic, and is externally applied to stop bleeding and heal wounds.

Practical Uses

Opens the breathing passages

Mood uplifting

Documented Properties

Analgesic, carminative, decongestant, diaphoretic, febrifuge, stimulant, tonic

Aromatherapy Methods of Use

Fragrancing

MANDARIN
TANGERINE
CLEMENTINE

Botanical Name: *Citrus clementine* (Clementine), *Citrus nobilis* (Mandarin), *Citrus reticulata* (Mandarin, Tangerine, and Clementine)

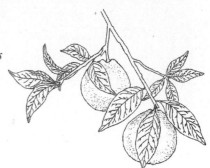

Family: *Rutaceae*

The essential oil is obtained from the peel of the fruit.

History and Information

- Mandarin and tangerine are evergreen citrus trees native to Asia. The trees grow to a height of about 10–25 feet (3–7.5 meters) and have fragrant white flowers that develop into orange fruits.

- Clementine is thought to be a hybrid fruit named after P'ere Clement, who discovered the tree in the early 1900s.

- The oils are used to flavor confectionery, beverages, chewing gum, and baked goods. They are also valued in perfumery.

Practical Uses

Cooling

Purifying; helps in the reduction of cellulite

Calming; promotes a restful sleep

Encourages dreaming

Mood uplifting; improves mental clarity, and alertness, sharpens the mind, relieves emotional tension and stress, calms angry and irritable children

Documented Properties

Antidepressant, antiemetic, antiseptic, antispasmodic, antistress, antitussive, aperitive, astringent, calmative, carminative, cholagogue, cytophylactic, decongestant, depurative, digestive, diuretic, emollient, hypnotic,

137

THE AROMATHERAPY ENCYCLOPEDIA

revitalizing, sedative, stimulant (digestive and lymphatic systems), stomachic, tonic, tranquilizer, uplifting

Aromatherapy Methods of Use

Application, aroma lamp, bath, diffusor, inhaler, lightbulb ring, massage, mist spray

Caution: People with dry or sensitive skin may require additional carrier oil when using mandarin, tangerine, or clementine essential oil topically. Use small amounts. These oils are phototoxic. Avoid exposure to direct sunlight for several hours after applying the oils on the skin.

MANUKA *(New Zealand Tea Tree)*

Botanical Name: *Leptospermum scoparium*

Family: *Myrtaceae*

The essential oil is obtained from the leaves and branches.

History and Information

- Manuka is an evergreen shrub native to New Zealand and Australia, where it is found on moist sandy soil along riverbanks. The shrub grows to a height of about 6–10 feet (2–3 meters), has small leaves and white or, occasionally, pink or red flowers. Manuka is also known as broom tea tree and kahikatoa.

- The Maori people of New Zealand have used all parts of this valuable shrub to produce healing remedies. The leaves were used to reduce fever and help with colds. The bark was brewed into a tea for a sedative.

- When Captain Cook and his crew discovered New Zealand in the eighteenth century, they made a tea with the leptospermum leaves. As a result, the tree became known as New Zealand tea tree.

Practical Uses

Calming, reduces stress and tension

Helps to breathe easier

Mood uplifting, aphrodisiac, euphoric; improves mental clarity

Loosens tight muscles, relieves aches and pains

Deodorant

Disinfectant

Healing to the skin

Documented Properties

Analgesic, antibacterial, antidepressant, antifungal, anti-inflammatory, antiseptic, disinfectant, sedative, vulnerary

Aromatherapy Methods of Use

Application, massage, mist spray

MARJORAM *(Spanish)*
MARJORAM *(Sweet)*

Botanical Name: *Thymus mastichina* (Spanish marjoram); *Majorana hortensis, Origanum majorana* (Sweet marjoram)

Family: *Lamiaceae*

The essential oil is obtained from the flowering tops and leaves.

The CO_2 extract is obtained from the leaves.

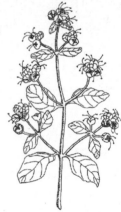

History and Information

- Spanish marjoram is native to Spain. The plant grows to a height of about 1 foot (.5 meter).

- Sweet marjoram is a bushy plant native to the Mediterranean area. The plant grows to a height of about 2 feet (.5 meter), has light-green leaves and white or purple flowers.

- Before the discovery of hops, marjoram was said to be used as an essential ingredient in the brewing of beer.

- Marjoram was cultivated by the Egyptians in 1000 B.C.

- The herb was used by the Egyptians, Greeks, and Romans for common colds and sore throats. The Romans also grew the herb for a digestive aid, to promote menstruation, heal bruises, and for perfume. The Greeks used it in perfumes and toiletries, for snakebites, and muscle and joint pains.

- The Romans and Greeks crowned young couples at weddings with marjoram.

- Dioscorides, the Greek physician, recommended marjoram for nervous disorders, while Pliny, the Roman herbalist, used it for digestive problems.

- European singers drink marjoram tea to maintain their voices.

- The flowering tops and leaves yield 0.2 to 0.8 percent essential oil.

Practical Uses

Warming; improves circulation, dilates the blood vessels

Improves digestion

Relaxing, calms nervous tension; promotes restful sleep

Vapors open the sinus and breathing passages; deepens the breathing; especially helpful during colds and nasal congestion

Relieves tense muscles, aches, pains, painful menstruation, inflammation, spasms

Disinfectant

Documented Properties

Analgesic, anaphrodisiac, antibacterial, antifungal, antioxidant, antiseptic, antispasmodic, antistress, antitussive, antiviral, calmative, carminative, cephalic, cordial, decongestant, detoxifier, diaphoretic, digestive, diuretic, emmenagogue, expectorant, febrifuge, galactagogue, hypotensor, laxative, nervine, restorative, sedative, stomachic, tonic (heart), vasodilator (arterial), vulnerary, warming

Aromatherapy Methods of Use

Application, aroma lamp, bath, diffusor, inhaler, lightbulb ring, massage, mist spray, steam inhalation, steam room and sauna

Caution: Due to the relaxing effect of the essential oil, marjoram should not be used before driving or doing anything that requires full attention. In large amounts, marjoram can dull the senses. Use small amounts.

MASSOIA BARK

Botanical Name: *Cryptocarya massoia*

Family: *Lauraceae*

The essential oil and CO_2 extract are obtained from the bark.

History and Information

- Massoia belongs to a species of two hundred evergreen trees and shrubs that thrive in tropical and subtropical regions of South America, Asia, and the southern part of Africa. The tree has leathery leaves and small flowers.

Practical Uses

Warming; improves circulation

Calming, relaxing

Mood uplifting, aphrodisiac, euphoric; reviving, improves mental clarity and concentration; heightens the senses

Aromatherapy Methods of Use

Application, aroma lamp, lightbulb ring, inhaler, massage, mist spray

Caution: Massoia bark oil can irritate the skin and should be used with extra care. People with sensitive skin should avoid using the essential oil.

MASTIC

Botanical Name: *Pistacia lentiscus*

Family: *Anacardiaceae*

The resin and essential oil are obtained from the bark.

History and Information

- Mastic is an evergreen tree native to the Mediterranean area. The small aromatic tree grows to a height of about 10 feet (3 meters), has shiny dark-green leathery leaves and clusters of green fragrant flowers that develop into small red to black berries. The bark sap is mastic.

- The ancient people chewed on the twigs and bark to strengthen their gums and teeth. This is the origin of the word "masticate."

- The Egyptians burned the resin for incense.

- The fruits and bark were used as a spice.

- In the Middle East, the resin is chewed to stimulate appetite and freshen the breath.

- The Turkish people chew mastic to sweeten the breath and maintain healthy gums.

- The resin and essential oil have similar properties to terebinth. The resin is used in baked goods, to freshen the breath, fill dental cavities, and in varnishes. Mastic is also known as lentisque oil.

Practical Uses

Calming, reduces stress and tension; promotes deep sleep

Vapors open the sinus and breathing passages

Encourages dreaming

Disinfectant

Documented Properties

Analgesic, antioxidant, antiseptic, antispasmodic, antitumor, antitussive, aphrodisiac, astringent, cardiotonic, carminative, diuretic, emmenagogue, expectorant, hemostatic, hepatic, hypotensor, sedative, stimulant, stomachic

Aromatherapy Methods of Use

Application, inhaler, massage, mist spray, steam inhalation, steam room and sauna

MELISSA *(Lemon Balm)*

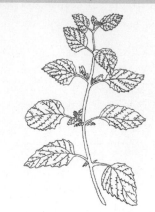

Botanical Name:
Melissa officinalis

Family: *Lamiaceae*

The essential oil and CO_2 extract are obtained from the leaves.

History and Information

- Melissa is native to Europe and the Mediterranean region. The plant grows to a height of about 1–3 feet (.5–1 meter) and has clusters of small light-blue, yellow, or white flowers.

- Melissa was mentioned by Theophrastus, the father of botany, and Arab and Persian physicans wrote about the plant's mood-elevating and digestive properties.

- The ancient Greeks placed the twigs of melissa in beehives to attract bees.

- Melissa became very popular as a remedy for nervousness and anxiety that Emperor Charlemagne ordered the herb grown in all of his gardens to guarantee an adequate supply.

- The Arabs found melissa to be a beneficial remedy for depression and anxiety, and believed it was also helpful for heart disorders. Avicenna, an Arab physician of the eleventh century, recognized the benefits of the herb and used it to relieve melancholy.

- In the Middle Ages, herbalists greatly expanded on earlier uses of melissa and recommended it for insomnia, pain, digestive problems, and menstrual cramps. Melissa became known as a cure-all. The herb was also strewn around the house to provide a clean and festive atmosphere.

- Paracelsus, a Swiss physician of the sixteenth century, highly valued melissa for its ability to revive and rejuvenate the body and uplift the mood.

- Charles V, the King of France, drank lemon balm

ESSENTIAL OILS

tea daily to maintain good health. The popularity of the tea was so widespread that it became known as the "tea of France."

- In Germany, the herb is widely used as a tranquilizer. It is also an active ingredient in Lomaherpan Creme, an ointment applied to cold sores and genital herpes.

- In the Amazon region, the leaves are made into a tea and taken for calming, as a tonic for the nervous system, to help digestion and sleep, and alleviate headaches. A hot poultice is applied on the abdomen for stomach and intestinal discomfort. The fresh leaves are placed on the eyelids and the tea taken to relieve eye inflammations.

- Melissa yields a small quantity of essential oil. Litsea cubeba, lemongrass, and citronella are often blended with or substituted for melissa, and then sold falsely as true melissa oil.

Practical Uses

Improves digestion

Calming, relieves nervousness and nervous conditions such as stress, tension and anxiety; promotes a restful sleep

Mood uplifting

Relieves aches, pains, and menstrual pain

Documented Properties

Analgesic, antibacterial, anticonvulsive, antidepressant, anti-inflammatory, antioxidant, antiputrid, antiseptic, antispasmodic, antistress, antiviral, aperitive, calmative, carminative, cephalic, choleretic, cordial, cytophylactic, diaphoretic, digestive, emmenagogue, febrifuge, galactagogue, hypotensor, insect repellent, nervine, sedative, stomachic, tonic, uplifting, vermifuge, vulnerary

Aromatherapy Methods of Use

Application, aroma lamp, diffusor, inhaler, lightbulb ring, massage, mist spray

Caution: People with dry or sensitive skin may require additional carrier oil when applying melissa essential oil topically. Use small amounts.

MIMOSA

Botanical Name: *Acacia dealbata, Acacia decurrens*
Family: *Mimosaceae*
The absolute/essential oil is obtained from the flowers.

History and Information

- Mimosa is native to Australia. The tree grows to a height of about 40–65 feet (12–20 meters), has small silver-grey feathery leaves and clusters of small, yellow, fragrant flowers followed by reddish-brown pods. The tree thrives in dry climates by storing a large quantity of water in the roots. There are about six hundred species of acacia trees. Mimosa is a wattle tree. The wattle tree is the national emblem of Australia. The picture of the tree is on coinage.

- Mimosa has been used for skin inflammations, bacterial infections, and to improve sleep.

- The tree is prized for gum arabic, which is secreted from the branches.

- The tree pods are a favorite food of elephants.

Practical Uses

Mood uplifting

Fragrancing

Documented Properties

Antidepressant, anti-inflammatory, antiseptic, astringent, moisturizer (skin), uplifting

Aromatherapy Methods of Use

Application, aroma lamp, fragrancing, lightbulb ring, massage, mist spray

MONARDA

Botanical Name: *Monarda fistulosa*
Family: *Lamiaceae*
The essential oil is obtained from the whole plant.

141

History and Information

- Monarda is a bushy plant native to the United States. The plant grows to a height of about 4 feet (1 meter) and has whorls of lavender-colored flowers. The entire plant smells similar to citrus.

- American Indians and early American settlers made a tea from the plant for headaches, fevers, colds, sore throats, intestinal troubles, and congestion. A tea made from the flowerheads and leaves was used to induce sweating to break fevers and encourage a restful sleep. Monarda was also added to flavor foods.

- The herb was popular during the Boston Tea Party era because it was used as a substitute for "black tea."

Practical Uses

Calming, relaxing; reduces stress

Helps the breathing

Mood uplifting; improves mental clarity; brings out feelings

Documented Properties

Anthelmintic, antibacterial, antifungal, antiseptic, antispasmodic, antiviral, carminative, diuretic, expectorant, stimulant, tonic

Aromatherapy Methods of Use

Application, aroma lamp, diffusor, inhaler, lightbulb ring, massage, mist spray

Caution: People with dry or sensitive skin may require additional carrier oil when applying monarda essential oil topically. Use small amounts.

MUGWORT (Armoise)

Botanical Name: *Artemisia vulgaris*

Family: *Asteraceae*

The essential oil is obtained from the whole plant.

History and Information

- Mugwort is native to Europe, Asia, and the Mediterranean region. The bushy plant grows to a height of about 2–8 feet (.5–2.5 meters) and has small reddish, yellow, or white flowers.

- Mugwort was used as a spice in China 4,000 years ago.

- In Rome, chewing the leaves was said to help fatigue.

- Europeans stuffed mugwort into their pillows to inhale all night because they believed that it helped them dream vividly.

- In Latin America, the plant infusion is used for intestinal parasites, menstrual problems, and nervous disorders.

- Oriental medicine uses the herb to treat malaria and anemia. In China, a compress of mugwort is applied to facilitate childbirth.

- American Indians used the leaves for respiratory congestion, digestive problems, and joint and muscle pains.

- Mugwort is known to regulate the female cycles and is referred to as a magical plant for its ability to increase one's psychic powers.

- A bath with the herb was helpful for muscle and joint pain, gout, and a general feeling of weakness.

- In Europe, the herb is added to flavor foods.

Practical Uses

Calming

Encourages dreaming

Relieves menstrual cramps

Documented Properties

Abortifacient, analgesic, anthelmintic, anti-inflammatory, antirheumatic, antispasmodic, aperitif, aperitive, carminative, cholagogue, diaphoretic, digestive, diuretic, emmenagogue, febrifuge, insect repellent, nervine, purgative (mild), regulator (menstrual cycle), sedative, stimulant (uterine), sudorific, tonic (uterine), vermifuge

Aromatherapy Methods of Use

Application

Caution: Mugwort oil contains a toxic component called thujone, which can interfere with the brain and nervous system functions.

MULLEIN

Botanical Name: *Verbascum thapsus*

Family: *Scrophulariaceae*

The essential oil is obtained from the leaves.

History and Information

- Mullein is a biennial plant native to Europe, where it is found on hillsides and open land. The plant likes full sun and reaches a height of about 6 feet (2 meters). The leaves are large, soft and velvety green. The flowers are yellow and grow in clusters. Mullein is also known as velvet plant, flannel flower, blanket herb, and feltwort.

- Ancients used the leaves for breathing problems, coughs, and congestion. The flowers were made into a tea to improve respiratory functions.

- Dioscorides, the Greek physician, recommended mullein for throat problems, coughs, poor eyesight, and toothaches.

- Native American Indians smoked the leaves to open the breathing passages by breaking up congestion.

- The leaves have been used to relieve irritation in the mucous membranes, respiratory system, and urinary tract, for hemorrhoids, digestive problems, wound healing, insect bites, and skin problems.

Practical Uses

Warming

Improves digestion

Helps reduce congestion of the breathing passages; soothing

Calming, reduces stress

Mood uplifting; energizing, improves mental clarity

Loosens tight muscles

Documented Properties

Anti-inflammatory, antiviral, astringent, demulcent, diuretic, expectorant, vulnerary

Aromatherapy Methods of Use

Application, aroma lamp, bath, diffusor, inhaler, lightbulb ring, massage, mist spray, steam inhalation, steam room and sauna

MUSTARD *(Black)*

Botanical Name: *Brassica nigra*

Family: *Brassicaceae*

The essential oil is obtained from the seeds.

History and Information

- Black mustard is native to Europe, Africa, Asia, and the Americas. The plant grows to a height of about 2–6 feet (.5–2 meters), has yellow flowers and seed pods that contain brown seeds.

- The Greeks and Romans valued mustard for medicinal uses and as a spice.

- Pliny, the Roman naturalist, used mustard as a main ingredient for many of his remedies.

- The early American settlers and Indians used mustard for sprains, headaches, and toothaches. They also consumed the greens as a vegetable and the seeds as a spice.

- In China, brown mustard seeds are favored over the black seeds, since the brown seeds are milder. The seeds are used for digestive problems, tight joints, and colds.

- Mustard plasters, applied on the chest, have long been relied upon to relieve congestion through their heat. Due to the ability of the seeds to stimulate circulation, they were used to treat coldness of the body and added to love potions.

- In Europe and Asia, the young leaves are used to flavor salads.

Documented Properties

Antirheumatic, antiseptic, aperitive, diuretic, emetic, febrifuge, laxative, stimulant (salivary glands), tonic

Caution: Black mustard oil is a strong irritant and can blister the skin when used topically. It is added to foods as a flavor ingredient and not used in aromatherapy.

MYRRH

Botanical Name: *Balsamodendron myrrha,*
Commiphora myrrha

Family: *Burseraceae*

The resin and essential oil are obtained from the bark.

The CO_2 extract is obtained from the resin.

History and Information

- Myrrh is native to Africa and Asia. The tree grows to a height of about 9–15 feet (2.5–4.5 meters) and has yellow-red flowers followed by small fruits.

- In ancient times, myrrh was highly prized and more widely used than any other aromatic oil in perfumes, anointing oils, incense, ointments, medicines, and for embalming purposes.

- The Egyptians believed that the fragrant odor pleased the gods and, therefore, burned the oil during religious ceremonies.

- The Ebers Papyrus, dated 1550 B.C., contains information on the use of myrrh for facial masks.

- The Greeks used the resin on wounded soldiers to promote healing.

- Myrrh has been used throughout history to maintain healthy teeth and gums.

- The bark contains approximately 8 percent essential oil.

Practical Uses

Cooling

Calming; promotes a restful sleep

Helpful for meditation

Mood uplifting

Soothes inflamed tissue

Healing to the skin

A fixative to hold the scent of a fragrance

Documented Properties

Analgesic, antidiabetic, antifungal, anti-inflammatory, antiputrid, antiseptic (strong) (infected gums), antispasmodic, antitussive, aperitive, astringent, balsamic, carminative, cicatrizant, cooling, deodorant, depurative, disinfectant, diuretic, drying, emmenagogue, expectorant, fixative, healing (traumatic injuries), hemostatic, invigorating (immune system), moisturizer, pectoral, rejuvenator (skin cells), revitalizing (skin), sedative, stimulant (digestive system), stomachic, sudorific, tonic (stomach), tonifying (cleanses and tightens the skin), vulnerary

Aromatherapy Methods of Use

Application, aroma lamp, bath, inhaler, lightbulb ring, massage, mist spray

MYRTLE

Botanical Name:
Myrtus communis

Family: *Myrtaceae*

The essential oil is obtained from the leaves, twigs, and flowering tops.

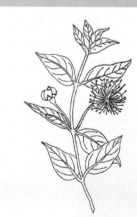

History and Information

- Myrtle is an evergreen shrub native to Europe and Asia. The shrub grows to a height of about 10–18 feet (3–5.5 meters), has scented dark-green leaves and small aromatic white or pink blossoms. The flowers develop into bluish-black berries that are edible fresh or dried. The fruit is aromatic and contains many small kidney-shaped seeds. There are sixteen species of the tree.

- Myrtle was always considered to represent peace.

- The ancient Egyptians and, later, Dioscorides, the Greek physician, macerated myrtle leaves to make a wine for respiratory and bladder afflictions.

- Greek and Roman folklore claimed that a tea made from myrtle had the virtue of preserving love and youth. They also used myrtle for its tonic and astringent effect on the skin.

- In Great Britain, it was customary to have myrtle sprigs in the bridal bouquets and for the bridesmaid to plant the sprigs. This connection with weddings has associated myrtle as a symbol of love.

- Traditionally, myrtle has been used to help intestinal conditions, alleviate parasites, treat urinary tract problems, and open the breathing passages.

- Myrtle berries have been used over the years to flavor wines. The leaves are added to potpourri, and the branches, twigs, leaves, and berries flavor foods and repel insects.

- In Africa, the people drink a tea made from the leaves for breathing problems.

- In the Middle East, the leaves are taken to help relieve nose bleeding.

- The oil is used to help with infections and breathing problems, as well as to fragrance cosmetics and perfumes.

Practical Uses

Calming

Helpful for meditation

Vapors open the sinus and breathing passages

Mood uplifting; refreshing

Relieves pain

Documented Properties

Antibacterial, antidiabetic, antifungal, anti-inflammatory, antimicrobial, antioxidant, antiseptic, anti-spasmodic, antitumor, astringent, balsamic, carminative, decongestant, deodorant, digestive, diuretic, emmenagogue, expectorant, hemostatic, laxative, nervine, parasiticide, sedative, tonic (skin)

Aromatherapy Methods of Use

Application, aroma lamp, bath, diffusor, inhaler, lightbulb ring, massage, mist spray, steam inhalation, steam room and sauna

MYRTLE (Anise)

Botanical Name: *Backhousia anisata*

Family: *Myrtaceae*

The essential oil is obtained from the leaves and branches.

History and Information

- Anise myrtle is native to Australia, and is found in the rainforest. The tree grows to a height of about 80–150 feet (24.5–45.5 meters), has aromatic anise-scented leaves, and fragrant white flowers.

Practical Uses

Soothes the intestines

Calming, reduces stress; promotes a restful sleep

Vapors open the sinus and breathing passages

Mood uplifting; improves mental clarity; encourages communication

Loosens tight muscles, relieves aches, pains, and menstrual discomfort

Documented Properties

Antibacterial, antifungal, carminative, insect repellent, sedative

Aromatherapy Methods of Use

Application, aroma lamp, bath, diffusor, inhaler, lightbulb ring, massage, mist spray, steam inhalation, steam room and sauna

MYRTLE (Lemon)

Botanical Name: *Backhousia citriodora*

Family: *Myrtaceae*

The essential oil is obtained from the leaves and branches.

History and Information

- Lemon myrtle is a bushy evergreen rainforest tree native to Australia, and is found in the costal forests. The tree grows to a height of about 30–50 feet (9–15 meters), has fragrant, lemon-scented, elliptical, green leaves and profuse clusters of cream-colored flowers. The tree is also known as lemon ironwood, lemon-scented myrtle, and sweet verbena tree. There are eight species in the Backhousia family.

- In Australia, the leaves are brewed to make a lemon-tasting herbal tea and the powdered leaves are sprinkled on foods to add flavor.

- Lemon myrtle is also an ingredient in personal care products.

Practical Uses

Warming

Improves digestion

Calming, relaxes the nerves, reduces stress and tension

Helpful for meditation

Vapors help open the sinus and breathing passages

Mood uplifting, euphoric; refreshing, improves mental clarity and alertness

Loosens tight muscles, relieves pain

Documented Properties

Antibacterial, antifungal, antiviral, carminative, sedative

Aromatherapy Methods of Use

Application, aroma lamp, diffusor, inhaler, lightbulb ring, massage, mist spray, steam inhalation

Caution: People with dry or sensitive skin may require additional carrier oil when using lemon myrtle essential oil topically.

NEROLI

Botanical Name: *Citrus aurantium*

Family: *Rutaceae*

The essential oil is obtained from the blossoms.

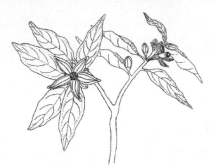

History and Information

- The oil of neroli is produced from the fragrant white blossoms of the bitter orange tree. Bitter orange is an evergreen citrus tree native to Asia.

- Neroli was named in 1680 when the princess of Nerole perfumed her gloves, stationery, shawls, and bathwater with the scent. For centuries, neroli has been added to cosmetic preparations, colognes, and perfumes.

- Neroli is often adulterated with the essential oil of petitgrain, which has similar properties and is relatively inexpensive.

Practical Uses

Soothes the intestines

Calms nervous tension, relaxes hyperactive children; promotes a restful sleep

Mood uplifting; boosts confidence, helps to face emotional fear

Helps to relieve menstrual discomfort

Documented Properties

Analgesic, antibacterial, antidepressant, antifungal, antiseptic, antispasmodic, antistress, aphrodisiac, astringent, blood purifier, calmative, carminative, cicatrizant, cordial, cytophylactic, deodorant, digestive, emollient, euphoriant, hypnotic, hypotensor, regenerator (skin cells), sedative, tonic, tranquilizer, uplifting

Aromatherapy Methods of Use

Application, aroma lamp, bath, inhaler, lightbulb ring, massage, mist spray

NEROLINA

Botanical Name: *Melaleuca quinquenervia* (chemotype nerolidol)

Family: *Myrtaceae*

The essential oil is obtained from the leaves and stems.

History and Information

- Nerolina is an evergreen tree native to Australia, where it is found along coastal regions. The tree grows to a height of about 35 feet (10.5 meters), has a white papery bark, aromatic leathery leaves and white, sometimes green or red, flowers. The tree is also known as broad-leafed paperbark tree.

Practical Uses

Cooling

Calming, reduces stress, soothing, promotes a peaceful state

Vapors open the sinus and breathing passages; deepens the breathing

Mood uplifting; improves mental clarity

Reduces pain and discomfort; soothing, comforting

Deodorant

Documented Properties

Antibacterial, anti-inflammatory, antiviral, hypotensor

Aromatherapy Methods of Use

Application, aroma lamp, bath, diffusor, inhaler, lightbulb ring, massage, mist spray, steam inhalation, steam room and sauna

NIAOULI

Botanical Name: *Melaleuca quinquenervia, Melaleuca viridiflora*

Family: *Myrtaceae*

The essential oil is obtained from the leaves and twigs.

History and Information

- Niaouli is an evergreen tree native to Australia, and is found along streams and swamps. The tree grows to a height of about 30–60 feet (9–18 meters), has leathery leaves and white or yellow-green flowers in the shape of a bottlebrush. The tree is also known as broad-leafed paperbark.

- In Madagascar, niaouli is used for headaches, fevers, breathing congestion, and muscle and joint aches.

- The oil of niaouli is also known as gomenol oil.

Practical Uses

Vapors open the sinus and breathing passages; deepens the breathing

Relieves aches and pains

Documented Properties

Analgesic, anthelmintic, antibacterial, antirheumatic, antiseptic, antispasmodic, balsamic, cicatrizant, decongestant, diaphoretic, expectorant, febrifuge, insecticide, regenerator (skin tissue), reviving, stimulant (circulation to the tissues), tonic (respiratory system), vermifuge, vulnerary

Aromatherapy Methods of Use

Application, aroma lamp, bath, diffusor, inhaler, lightbulb ring, massage, mist spray, steam inhalation, steam room and sauna

NUTMEG

Botanical Name:
Myristica aromata,
Myristica fragrans,
Myristica officinalis

Family: *Myristicaceae*

The essential oil and
CO_2 extract are
obtained from the seeds.

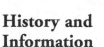

History and Information

- Nutmeg is an evergreen tree native to the Molucca Islands, and is found in humid locations. The tree grows to a height of about 60–100 feet (18–30.5 meters), has large, fragrant, dark-green leaves and small yellow flowers that develop into yellow fruits resembling apricots. The fruit contains a dark-brown seed inside. The seed is surrounded by a netlike substance, which is known as mace. The male and female flowers are on different trees. The male flowers are white in color.

- Nutmeg was recommended in Arabian writings to treat urinary and digestive disorders and as an aphrodisiac.

- Hindu practitioners in India have used nutmeg since early times. The spice was taken for pain, bad breath, and intestinal disorders.

- In Africa, nutmeg has been externally applied to help muscle and joint aches. The seeds are eaten for an aphrodisiac effect.

- In Europe, the seeds are used for menstrual problems and to abort a fetus.

- The seeds contain approximately 10 percent essential oil.

- The fruit is made into jams. The dried aril is used as a spice known as mace.

Practical Uses

Slightly warming

Improves digestion

Calming and promotes a restful sleep in small amounts

Encourages dreaming

Mood uplifting; reviving, mental stimulant, improves mental clarity and alertness

Loosens tight muscles, relieves aches, pains, sore muscles and menstrual pains

Documented Properties

Abortifacient, analgesic, antibacterial, antiemetic, antioxidant, antirheumatic, antiseptic, antispasmodic, aperitive, aphrodisiac, astringent, calmative, cardiac, carminative, digestive, emmenagogue, estrogenic, expectorant, invigorating, laxative, reviving, sedative, stimulant (circulatory system), stomachic, tonic, uplifting, warming

Aromatherapy Methods of Use

Application, aroma lamp, bath, inhaler, lightbulb ring, massage, mist spray

Caution: Nutmeg oil can dull the senses. Use small amounts.

ONION

Botanical Name: *Allium cepa*

Family: *Liliaceae*

The essential oil is obtained from the plant.

History and Information

- Onion is native to Asia. The plant grows to a height of about 2 feet (.5 meter) and has white flowerheads.

- Dioscorides, the Greek physician, recommended onions as a tonic, diuretic, and for infections.

- As a folk remedy, onions have been used to draw toxins out of the body by slicing and placing them on the inflamed area.

- The American Indians used onion juice to soothe insect stings.

- Onions are eaten regularly by the Bulgarian people, many of whom live to be over 100 years old.

Documented Properties

Analgesic, antibacterial, antirheumatic, antisclerotic, antiscorbutic, antiseptic, aphrodisiac, digestive, diuretic, emollient, expectorant, hypoglycemient, hypnotic, hypotensor, insect repellent, resolvent, stimulant, vermifuge, vulnerary

Comments: Onion oil is not used in aromatherapy because of its disagreeable odor. It is added to foods as a flavoring ingredient.

OPOPANAX

Botanical Name: *Commiphora erythraea, Opopanax chironium*

Family: *Burseraceae*

The resin/essential oil is obtained from the bark.

History and Information

- Opopanax is a tall tree native to Asia and Africa belonging to the same family as myrrh and frankincense.

- Opopanax resin is also produced from Opopanax chironium, which is in the Apiaceae family. This herbaceous plant is native to Greece.

- The resin is solid at room temperature and is usually mixed with solvents to keep it liquified.

- Opopanax is used as a fixative in perfumes.

Practical Uses

Fragrancing
A fixative to hold the scent of a fragrance

Documented Properties

Anti-inflammatory, antiseptic, antispasmodic, expectorant, fixative

Aromatherapy Methods of Use

Fragrancing

ORANGE *(Bitter)*
ORANGE *(Blood)*
ORANGE *(Sweet)*
TANGELO
TEMPLE ORANGE

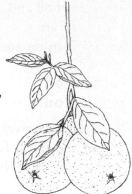

Botanical Name: *Citrus aurantium* (Bitter orange), *Citrus reticulata* (Temple orange), *Citrus sinensis* (Blood orange, Sweet orange), *Citrus tangelo* (Tangelo)

Family: *Rutaceae*

The essential oil is obtained from the peel of the fruit.

History and Information

- Orange, tangelo, and temple orange are evergreen citrus trees native to Asia. The trees grow to a height of about 20–30 feet (6–9 meters), have glossy leaves and fragrant white flowers that develop into edible orange-colored citrus fruit. However, bitter orange is not edible when fresh.

- The tangelo tree was first produced in 1897 by the United States Agriculture Department. The tangelo fruit is a hybrid cross between a tangerine and a grapefruit.

- Temple orange is a cross between a tangerine and an orange hybrid. The tree was propagated in 1917 in Florida and named after William Chace Temple, who was a prominent person in the citrus field.

- In Chinese medicine, the dried orange fruit was taken as a remedy for swelling in the stomach and indigestion; the peel was taken for coughs, to help the spleen and stomach, and as a tonic to the body.

- Oranges are one of the most popular of all the fruits. The seeds yield an oil that is used for cooking and as an ingredient in soaps and plastics. The oil from the rind is used in food flavorings, cosmetics, and perfumes, and is added to wood-care products to protect against insect damage.

Practical Uses

Cooling

Improves digestion

Purifying; helps in the reduction of cellulite

Calming, reduces stress; promotes a restful sleep

Mood uplifting; improves mental clarity and alertness; relieves emotional tension and stress, calms angry and irritable children

Relieves spasms

Documented Properties

Antibacterial, anticoagulant, antidepressant, antiemetic, antifungal, anti-inflammatory, antipyorrhea, antiscorbutic, antiseptic, antispasmodic, antistress, antitoxic, antitussive, antiviral, aperitif, aperitive, astringent, calmative, carminative, cholagogue, choleretic, depurative, digestive, disinfectant, diuretic, expectorant, febrifuge, hemostatic, hepatic, hypotensor, hypnotic, laxative, nervine, refreshing, sedative, stimulant (digestive and lymphatic systems), stomachic, tonic, vasoconstrictor, vulnerary

Aromatherapy Methods of Use

Application, aroma lamp, bath, diffusor, inhaler, lightbulb ring, massage, mist spray

Caution: People with dry or sensitive skin may require additional carrier oil when using orange, tangelo, or temple orange essential oil topically. Use small amounts. These oils are phototoxic. Avoid exposure to direct sunlight for several hours after applying the oils on the skin.

OREGANO

Botanical Name: *Origanum vulgare*

Family: *Lamiaceae*

The essential oil is obtained from the flowering plant. The CO_2 extract is obtained from the leaves.

History and Information

- Oregano is native to Europe and America. The plant grows to a height of about 1–2 feet (.5 meter), has dark-green leaves and purple buds that blossom into white, pink, or lilac-colored flowers. The entire plant is aromatic. There are about twenty species of oregano.

- The Greeks used oregano to heal wounds and placed the leaves on sore and aching muscles to relieve discomfort. Dioscorides, the Greek physician, used oregano for poisonous animal bites.

- Pliny, the Roman herbalist, recommended oregano to improve digestion and for poisonous spider bites.

- During the Middle Ages, oregano was used by herbalists to aid digestion, improve eyesight, and for poisonous bites.

- Modern herbalists use oregano for digestion, headaches, coughs, to promote menstruation, and prevent sea sickness.

- The common name of the plant is wild marjoram. The essential oil is one of the most antiseptic of all the oils. It is also known as origanum oil.

Practical Uses

Heating; improves circulation, promotes perspiration

Improves digestion

Purifying; helps in the reduction of cellulite, waste material and excessive fluids from the body

Vapors open the sinus and breathing passages

Mood uplifting; improves mental clarity and alertness

Loosens tight muscles, relieves muscle aches and pains

Increases physical endurance and energy

Disinfectant

Repels insects

Documented Properties

Analgesic, anaphrodisiac, anthelmintic, antibacterial, antifungal, anti-inflammatory, antirheumatic, antiseptic, antispasmodic, antitoxic, antiviral, aperitif, aperitive, balsamic, carminative, cholagogue, choleretic, cytophylactic, diaphoretic, disinfectant, diuretic, emmenagogue, expectorant, febrifuge, hepatic, hypnotic, laxative, parasiticide, rubefacient, stimulant (nerves), stomachic, sudorific, tonic, vulnerary, warming

Aromatherapy Methods of Use

Application, aroma lamp, diffusor, inhaler, lightbulb ring, massage, mist spray

Caution: Oregano oil is heating. People with dry or sensitive skin may require additional carrier oil when using the essential oil topically. Use small amounts.

ORRIS ROOT

Botanical Name: *Iris florentina, Iris pallida*

Family: *Iridaceae*

The concrete, absolute, essential oil, CO_2 extract, and powder are obtained from the roots.

History and Information

- Orris is native to the Mediterranean area. The plant grows to a height of about 2 feet (.5 meter), has swordlike silver-white leaves and large scented flowers ranging in various colors, depending on the variety, followed by seeds.

- The Egyptians, Greeks, and Romans used orris root as an ingredient in their perfumes. The plant was found depicted on the walls of an Egyptian temple dated about 1500 B.C.

- Theophrastus, Dioscorides, and Pliny wrote about the medicinal value of the plant.

- In Europe, orris root was used for culinary purposes, but its popularity in perfumery was far greater than any other use.

- Orris root was used as a dry shampoo in the eighteenth century and, up until the twentieth century, as a face powder.

- The root requires a three-year growing period before it can be harvested; it is then left to dry for two to three years until it acquires a scent similar to violets.

- The oil is extensively used in perfumery, and added to fragrance soaps, powders, and toothpastes.

Practical Uses

Fragrancing

A fixative to hold the scent of a fragrance

Documented Properties

Analgesic, anthelmintic, diuretic, expectorant, fixative, purgative, stomachic

Aromatherapy Methods of Use

Fragrancing

Caution: Orris root is toxic.

OSMANTHUS

Botanical Name: *Osmanthus fragrans*

Family: *Oleaceae*

The absolute and essential oil are obtained from the flowers.

History and Information

- Osmanthus is an evergreen tree native to Asia. The tree grows to a height of about 40 feet (12 meters), has long leathery leaves and clusters of white or yellow flowers with a jasminelike scent. The flowers develop into black, blue, or violet-colored oval fruits. Osmanthus belongs to the olive family.

- In China, osmanthus flowers are added to foods and beverages, and the oil is used in expensive perfumes.

Practical Uses

Calming, reduces stress

Fragrancing

Documented Properties

Antidepressant, calmative, sedative

Aromatherapy Methods of Use

Application, fragrancing, massage

PALMAROSA

Botanical Name: *Andropogon martinii, Cymbopogon martinii var. motia*

Family: *Poaceae*

The essential oil is obtained from the plant.

History and Information

- Palmarosa is a fragrant grass native to Asia. The plant grows to a height of about 9 feet (2.5 meters) and has clusters of flowers that turn red when they mature.

- The expensive oil of rose is often adulterated with palmarosa, which is cheaper in price.

- Palmarosa is also known as rosha or rusha. The oil is widely used in perfumery and cosmetology.

Practical Uses

Warming; improves circulation

Calming, reduces stress

Mood uplifting; refreshing

Reduces aches, pains, and inflammation

Moisturizing and regenerating to the skin

Documented Properties

Abortifacient, analgesic, anthelmintic, antibacterial, antifungal, antiseptic, antispasmodic, antistress, antiviral, aperitive, aphrodisiac, astringent, calmative, carminative, cicatrizant, cytophylactic, digestive, emmenagogue, emollient, febrifuge, moisturizer, nervine, refreshing, regenerator (skin cells), sudorific, stimulant (circulatory and digestive systems), tonic, uplifting, vermifuge

Aromatherapy Methods of Use

Application, aroma lamp, bath, diffusor, inhaler, light-bulb ring, massage, mist spray

PARSLEY

Botanical Name: *Apium petroselinum, Carum petroselinum, Petroselinum crispum, Petroselinum hortense, Petroselinum sativum*

Family: *Apiaceae*

The essential oil and CO_2 extract are obtained from the seeds.

History and Information

- Parsley is native to the Mediterranean area and Africa. The plant grows to a height of about 3 feet (1 meter) and has green-yellow flowers.

- Theophrastus, the father of botany, claimed parsley benefited the heart.

- Galen, the Greek physician, prescribed parsley for water retention and sleeping sickness.

- The Greeks used parsley to crown victors at their games and decorate tombs.

- The Romans were the first people to use parsley for food and to counter bad odors.

- Emperor Charlemagne ordered parsley grown in his imperial gardens to ensure that he had an adequate supply for each meal.

- Female peasants in the Mediterranean area used parsley leaves to relieve breast soreness and curtail lactation of nursing mothers.

- Nicholas Culpeper, the seventeenth century herbalist, recommended parsley for menstrual conditions, urinary problems, and edemas.

- Parsley tea was consumed in World War I for kidney problems caused by dysentery.

- The herb was taken in large doses by pregnant women to abort the fetus. In France, apiol, a constituent of parsley, was used for contraception before birth control pills were available. Apiol is also used in South America as a contraceptive. The oil is a powerful uterine stimulant and must be avoided during pregnancy.

- The root has been used to reduce thyroid activity.

- In Latin America, the tea is made to facilitate childbirth, eliminate uric acid retention, and regulate blood pressure.

- In Germany, parsley tea is taken to reduce high blood pressure. Due to its diuretic property, it is used for treating the heart.

- In Russia, parsley juice is used to help quicken childbirth delivery.

- The parsley plant is a rich source of protein, potassium, calcium, and vitamin C, which are valuable in the mending of bones, strengthening blood vessels, and keeping the skin and muscles healthy. A deficiency of vitamin C is known to result in easy bruising of the skin and slow healing of broken bones.

- The seeds yield 3 to 6 percent essential oil and the leaves yield 0.25 percent.

- Parsley seeds have been known to be deadly to birds.

Practical Uses

Improves digestion

Calms the nerves

Eliminates excess water from the body

Documented Properties

Abortifacient, antianemia, antibacterial, antifungal, antigalactagogue, anti-inflammatory, antilithic, antioxidant, antirheumatic, antiseptic, antispasmodic, aperient, aperitive (in small amounts), aphrodisiac, blood builder, blood purifier, calmative, carminative, cooling, depurative, digestive, diuretic (strong), emmenagogue (strong), estrogenic, expectorant, febrifuge, hepatic, insect repellent, laxative, lithotriptic, parasiticide (intestinal), parturient, purgative, sedative, stimulant (kidneys; uterine contractions), stomachic, tonic (female reproductive and circulatory systems), vasodilator, vermifuge

Aromatherapy Methods of Use

Application, aroma lamp, inhaler, lightbulb ring, massage, mist spray

Caution: People with dry or sensitive skin may require additional carrier oil when using parsley essential oil topically. Use small amounts. Parsley is phototoxic. Avoid exposure to direct sunlight for several hours after applying the oil on the skin.

PATCHOULI

Botanical Name: *Pogostemon cablin, Pogostemon patchouli*

Family: *Lamiaceae*

The essential oil is obtained from the leaves.

History and Information

- Patchouli is native to Asia. The plant grows to a height of about 3 feet (1 meter), has oblong leaves and whorls of light-purple or lavender flowers. Patchouli requires full sun to bring out its fragrance.

- The Arabs used patchouli to repel fleas and lice from their bedding.

- In the Philippines, an infusion of the leaves is taken for menstrual cramps.

- In Asia, patchouli is used for snakebite, as an insect repellent, for menstrual discomforts, colds, nausea, abdominal cramps, and headache.

- In Latin America, a leaf tea is taken for flu, colds and congestion.

- In India, patchouli is used to scent inks.

- The leaves yield approximately 2.5 percent essential oil.

- Because the oil makes a great base note, it is used in more than one out of three perfume blends.

- The oil improves with age, becoming sweeter and milder the longer it matures.

- Patchouli oil is a flavoring agent for chewing gum, baked goods, candy, and beverages.

- The color of the essential oil is determined by the type of metal used in the distillation process. If the oil is produced in a stainless steel container, the color of the oil will be light. If the oil is distilled in an iron vessel, the color will be darker due to the iron leeching into the oil.

Practical Uses

Nerve stimulant; prevents sleep

Mood uplifting, euphoric, aphrodisiac

Repels insects

Healing to the skin

A fixative to hold the scent of a fragrance

Documented Properties

Alterative, analgesic, antibacterial, antidepressant, antiemetic, antifungal, anti-inflammatory, antiphlogistic, antiseptic, antistress, antitoxic, antiviral, aphrodisiac, astringent (strong), calmative, carminative, cicatrizant (strong), cytophylactic, decongestant, deodorant, diaphoretic, digestive, diuretic, febrifuge, fixative, insect repellent, insecticide, laxative, nervine, parasiticide, regenerator (skin tissue), sedative (large amounts), stimulant (small amounts) (nerves), stomachic, tonic (uterus)

Aromatherapy Methods of Use

Application, aroma lamp, bath, inhaler, lightbulb ring, massage, mist spray

PENNYROYAL

Botanical Name: *Mentha pulegium*

Family: *Lamiaceae*

The essential oil is obtained from the flowering plant.

History and Information

- Pennyroyal is native to England. The plant grows to a height of about 1 foot (.5 meter) and has purple aromatic flowers.

- The Romans used the leaves to repel fleas and insects.

- During medieval times, the plant was strewn throughout households to freshen the air and provide a pleasant fragrance.

- Pennyroyal was used by sailors in the sixteenth century to purify drinking water.

- In the nineteenth century, the herb was commonly used in folk medicine to promote perspiration during the onset of a cold and stimulate menstruation. Pennyroyal tea was given to babies to help with stomach problems.

- From 1831 through 1916, the herb was listed in the United States Pharmacopoeia as a carminative, emmenagogue, and stimulant.

Practical Uses

Repels insects

Fragrancing

Documented Properties

Abortifacient, analgesic, antipruritic, antiseptic, antispasmodic, blood purifier, carminative, diaphoretic, digestive, emmenagogue, expectorant, febrifuge, insect repellent, sedative (mild), stimulant (circulatory system), stomachic, warming

Aromatherapy Methods of Use

Mist spray

Caution: Pennyroyal oil is toxic due to the thujone content.

PEPPER *(Black)*

Botanical Name: *Piper nigrum*

Family: *Piperaceae*

The essential oil and CO_2 extract are obtained from the berries.

History and Information

- Black pepper is a tropical climbing vine native to India. The plant grows to a height of about 10 feet (3 meters) and has clusters of small white flowers. As the berries ripen, they turn from green to orange to red. After the berries are picked, they are left in the sun to dry, which turns their color to black.

- Black pepper is one of the oldest known spices, used in India, ancient Greece, and Rome for thousands of years.

- Hippocrates claimed that pepper assisted digestion.

- Throughout medieval Europe, this precious spice was commonly traded ounce for ounce for gold. During the Middle Ages and the siege of Rome in 400 A.D., the spice was used as currency. Owners kept it under lock and key.

- During the Middle Ages, pepper was the most important commodity traded between India and Europe. Rents and taxes were frequently paid with pepper.

- Workers unloading black pepper from ships were forbidden to wear clothes with pockets to ensure that they did not steal the valuable peppercorns.

- Over the years, black pepper was highly valued by many of the immigrants that settled in the United States from Europe. At the onset of a cold or flu, a tea was made from a small amount of the powdered spice. Pepper was added as a seasoning to practically every meal. Even for breakfast, scrambled eggs and baked goods contained pepper. These people not only enjoyed the taste of the spice, but also treasured its ability to control bacterial organisms in the human body and in the food. This property of pepper had tremendous significance since there was no refrigeration to preserve the freshness of foods.

- In India, pepper is used for liver problems and hemorrhoids.

- The fruits yield approximately 3 percent essential oil. Pepper is one of the most consumed spices throughout the world. White pepper is produced by removing the dark outer skin of the black pepper, which gives it a milder taste. Powdered peppercorns lose their spicy flavor rapidly after being ground.

Practical Uses

Warming; increases circulation

Improves digestion in small amounts

Reviving, stimulating, improves mental clarity

Loosens tight muscles

Improves the benefits of other oils that are used together with black pepper

Documented Properties

Analgesic, antibacterial, anticholeric, anticonvulsive, antidote, antiemetic, antiseptic, antispasmodic, antitoxic, antitussive, aperitive, aphrodisiac, cardiac, carminative, detoxifier, diaphoretic, digestive, diuretic, drying, expectorant, febrifuge, heating, insect repellent, insecticide, laxative, rubefacient, sedative, stimulant (circulation; kidneys), stomachic, tonic, tonifying (muscles), vasodilator

Aromatherapy Methods of Use

Application, massage, mist spray

Caution: People with dry or sensitive skin may require additional carrier oil when applying black pepper essential oil topically. Use small amounts.

PEPPER (Red) (Cayenne Pepper)

Botanical Name: *Capsicum frutescens*

Family: *Solanaceae*

The essential oil and CO_2 extract are obtained from the fruits.

History and Information

- Red pepper is native to the Americas. The plant grows to a height of about 2–5 feet (.5–1.5 meters), has elliptical green leaves and white or green flowers followed by a long red, purple, yellow, or green fruit containing many seeds.

- In Mexico, red pepper was added to foods before 3000 B.C.

- Chinese texts mention cayenne's use a few thousand years ago.

155

- In Ayurvedic medicine, red pepper was used as a digestive aid and to help paralysis.

- During the Middle Ages cayenne was highly valued and used as currency.

- In folk medicine, the herb was taken for muscle and joint aches, toothaches, cramps, to help circulation, and as a gargle for sore throats and colds.

- Native Americans used cayenne to relieve pain, muscle and joint aches, increase circulation, treat infections, menstrual discomforts, and sore throats. The fruits were mixed into foods for flavoring.

- In the Pacific region, the fruit was taken to relieve muscle and joint aches, backaches, and other painful areas.

- Red pepper has been added to foods to help with shingles.

- The hotter the pepper is, the more capsaicin it contains. Capsaicin plays a major role in the healing power of cayenne pepper.

Practical Uses

Heating; increases circulation

Stops bleeding

Documented Properties

Analgesic, antibacterial, anti-inflammatory, antimicrobial, antiseptic, antispasmodic, aperitive, astringent, carminative, depurative, diaphoretic, digestive, expectorant, febrifuge, heating, hemostatic, irritant, regulator (blood pressure and blood flow), restorative, rubefacient, stimulant (kidneys, excretion of waste in the sweat; circulatory system), stomachic, sudorific, tonic

Caution: Red pepper is a hot oil and can burn the skin. For this reason, it is advisable not to use the oil on the body.

PEPPERMINT

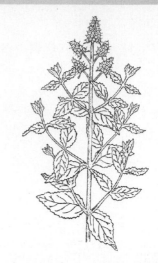

Botanical Name:
Mentha piperita

Family: *Lamiaceae*

The essential oil is obtained from the whole plant.

The CO_2 extract is obtained from the leaves.

History and Information

- Peppermint is a cross between a number of wild mints, and has been known since the seventeenth century. The true peppermint plant cannot reproduce; therefore, propagation through the root system below the soil is needed. The plant grows to a height of about 1–3 feet (.5–1 meter), has a purplish stem and pale-violet flowers.

- Peppermint capsules are used in Europe for irritated bowels. The extract is said to be effective against herpes simplex and other viral organisms. The oil stops spasms of smooth muscles. It is also an important ingredient in many personal hygiene products such as aftershave lotions, colognes, and dental toothpastes.

- The leaves yield 0.1 to 0.8 percent essential oil.

Practical Uses

Cooling

Improves digestion, soothes the intestines, relieves flatulence and nausea, increases appetite; freshens bad breath

Vapors open the sinus and breathing passages; deepens the breathing

Mood uplifting especially to people who have a slow metabolism, aphrodisiac; refreshing, reviving, stimulates the brain, nerves, and metabolism, increases mental clarity, alertness, and the ability to concentrate, sharpens the senses; encourages communication; helps to revive a person from a fainting spell or shock

Increases physical strength and endurance

Relieves pain, inflammation, menstrual pain, and cramps

Reduces lactation

Repels insects, kills parasites

Soothes itching skin

Documented Properties

Alterative (mild), analgesic, anesthetic, antibacterial, anticonvulsive, antidepressant, antidiarrhoeic, antigalactagogue, anti-inflammatory, antineuralgic, antiphlogistic, antipruritic, antiseptic, antispasmodic (digestive system), antitoxic (gastrointestinal poisoning), antitussive, antiviral, aperitive, aphrodisiac, astringent, carminative, cephalic, cholagogue, cordial, decongestant, depurative, digestive, emmenagogue, expectorant, febrifuge, hepatic, insect repellent, invigorating, nervine, parasiticide, refreshing, refrigerant, restorative, stimulant (nervous system), stomachic, sudorific, tonic (heart), uplifting, vasoconstrictor, vermifuge

Aromatherapy Methods of Use

Application, aroma lamp, diffusor, inhaler, lightbulb ring, massage, mist spray, steam inhalation, steam room and sauna

Caution: People with dry or sensitive skin may require additional carrier oil when applying peppermint essential oil topically. Use small amounts. Avoid using before bedtime since the oil can overstimulate the nervous system.

PERILLA

Botanical Name: *Perilla frutescens, Perilla ocimoides*

Family: *Lamiaceae*

The essential oil is obtained from the leaves and flower stems.

History and Information

- The essential oil from the leaves contains a major component known as perillaldehyde that has an herbaceous scent and a sweet herbaceous taste. It is 2,000 times sweeter than sugar and increases the appetite. The leaves are edible.

- Perilla is used in the food and flavor industry to flavor foods, mask fishy odors, and to inhibit the growth of micro-organisms.

- In Japan, the essential oil is called ao-jiso.

For more information on Perilla, see Perilla Seed in Chapter 2, page 49.

Practical Uses

Cooling

Improves digestion

Vapors open the sinus and breathing passages; deepens the breathing

Mood uplifting; energizing, improves mental clarity

Documented Properties

Antitumor, sedative

Aromatherapy Methods of Use

Application, aroma lamp, diffusor, inhaler, lightbulb ring, massage, mist spray, steam inhalation, steam room and sauna

PERU BALSAM

Botanical Name: *Myrospermum pereirae, Myroxylon pereirae, Toluifera pereirae*

Family: *Fabaceae*

The resin and essential oil are obtained from the bark.

History and Information

- Peru balsam is a slow-growing evergreen tree native to Central America. The tree grows to a height of about 60–120 feet (18–36.5 meters) and has fragrant flowers. Peru balsam is also known as black balsam and Indian balsam.

- The tree thrives in El Salvador. However, the resin was exported to Europe from ports in Peru, and thus derived the name Peru balsam.

- In the seventeenth century, the Germans used Peru balsam in their medicine and, thereafter, its use spread universally.

- In the Amazon, the powdered bark was used for incense and the resin for colds, congestion, wounds, and muscle and joint aches.

- The Indians in Central and South America consider the Peru bark to be effective to stop bleeding and promote healing. The leaves are taken as a diuretic and to expel parasitic worms. The dried fruits are used to relieve itching and the resin applied to heal skin bruises and cuts.

- The leaves are used to ease breathing problems, for muscle and joint aches, and wounds.

- In China, Peru balsam is used as a fragrance and fixative in oriental-type perfumes and cosmetics.

- Peru balsam has been in the United States Pharmacopeia since 1820.

- In the United States, the resin is used as an ingredient in dental cements and suppositories (to relieve itching of hemorrhoids); as a flavor additive; to fragrance detergents, soaps, skin care, and perfumes; and as a fungicide. It is also extensively added to topical preparations to heal skin tissue.

- An aromatic dark-brown resin begins to flow when the tree trunk is wounded. The fruit also yields a balsam, which is extracted.

Practical Uses

Warming; increases circulation, helps to move stagnant blood

Purifying

Calming, reduces stress; promotes a restful sleep

Helpful for meditation

Mood uplifting

Loosens tight muscles

Healing to the skin, improves poor skin conditions

A fixative to hold the scent of a fragrance

Documented Properties

Antibacterial, antifungal, anti-inflammatory, antipruritic, antiseptic, antitussive, balsamic, emollient, expectorant, healing, parasiticide (skin), rubefacient, stimulant, vulnerary

Aromatherapy Methods of Use

Application, aroma lamp, lightbulb ring, inhaler, massage, mist spray

Caution: People with dry or sensitive skin may require additional carrier oil when applying Peru balsam resin or essential oil topically. Use small amounts.

PETITGRAIN

Botanical Name: *Citrus bigaradia*

Family: *Rutaceae*

The essential oil is obtained from the leaves and twigs.

History and Information

- Petitgrain oil is derived from the leaves and twigs of the orange, lemon, or tangerine tree. The citrus evergreen trees are native to Asia.

- The oil is widely used in perfumery.

Practical Uses

Cooling

Calms the nerves, relieves anxiety, tension and mental stress; promotes a restful sleep

Helpful for meditation

Mood uplifting; improves mental clarity and alertness

Soothes inflamed and irritated skin tissue

Documented Properties

Antidepressant, antiseptic, antispasmodic, antistress, astringent, calmative, deodorant, digestive, fixative, nervine, refreshing, sedative, stimulant (digestive system), stomachic, tonic, uplifting

Aromatherapy Methods of Use

Application, aroma lamp, bath, diffusor, inhaler, lightbulb ring, massage, mist spray

PINE

Botanical Name: *Pinus sylvestris*

Family: *Pinaceae*

The essential oil is obtained from the needles and small branches.

History and Information

- Pine is an evergreen tree native to Asia and Europe. The tree grows to a height of about 115–130 feet (35–39.5 meters), and has greenish-blue needle-like leaves and cones. There are ninety species of trees in the pine family. It is estimated that a pine can live to 1,200 years.

- The American Indians used pine needles to prevent scurvy and the bark and berries for rheumatism, broken bones, bruises, sores, inflammation, colds, coughs, lung ailments, headaches, and to fight infection.

- The major uses of the pine tree are wood for construction, furniture, boats, paper products, turpentine, pine oil, and pine nuts for food. Turpentine, the largest produced oil in the United States, is extracted from lumber byproducts of the pine tree.

Practical Uses

Purifying; removes lymphatic deposits from the body, helps in the reduction of cellulite

Vapors open the sinus and breathing passages

Mood uplifting; refreshing, reviving, improves mental clarity, alertness, and memory

Lessens pain

Stimulates the adrenal glands; promotes vitality

Disinfectant

Documented Properties

Analgesic, antibacterial, antifungal, antineuralgic, antiphlogistic, antirheumatic, antiscorbutic, antiseptic (strong), antispasmodic, antitussive, antiviral, balsamic, cholagogue, choleretic, decongestant, deodorant, depurative (kidneys), disinfectant, diuretic, expectorant, hypertensor, insecticide, laxative, pectoral, refreshing, restorative, reviving, rubefacient, stimulant (circulatory and nervous systems; adrenal glands), sudorific, tonic, vermifuge, vulnerary

Aromatherapy Methods of Use

Application, aroma lamp, bath, diffusor, inhaler, lightbulb ring, massage, mist spray, steam inhalation, steam room and sauna

Caution: Pine oil has a strong diuretic effect on the kidneys. Use small amounts with care. People with dry or sensitive skin may require additional carrier oil when applying the essential oil topically.

RAMBIAZANA (*Rambiaze*)

Botanical Name: *Helichrysum gymnocephalum*

Family: *Asteraceae*

The essential oil is obtained from the whole plant.

History and Information

- Rambiazina is native to Madagascar and is found in high altitudes. The shrub grows to a height of about 4–12 feet (1.5–3.5 meters) and has large leaves. The genus consists of six hundred species of plants.

- The whole plant was used to alleviate discomfort in the urinary tract and help with incontinence.

- A footbath was made with the leaves to help with menstrual problems.

- In Africa, the roots are used to soothe coughs.

- In Madagascar, the leaf tea is used for liver difficulties, wounds, fevers, colds, coughs, congestion, muscle and joint aches, skin problems, and insect bites.

- The leaves, dried flowers and seeds are smoked in a pipe. The leaves are used for head colds, and the flowers and seeds for lung conditions. A poultice made from the leaves is applied for gout and joint pain.

- The plant is helpful for chest congestion and has been used for gingivitis, as well as for skin care.

Practical Uses

Cooling

Opens the sinus and breathing passages; deepens the breathing

Promotes alertness

Documented Properties

Antibacterial, antimicrobial, antiviral, astringent, diuretic

Aromatherapy Methods of Use

Application, bath, diffusor, inhaler, massage, mist spray, steam inhalation, steam room and sauna

RAVENSARA ANISATA
(Havozo Bark)

Botanical Name: *Cinnamonum camphora, Ravensara anisata*

Family: *Lauraceae*

The essential oil is obtained from the bark.

History and Information

- Ravensara is native to Madagascar and is found in high mountainous altitudes and dense forests. The tree grows to a height of about 60 feet (18 meters), has an anise-scented bark, shiny aromatic green leaves, and green flowers followed by fleshy aromatic fruits. There are eighteen species of the tree. It is also known as ravintsara, avozo, havozomamy, and morindrano.

- In Madagascar, the dried leaves are made into a syrup for coughs and breathing congestion. The leaves are brewed into a tea for colds, flu, headaches, and digestive upsets. The dried fruits are taken as a stimulant.

- The seeds, leaves, and bark taste like cloves and are used as a spice known as Madagascar clove

nutmeg. The bark is used in making an alcoholic rum drink.

- Havozo essential oil is highly valued in cosmetics, perfumes, and for flavorings.

Practical Uses

Warming

Soothes the intestines

Calming, reduces stress; promotes a restful sleep

Vapors open the sinus and breathing passages

Mood uplifting, aphrodisiac, euphoric; improves mental clarity; encourages communication

Loosens tight muscles, relieves aches, pains, and menstrual discomfort

Documented Properties

Antifungal, antiseptic, antispasmodic, carminative, cholagogue, choleretic, emmenagogue, estrogenic, galactagogue, stomachic, tonic

Aromatherapy Methods of Use

Application, aroma lamp, bath, diffusor, inhaler, lightbulb ring, massage, mist spray, steam inhalation, steam room and sauna

RAVENSARA AROMATICA

Botanical Name: *Cinnamonum camphora, Ravensara aromatica*

Family: *Lauraceae*

The essential oil is obtained from the leaves.

History and Information

See Ravensara Anisata

Practical Uses

Calming, reduces stress

Vapors open the sinus and breathing passages; deepens the breathing

Mood uplifting; refreshing, improves mental clarity

Relieves aches and pains

Documented Properties

Analgesic, antibacterial, antiseptic, antispasmodic, antitoxic, antitussive, antiviral, carminative, cholagogue, choleretic, expectorant, febrifuge, sedative, tonic

Aromatherapy Methods of Use

Application, aroma lamp, bath, diffusor, inhaler, lightbulb ring, massage, mist spray, steam inhalation, steam room and sauna

RED BERRY *(Pepper Tree)*

Botanical Name: *Schinus molle, Schinus terebinthifolius*

Family: *Anacardiaceae*

The essential oil and CO_2 extract are obtained from the berries.

History and Information

- Pepper tree is an evergreen native to South America. The small tree grows to a height of about 12–30 feet (3.5–9 meters) with drooping branches, narrow, spiky, long leaves, and small yellow or white flowers. The fruits, when ripe, are soft and red and have a peppery aroma and taste. The tree is also known as peppercorn tree, Brazilian mastic tree, mastic tree, pili pili, and castilla.

- The bark, leaves, fruit, seeds, and resin are all used in various forms throughout the world in herbal medicine to treat bronchitis, cataracts, gingivitis, gout, rheumatism, swellings, ulcers, and wounds.

- In Latin American countries, the leaves are used for flavoring food and brewing an alcoholic drink, and the fruit as pepper. The white sap is chewed as a gum in South America.

- In Africa, pepper tree leaf extract and essential oil are used for colds, respiratory problems, sore joints, and rheumatism.

- In Mexico, a syrup is made with the berries for chest congestion.

- The gum from the tree trunk, known as Jesuits'

balm, is said to be a purgative; it also has healing properties for the skin.

- The leaves are chewed to heal ulcers of the mouth.

- The berries are added to foods, beverages, vinegar, and wine as a flavor ingredient.

- The seeds are used to adulterate pepper.

Practical Uses

Warming; increases circulation

Balancing; reduces tension

Helps to breathe easier

Refreshing, stimulating, energizing, improves mental clarity

Loosens tight muscles, penetrating and soothing; helps to relieve discomfort

Documented Properties

Antibacterial, antifungal, antirheumatic, antiseptic, antispasmodic, antiviral, astringent, balsamic, diuretic, emmenagogue, purgative, stimulant, tonic, vulnerary

Aromatherapy Methods of Use

Application, aroma lamp, diffusor, inhaler, lightbulb ring, massage, mist spray, steam inhalation, steam room and sauna

RHODODENDRON

Botanical Name: *Rhododendron anthopogon*

Family: *Ericaceae*

The essential oil is obtained from the leaves and flowers.

History and Information

- Rhododendron is native to the Northern Hemisphere. The aromatic plant grows to a height of about 2 feet (.5 meter), has glossy leaves and white or pink flowers. The plant belongs to a species of 850 trees and shrubs.

- In Russia, a tea made from the leaves is said to improve circulation and heart function.

Practical Uses

Calming, reduces stress

Vapors help open the sinus and breathing passages

Mood uplifting; improves mental clarity, mentally energizing

Documented Properties

Antibacterial, antioxidant, cardiotonic

Aromatherapy Methods of Use

Application, aroma lamp, bath, diffusor, inhaler, lightbulb ring, massage, mist spray, steam inhalation

ROSALINA *(Lavender Tea Tree)*

Botanical Name: *Melaleuca ericifolia*

Family: *Myrtaceae*

The essential oil is obtained from the leaves and branches.

History and Information

- Rosalina is an evergreen shrub native to Australia. The shrub grows to a height of about 15–30 feet (4.5–9 meters), has a papery white bark, narrow grey-green leaves, and white or yellow-white flowers.

Practical Uses

Calming, relaxing, reduces stress and tension

Vapors open the sinus and breathing passages; deepens the breathing

Mood uplifting; improves mental clarity

Documented Properties

Antibacterial, anticonvulsant, antifungal, carminative, decongestant, immunostimulant, sedative

Aromatherapy Methods of Use

Application, aroma lamp, bath, diffusor, inhaler, lightbulb ring, massage, mist spray, steam inhalation, steam room and sauna

ROSE

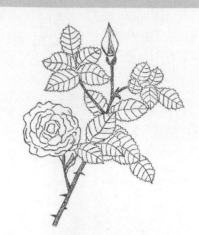

Botanical Name:
Rosa centifolia,
Rosa damascena

Family: *Rosaceae*

The absolute and essential oil are obtained from the flowers.

History and Information

- Rose is native to the Mediterranean area. The different varieties of bushes grow to various heights and produce sweet, fragrant flowers.

- Roses have been used throughout history for their appearance, scent, and therapeutic properties. The oil was considered more precious and valuable than gold.

- Hippocrates recommended rose flowers mixed with oil for uterine problems.

- Ayurvedic practitioners used rose petals for skin wounds, inflammations, and as a laxative.

- The Romans greatly favored the rose and introduced its use to all the people they conquered.

- The Persians were thought to have originated the distillation of rose oil before the Christian era.

- The fragrance symbolizes the love and beauty that was offered to the kings and gods. Cleopatra strewed red rose pedals to a height of 18 inches (45 centimeters) when she first met Mark Anthony.

- The Persians, Greeks, and Romans bathed their bodies in rose fragrance and used the perfume lavishly during religious ceremonies, burials, and sacrifices.

- Wines and drinks were fragranced with roses by the Persians, Romans, and British.

- Arabic doctors were the first to use rose as a remedy in the form of a jam, while Arabian women used rose as an ingredient in their eye cosmetics.

- American Indians healed mouth sores, fever sores, and blisters with rose. A tea was made from the flowers to strengthen the heart, soothe coughs and sore throats, and for stomach and liver disorders.

- The most expensive oil is damask rose, which comes from Bulgaria.

Practical Uses

Cooling

Purifying

Calming, reduces stress

Mood uplifting, aphrodisiac; calms emotional shock and grief

Lessens aches, pains, and inflammation

Balances the female hormonal and reproductive system

Regenerates the skin cells; especially beneficial for dry, sensitive, inflamed, red, aging skin

Fragrancing

Documented Properties

Antibacterial, antidepressant, anti-inflammatory, antiphlogistic, antiseptic, antispasmodic, antistress, antiviral, aperient, aphrodisiac, astringent (mild), calmative, carminative, cephalic, cholagogue, choleretic, cicatrizant, cytophylactic, depurative, digestive, diuretic, emmenagogue, emollient, hemostatic, hepatic, laxative, nervine, nutritive, pectoral, regenerator (skin cells), sedative, stimulant (circulatory system), stomachic, tonic (nerves), tonifying, uplifting

Aromatherapy Methods of Use

Application, aroma lamp, bath, fragrancing, inhaler, lightbulb ring, massage, mist spray

ROSEMARY

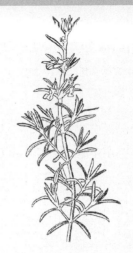

Botanical Name:
Rosmarinus officinalis

Family: *Lamiaceae*

The essential oil is obtained from the flowers and leaves.

The CO_2 extract is obtained from the leaves.

History and Information

- Rosemary is an evergreen shrub native to the Mediterranean region. The bushy plant grows to a height of about 2–6 feet (.5–2 meters), has needle-shaped leathery leaves and blue flowers. The entire plant is aromatic.

- Rosemary has long been a symbol of love, loyalty, and eternity. The plant also became known as a symbol of remembrance. Brides wore rosemary wreaths and carried rosemary bouquets to show that they would always remember their families. During funerals, mourners threw fresh rosemary into the grave to signify that the dead would not be forgotten.

- The ancients honored their gods by decorating the statues with the aromatic plant. They also planted rosemary around tombs.

- In ancient Greece, students wore the sprigs of rosemary in their hair and around their neck while they studied to strengthen their memory.

- Dioscorides, the Greek physician, recommended a tea made from rosemary as a remedy for jaundice.

- The Arabians claimed rosemary helped the brain and memory.

- Rosemary oil was one of the first essential oils to be distilled, in the year 1330.

- In the Middle Ages, the plant was burned to fumigate sickrooms to protect against rampant diseases, and as incense for funeral services. Rosemary was also used in the judicial courts to prevent the spread of jail fever.

- In the sixteenth century, wealthy families hired perfumers to fragrance their homes with rosemary incense.

- During the plague of 1665, the herb was carried along in the handles of walking sticks and pouches so the vapors could be inhaled when traveling through infected areas.

- From the 1800s until 1950, rosemary was listed in the United States Pharmacopoeia.

- Rosemary oil was recommended by many apothecaries to prevent baldness.

- Gypsies valued the herb for its beneficial effect on the hair and skin.

- During World War II, a mixture of rosemary leaves and juniper berries was burned in the hospitals in France to kill germs.

- The Europeans combine rosemary with white wine as a remedy for poor circulation.

- The plant yields 0.5 to 1.5 percent essential oil, which is used in cosmetics, soaps, perfumes, deodorants, and hair tonics.

Practical Uses

Warming; improves circulation

Improves digestion

Purifying; removes cellulite and lymphatic deposits out of the body

Vapors open the sinus and breathing passages; deepens the breathing

Mood uplifting to people who tend to have a slower metabolism; stimulates the nerves, metabolism, and all other body functions; refreshing, improves mental clarity, alertness, and the memory

Relieves aches and pains

Disinfectant

Repels insects

Documented Properties

Analgesic, antibacterial, antidepressant, antifungal, antineuralgic, antioxidant, antirheumatic, antiseptic, antispasmodic, antitoxic, antitussive, antiviral, aphrodisiac, astringent, carminative, cephalic, cholagogue, choleretic, cicatrizant, cordial, cytophylactic, decongestant (liver), detoxifier, diaphoretic, digestive, diuretic, emmenagogue, expectorant, hepatic, hypertensor, insecticide (strong), invigorating, laxative, nervine, parasiticide, pectoral, rejuvenator (skin cells), resolvent, reviving, rubefacient, stimulant (adrenal glands and nerves), stomachic, sudorific, tonic, vulnerary, warming

Aromatherapy Method of Use

Application, aroma lamp, bath, diffusor, inhaler, lightbulb ring, massage, mist spray, steam inhalation, steam room and sauna

Caution: Use small amounts. Rosemary oil should be avoided by people prone to epileptic seizures.

RUE

Botanical Name: *Ruta graveolens*

Family: *Rutaceae*

The essential oil is obtained from the plant.

History and Information

- Rue is an evergreen plant native to the Mediterranean region. The plant grows to about 3 feet (1 meter) high, has aromatic leaves and greenish-yellow flowers.

- The Greeks used rue as the main ingredient in a poison antidote.

- The early Romans recognized rue as a helpful remedy for more than eighty complaints.

- During the first century A.D., Pliny, the Roman herbalist, reported that rue helped improve eyesight.

- Herbalists in the sixteenth and seventeenth centuries suggested rue as an antidote for snakebites.

- According to the American Indians, the plant assisted in promoting fertility.

- Rue was used to expel poisons from the body from snakebites and poisonous insects.

- The herb was used for headaches and to ease menstrual discomfort; topically it was applied for skin injuries, poisonous snakebites, and stings from insects. The leaves and seeds were taken for tumors.

- In Africa, the leaves are used to lower fevers.

- Rue oil is an ingredient in beverages, baked goods, dairy, and other food products.

Practical Uses

Lessens pain

Documented Properties

Abortifacient, anthelmintic, antidote, antiseptic, antispasmodic, antitoxic, antitumor, antitussive, antiviral, aperitive, carminative, cephalic, cholagogue, detoxifier, digestive, diuretic, emetic, emmenagogue, expectorant, febrifuge, insecticide, nervine, rubefacient, sedative, stimulant (digestive system), stomachic, tonic, vasodilator, vermifuge

Caution: Rue oil is toxic, and is not used in aromatherapy.

SAFFRON

Botanical Name: *Crocus sativus*

Family: *Iridaceae*

The essential oil is obtained from the dried stigma.

History and Information

- Saffron is native to the Mediterranean. The plant grows to a height of about 1 foot (.5 meter), has grasslike leaves and fragrant purple flowers.

- Saffron has been known to be used since 1600 B.C.

- Saffron was added to cinnamon and cassia to anoint the Egyptian pharaohs.

- During ancient times, the plant symbolized beauty and youth, and was presented to newlyweds.

- Roman women colored their hair blonde with dye from the flowers. The Greeks and Romans used saffron to perfume their homes, public buildings, and baths.

- In the fourteenth through the eighteenth centuries, saffron was widely used in Europe as a spice and remedy for women's ailments.

- In Chinese medicine, saffron is used to alleviate mental depression and menstrual discomfort.

- The flowers are used as a yellow dye and the oil is an ingredient in expensive perfumes. Saffron is considered the most expensive spice today. To produce one pound of the spice, 35,000–40,000 flowers are required.

Documented Properties

Analgesic, antineuralgic, antispasmodic, aphrodisiac, diaphoretic, emmenagogue, expectorant, febrifuge, hepatic, hypotensor, nervine, sedative, stimulant

Aromatherapy Methods of Use

Fragrancing

Caution: Saffron contains toxic components that act on the nervous system; it can also damage the kidneys.

SAGE

SAGE *(Spanish)*

Botanical Name: *Salvia lavandulifolia* (Spanish sage), *Salvia officinalis* (Sage)

Family: *Lamiaceae*

The essential oil is obtained from the flowers and leaves.

The CO_2 extract is obtained from the leaves.

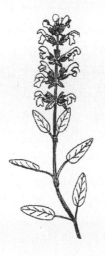

History and Information

- Sage is an evergreen plant native to the Mediterranean region. The plant grows to a height of about 2.5 feet (.5 meter), has aromatic greyish-green leaves and small light-blue to purple flowers.

- Spanish sage is an evergreen plant native to Spain. The plant grows to a height of about 2.5 feet (.5 meter) and has small purple flowers. There are about five hundred different varieties of sage.

- Ancient Egyptian women who were unable to bear children were given sage leaves to help them become pregnant. The herb was also used as a tonic for the brain.

- The Romans called sage, *herba sacra,* which means "sacred herb." The Romans and Greeks used sage for snakebites, to invigorate the mind and body, and promote longevity. According to Hippocrates, sage helped women become fertile.

- Sage was included among the herbs Emperor Charlemagne ordered to be grown in his imperial gardens.

- In the Middle Ages, sage was used for constipation, cholera, colds, fever, liver troubles, and epilepsy.

- The Chinese traded three times the amount of their best tea for the Dutch's European sage.

- In the early 1800s, the freshly crushed leaves were used to remove warts.

- Sage was associated with wisdom and consumed regularly with the belief that it made one wise and strengthened the memory.

- The herb was taken to regulate blood sugar, improve appetite, and help with confusion and dizziness.

- Mothers took the herb to wean the baby off nursing, since sage dries up breast milk.

- The American Indians used a salve from the leaves to heal skin sores.

- Many Swiss peasants and Bedouin Arabs rub sage leaves over their teeth to keep them clean and free of yellow film and stains.

- In Europe, sage has been used by women to regulate their menstrual cycle.

- In Latin America, the leaves are rubbed on insect bites to soothe the skin.

- Sage leaves yield 1.5 to 2.5 percent essential oil, which is used for its spicy flavor in foods, as well as to fragrance perfumes and personal care products.

Practical Uses

Improves circulation

Improves digestion

Purifying; helps in the reduction of cellulite

Reduces stress

Improves alertness

Relaxes sore muscles, lessens aches, pains, and menstrual pain; used for general weakness

Suppresses perspiration

Suppresses lactation

Documented Properties

Antibacterial, antidepressant, antidiabetic, antifungal, antigalactagogue, anti-inflammatory, antioxidant, antirheumatic, antiseptic, antispasmodic, antisudorific, antiviral, aperitif, aperitive, astringent, blood purifier, carminative, cholagogue, cicatrizant, depurative, digestive, disinfectant (strong), diuretic, emmenagogue, estrogenic, euphoriant, expectorant, febrifuge, healing, hemostatic (bleeding gums), hepatic, hypertensor, insect repellent, laxative, nervine, stimulant (brain, circulatory system, adrenal glands), stomachic, tonic (digestive system), vermifuge, vulnerary, warming

Aromatherapy Methods of Use

Application, aroma lamp, bath, diffusor, inhaler, lightbulb ring, massage, mist spray

Caution: Sage oil contains a toxic component called thujone, which can interfere with brain and nervous system functions. Spanish sage is less toxic and safer to use. Both common sage and Spanish sage should be avoided by people prone to epileptic seizures.

SANDALWOOD
SANDALWOOD (Australian)

Botanical Name: *Santalum album* (Sandalwood), *Santalum spicatum* (Australian sandalwood)

Family: *Santalaceae*

The essential oil is obtained from the inner wood.

History and Information

- Sandalwood is an evergreen tree native to Asia. The tree grows to a height of about 30 feet (9 meters), has small purple flowers and small fruits containing a seed. There are ten species of sandalwood trees.

- Australian sandalwood is an evergreen tree native to Australia. The tree grows to a height of about 18 feet (5.5 meters).

- Sandalwood has been used throughout history in medicine, perfumery, cosmetics, and incense. Since ancient times, sandalwood has been very sacred to the people of India, who used the wood to make furniture, caskets, and canes. Temples were built with the wood because of its fragrant scent and insect-resistant property.

- Today, the Indian government owns all the sandalwood trees grown in India to keep them from extinction. Government inspectors allow the extraction of the oil only after the tree has turned thirty years old and grown 30 feet (9 meters) in height.

- The oil is used extensively in Oriental funeral ceremonies and religious rites.

- Sandalwood is used as a fixative in perfumes, soaps, lotions, detergents, and is burned as incense. It is also used to flavor foods, candies, beverages, baked goods, and liqueurs.

- The roots and wood yield about 6 percent oil, while the leaves and shoots yield about 4 percent oil.

Practical Uses

Calming, relaxing, reduces stress; promotes a restful sleep

Encourages dreaming; helpful for meditation

Soothing to the breathing passages

Mood uplifting, aphrodisiac, euphoric; brings out emotions

Healing and moisturizing to the skin

A fixative to hold the scent of a fragrance

Documented Properties

Analgesic, antibacterial, antidepressant, antifungal, anti-inflammatory, antiphlogistic, antipruritic, antiseptic, antispasmodic, antistress, antiviral, aphrodisiac, astringent, calmative, carminative, cicatrizant, decongestant, deodorant, diaphoretic, diuretic, emollient, euphoriant, expectorant, febrifuge, fixative, healing (skin), insect repellent, relaxant, sedative, stimulant, stomachic, tonic

Aromatherapy Methods of Use

Application, aroma lamp, bath, inhaler, massage, mist spray, steam inhalation, steam room and sauna

SANTOLINA (Lavender Cotton)

Botanical Name: *Lavandula taemina, Santolina chamaecyparissus*

Family: *Asteraceae*

The essential oil is obtained from the seeds.

History and Information

- Santolina is an evergreen plant native to Italy. The plant grows to a height of about 2 feet (.5 meter), has silver-grey leaves and yellow daisylike flowers. The entire plant is fragrant. Santolina is a member of the daisy family and is not related to lavender, even though it is referred to as lavender cotton.

- Pliny, the Roman herbalist, recommended santolina for snakebites.

- During medieval times, santolina was used to promote menstruation, purify the kidneys, and for worms and jaundice.

- The plant was used as an air freshener in the Mediterranean area.

Documented Properties

Anthelmintic, antifungal, antiphlogistic, antiseptic, antispasmodic, antitoxic, diuretic, emmenagogue, hepatic, insect repellent, parasiticide, refreshing, stimulant, stomachic, tonic, vermifuge, vulnerary

Aromatherapy Methods of Use

Fragrancing

Caution: Santolina oil is toxic.

SASSAFRAS

Botanical Name:
Sassafras albidum,
Sassafras officinale

Family: *Lauraceae*

The essential oil is obtained from the bark.

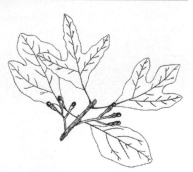

History and Information

- Sassafras is native to North America. The tree grows to a height of about 65–125 feet (20–38 meters), has green leaves, and clusters of small yellow flowers that develop into egg-shaped, dark-blue berries. The tree's powerful roots can penetrate rocks.

- Native American Indians made the leaves in soups.

- The bark was used as a folk remedy for stomachaches, gout, muscle and joint aches, colds, fevers, and to reduce lactation; the oil also helped warm muscles, and kill lice.

- Sassafras is added to flavor toothpastes, mouthwashes, root beer, chewing gum, and tobacco products, and to fragrance perfumes, candles, and soaps. The oil is also used as an antiseptic in dentistry.

- The bark contains approximately 7 percent essential oil.

- The young leaves are eaten in salads.

Practical Uses

Purifying, helps in the reduction of cellulite

Loosens tight muscles, relieves aches, pains, and inflammations

Stimulates the liver

Documented Properties

Alterative, antidote, antigalactagogue, antispasmodic, blood purifier, carminative, depurative, diaphoretic, digestive, diuretic, emmenagogue, febrifuge, hypotensor, insect repellent, stimulant (mild), tonic, warming

Caution: Sassafras oil is toxic.

SAVORY

Botanical Name: *Calamintha montana, Satureja montana, Satureja obovata* (Winter savory); *Calamintha hortensis, Satureja hortensis* (Summer savory)

Family: *Lamiaceae*

The essential oil is obtained from the plant.

History and Information

- Savory is native to Europe and Asia. The plant grows to a height of about 1 foot (.5 meter), has small aromatic greyish leaves that turn purple (in late summer) and white, pink, or violet flowers. There are thirty species of savory.

- The Egyptians and Romans used savory as an aphrodisiac in love potions. The Roman men mixed the herb with melted beeswax and made it into a massage lotion to help entice unromantic women (Hurley, Judith Benn. *The Good Herb.* William Morrow Company, 1995. p. 250).

- During medieval times, the plants were strewn throughout households to freshen the air.

- Savory was used in medications to treat mouth and throat ulcers.

- Herbalists recommended savory for insect stings and to aid digestion
- The leaves yield 1 percent essential oil.

Practical Uses

Heating; improves circulation, induces perspiration

Improves digestion

Purifying, removes cellulite, waste material and excessive fluids from the body

Vapors open the sinus and breathing passages

Loosen tight muscles, relieves pain

Soothes insect bites

Repels insects and kills lice

Documented Properties

Analgesic, antibacterial, antifungal, antiputrid, antiseptic, antispasmodic, antiviral, aperitive, aphrodisiac, astringent, carminative, cicatrizant, digestive, disinfectant, emmenagogue, expectorant, irritant (skin), parasiticide, resolvent, revitalizing, rubefacient, stimulant (circulatory, digestive, and nervous systems; adrenal glands), tonic, vermifuge

Aromatherapy Methods of Use

Application, aroma lamp, lightbulb ring, inhaler, massage, mist spray

Caution: People with dry or sensitive skin may require additional carrier oil when applying savory essential oil topically. Use small amounts.

SCHISANDRA

Botanical Name: *Kadsura chinensis, Schisandra chinensis, Schisandra japonica, Schisandra sphenanthera*

Family: *Schisandraceae*

The CO_2 extract is obtained from the berries.

History and Information

- Schisandra is native to Asia. The woody vine grows to 25 feet (7.5 meters) and has white, yellow, or pink fragrant flowers, followed by bunches of red berries with two seeds inside. The vine is also known as bay star vine, magnolia vine, and wu wei zi (Chinese).
- The healing value of schisandra was mentioned during the Han dynasty in China, 25–200 A.D. The plant was also used in Russia and Japan for many centuries. China, Russia, and Japan listed the herb in their pharmacopeias. The berries were helpful to treat breathing conditions, muscle and joint aches, diarrhea, kidney complaints, and to promote a restful sleep. It was also said to improve stamina, relieve fatigue, increase mental clarity, improve memory, and as a stress reducer.
- In China, the berries are used for blood-sugar problems, to help sleep, reduce frequent urination, ease coughs and breathing problems, reduce stress, and for night sweats, dehydration, endurance, and as a tonic to strengthen the body.
- In some areas, the leaves are cooked as a vegetable and the fruit is eaten fresh or made into jam. The flesh of the fruit is sour, while the skin is sweet.
- The CO_2 extract is used for stressed and overly sensitive skin.

Practical Uses

Warming

Calming, reduces stress, relieves tension; promotes a restful sleep

Helps to breathe easier

Mood uplifting; improves mental clarity

Healing to the skin

Documented Properties

Adaptogen, antibacterial, anticonvulsive, antidepressant, antidiabetic, anti-inflammatory, antimutagenic, antioxidant, antitussive, aphrodisiac, astringent, cardiotonic, digestive, emmenagogue, expectorant, hepatic, nervine, rejuvenator, relaxant, restorative, sedative, tonic (brain, immune and nervous system)

Aromatherapy Methods of Use

Application, inhaler, massage, mist spray

SPEARMINT

Botanical Name: *Mentha spicata, Mentha viridis*

Family: *Lamiaceae*

The essential oil is obtained from the leaves and flowering tops.

History and Information

- Spearmint is native to the Mediterranean region. The plant grows to a height of about 1–3 feet (.5–1 meter), has shiny green leaves, and white or lilac-colored flowers.

- Spearmint has been used for centuries by Egyptian, Greek, and Roman physicians. The Romans wore mint wreaths in their hair during banquets and decorated their tables with the twigs.

- Hippocrates mentioned mint for its diuretic and stimulant properties.

- Pliny, the Roman herbalist, mentioned spearmint in forty-one different potions. Specifically, he recommended its use as a restorative to vitalize the body and aid digestion.

- Spearmint leaves were strewn on the streets by the Romans to congratulate triumphant gladiators.

- Galen, the Greek physician, considered mint to be an aphrodisiac.

- During the Middle Ages, powdered mint leaves were used to heal mouth sores, animal and insect bites, whiten teeth, repel mice and rats, and prevent milk from curdling.

- The American Indians used the leaves to aid digestion, relieve headaches, fevers, sore throats, and diarrhea.

- Spearmint is renowned for its use to help overcome frigidity in both males and females. It is given to bulls and stallions to encourage sexual interest.

- It is said that the fresh leaves have a high content of vitamin C and more vitamin A than carrots.

Practical Uses

Cooling

Improves digestion, soothes the intestines, relieves flatulence, freshens the breath and the intestines; increases appetite

Stimulates and strengthens the nerves

Vapors open the sinus and breathing passages; deepens the breathing

Mood uplifting, aphrodisiac; refreshing, reviving, stimulates the metabolism, increases physical strength and endurance, improves mental clarity, alertness, and the memory, sharpens the senses; encourages communication

Relieves aches, pains, inflammation, and menstrual pain

Repels insects

Soothes itching skin

Documented Properties

Analgesic, antidepressant, antigalactagogue, antipruritic, antiseptic, antispasmodic, antitoxic, aperitive, aphrodisiac, astringent, carminative, cephalic, cholagogue, decongestant, diaphoretic, digestive, diuretic, emmenagogue, expectorant, febrifuge, hepatic, insecticide, nervine, refreshing, refrigerant, restorative, reviving, stimulant (nervous and digestive systems), stomachic, tonic

Aromatherapy Methods of Use

Application, aroma lamp, bath, diffusor, inhaler, lightbulb ring, massage, mist spray, steam inhalation, steam room and sauna

Caution: People with dry or sensitive skin may require additional carrier oil when applying spearmint essential oil topically. Use small amounts. Avoid using before bedtime since the oil can overstimulate the nervous system.

SPIKENARD

Botanical Name: *Nardostachys grandiflora, Nardostachys jatamansi*

Family: *Valerianaceae*

The essential oil is obtained from the roots.

History and Information

- Spikenard is native to the Himalaya Mountains and Asia. The aromatic plant grows to a height of about 2 feet (.5 meter) and has pink bell-shaped flowers. Spikenard is also known as musk root.

- Ancient people used the roots for nervous disorders.

- The herb was highly prized by the Romans as a perfume.

- In Ayurvedic medicine, the roots are taken for liver, ulcer, and skin conditions. It is said to facilitate childbirth and darken the color of hair and promote its growth.

- In India, the roots are used for sleeping sickness, hysteria, and convulsions.

- In the Middle East, the root tea is used for heart and nervous conditions.

- Spikenard oil is also referred to as nard oil. The properties of the oil are similar to valerian.

Practical Uses

Calming, relaxing, reduces stress; promotes a restful sleep

Mood uplifting

Reduces inflammation

A fixative to hold the scent of a fragrance

Documented Properties

Analgesic, anthelmintic, antibacterial, anticonvulsant, antifungal, anti-inflammatory, antioxidant, antiseptic, antispasmodic, aperitif, calmative, cardiotonic, carminative, deodorant, depurative, digestive, diuretic, emmenagogue, febrifuge, hepatic, laxative, nervine, sedative, tonic, tranquilizer

Aromatherapy Methods of Use

Application, aroma lamp, bath, inhaler, lightbulb ring, massage, mist spray

SPRUCE (Black)
SPRUCE (Sitka)
SPRUCE (White)
SPRUCE-HEMLOCK

Botanical Name: *Picea mariana* (Black spruce), *Picea sitchensis* (Sitka spruce), *Tsuga canadensis* (Spruce-hemlock and White spruce)

Family: *Pinaceae*

The essential oil is obtained from the bark and branches.

History and Information

- Spruce is an evergreen tree native to North America. Black spruce grows to a height of about 70–200 feet (9 meters), has blue-green needlelike leaves, red flowers, and male and female cones.

- Sitka spruce reaches 115–150 feet (35–45.5 meters).

- White spruce grows to a height of about 150 feet (45.5 meters), has shallow roots and can be easily blown over by strong winds. The tree has light-brown seed cones and red pollen cones.

- Spruce-hemlock grows to about 80 feet (24 meters).

- There are approximately fifty species in the spruce tree family. It is estimated that the trees can live to an age of 1,200 years.

- The American Indians heated the twigs in steam baths to induce sweating for relief of rheumatism, colds, and coughs, and applied the bark and twigs externally to stop bleeding wounds. They also made beer by boiling the spruce twigs and cones in maple syrup. A tea from the bark was taken for colds, painful joints, and as a laxative; a poultice applied to reduce inflammations; and a leaf tea to soothe breathing congestion.

- The resin that exudes from the branches of the black spruce is made into chewing gum. Spruce beer is produced by boiling the branches in water.

- The wood is used for the sounding boards in pianos and for the bodies of violins.

Practical Uses

Calming, reduces stress

Vapors open the sinus and breathing passages; deepens the breathing

Mood uplifting, euphoric; improves mental clarity; brings out inner feelings, encourages communication

Disinfectant

Documented Properties

Anti-inflammatory, antiseptic, antispasmodic, antitussive, astringent, diaphoretic, diuretic, expectorant, hemostatic, nervine, parasiticide, rubefacient, sedative, tonic, vulnerary, warming

Aromatherapy Methods of Use

Application, aroma lamp, bath, diffusor, inhaler, lightbulb ring, massage, mist spray, steam inhalation, steam room and sauna

ST. JOHN'S WORT

Botanical Name: *Hypericum perforatum*

Family: *Guttiferae*

The essential oil and CO_2 extract are obtained from the blossoms.

History and Information

- St. John's Wort is native to Europe, Asia, and Africa. The plant grows to a height of about 1–3 feet (.5–1 meter) and has star-shaped yellow flowers. When the flowers are pinched, the petals turn red.

- The Greeks and Romans used the herb as a remedy for wounds, sores, burns, bruises, inflammations, coughs, sleeplessness, melancholy, nervous exhaustion, menstrual problems, and to lower fevers.

- In the Middle Ages, St. John's Wort was frequently applied to heal wounds, and taken for depression, despair, and nerve problems. It was also widely believed to ward off evil spirits and demonic possession.

- The American Indians made a tea from the plant to help respiratory problems. The root was used internally and also applied externally on snakebites.

- Herbalists used St. John's Wort to heal nerve damage, reduce pain and inflammation, and for sleep, anxiety, depression, nervous problems, fevers, digestive discomfort, and suppressed menstruation.

- An infusion of the fresh flowers, called hypericum oil, was used to heal skin problems. It was sold in pharmacies in the early twentieth century.

- In Europe, a leaf extract is applied topically to stimulate hair growth and for wounds and skin abrasions. The leaf tea is taken for menstrual cramps, to neutralize poisonous bites, and rid the body of intestinal parasites. The fresh leaves are eaten to help calm the nerves and improve sleep. A flower infusion is applied to heal skin tissue.

Practical Uses

Cooling

Soothes the intestines

Calming, reduces stress

Helps to breathe easier

Mood uplifting, euphoric; improves mental clarity

Relieves aches, pains, and menstrual discomfort

Documented Properties

Abortifacient, alterative, analgesic, antibacterial, antidepressant, antifungal, anti-inflammatory, antiseptic, antispasmodic (menstrual cramps), antiviral, astringent, blood purifier, calmative, carminative, diuretic, emmenagogue, euphoric, expectorant, febrifuge, hemostatic, nervine, sedative, stomachic, tonic (nervous system), tranquilizer, vermifuge, vulnerary

Aromatherapy Methods of Use

Application, aroma lamp, bath, diffusor, inhaler, light-bulb ring, massage, mist spray

Caution: St. John's Wort is phototoxic. Avoid exposure to direct sunlight for several hours after applying the essential oil on the skin.

STYRAX *(American)*

STYRAX *(Asian)*

Botanical Name: *Balsam styracis, Liquidambar orientalis* (Asian styrax), *Liquidambar styraciflua* (American styrax)

Family: *Hamamelidaceae*

The resin, absolute, and essential oil are obtained from the inner bark.

History and Information

- Liquidambar styraciflua is native to America. The tree grows to a height of about 75–150 feet (23–45.5 meters), has glossy, five-pointed, star-shaped leaves and small yellow-green flowers that develop into brown fruit. The styrax resin is secreted under the bark and is referred to as storax. The tree is also known as sweet gum, red gum, and alligator tree.

- Styrax gum is also derived from the Liquidambar orientalis tree, which is native to Asia. The tree grows to a height of about 25–40 feet (7.5–12 meters), thrives in warm, hilly locations, and has clusters of male yellow flowers and greenish female flowers that develop into fruit. The gum is also known as Turkish sweet gum.

- Both trees are also known as liquidambar and storax.

- The American pioneers made an ointment from the balsam to relieve hemorrhoids, ringworm, and scalp and skin infections. The bark and leaves were used for diarrhea.

- The American Indians made a preparation of styrax to relieve fevers, inflammations, heal wounds, and for skin itch.

- Guatemala and Honduras are the main suppliers of styrax. It is used to flavor soft drinks, tobacco, candy, chewing gum; to fragrance perfumes, soaps, cosmetics; and as an incense. The tree is grown for its timber for furniture making.

Practical Uses

Helps break down cellulite, removes lymphatic deposits

Calming

Mood uplifting

Reduces inflammation

A fixative to hold the scent of a fragrance

Documented Properties

Antibacterial, anti-inflammatory, antiseptic, antispasmodic, antitussive, astringent, balsamic, diaphoretic, diuretic, expectorant, nervine, stimulant

Aromatherapy Methods of Use

Application, massage

TAGETES

Botanical Name: *Tagetes erecta, Tagetes minuta, Tagetes patula*

Family: *Asteraceae*

The essential oil is obtained from the plant.

History and Information

- Tagetes is native to America. The plant grows to a height of about 1–3 feet (.5–1 meter) and produces many flowers. The colors of the flowers on the different varieties of tagetes are yellow, orange, and reddish brown. The plant is also known as French marigold and African marigold.

- The Aztecs used the flowers to lower blood pressure, reduce inflammation, and calm the nerves.

- In China, the plant is used for coughs, colds, sores, and ulcers.

- Tagetes is added to chicken feed to give a yellow coloring to the skin of the chicken and the egg yolk.

- The oil is used in perfumery, cosmetics, and for food flavorings.

Practical Uses

Disinfectant

Healing to the skin

Documented Properties

Anthelmintic, antibacterial, antifungal, anti-inflammatory, antiphlogistic, antiseptic, antispasmodic, carminative, cytophylactic, decongestant, diaphoretic, dilator, emmenagogue, emollient, hypotensor, insect repellent, insecticide, parasiticide, sedative, stomachic, tranquilizer

Aromatherapy Methods of Use

Application, aroma lamp, lightbulb ring, massage, mist spray

Caution: People with dry or sensitive skin may require additional carrier oil when using tagetes essential oil topically. Use small amounts. Avoid exposure to direct sunlight for several hours after applying the oil on the skin.

TANA

Botanical Name: *Rhus taratana*

Family: *Anacardiaceae*

The essential oil is obtained from the whole plant.

History and Information

- Tana is a tree native to Africa that grows to a height of about 45–50 feet (13.5–15 meters) and has small flowers.

- Tana has been reported to be helpful for stomach problems, bad breath, and low energy.

Practical Uses

Cooling

Opens the sinus and breathing passages

Relaxing, reduces stress

Mood uplifting; refreshing, promotes alertness, helps to focus and concentrate, increases mental energy

Aromatherapy Methods of Use

Application, aroma lamp, bath, diffusor, inhaler, lightbulb ring, massage, mist spray

TANGELO

See Orange

TANGERINE

See Mandarin

TANSY

Botanical Name: *Tanacetum vulgare*

Family: *Asteraceae*

The essential oil is obtained from the whole plant.

History and Information

- Tansy is native to Europe. The plant grows to about 1–5 feet (.5–1.5 meters) high and has clusters of aromatic yellow flowers.

- The dried flowers and herb were used in the past for fever, muscle and joint pain, and to get rid of intestinal parasites.

Documented Properties

Abortificent, anthelmintic (mild), anti-inflammatory, antimicrobial, carminative, diaphoretic, digestive, emmenagogue, febrifuge, nervine, stimulant, tonic, vermifuge

Caution: Tansy oil contains a high concentration of the toxic component thujone, which can interfere with the brain and nervous system functions. The oil is not recommended for use in aromatherapy. The variety of *Tanacetum annuum* known as blue tansy is used in aromatherapy and is said by some people to be safe.

TARRAGON *(Estragon)*

Botanical Name: *Artemisia dracunculus*

Family: *Asteraceae*

The essential oil is obtained from the plant.

History and Information

- Tarragon is native to Russia. The shrubby plant grows to a height of about 2–3 feet (.5 meter) and has light-green flowers.

- Pliny, the Roman herbalist, claimed the herb prevented fatigue.

- In the Middle Ages, sprigs of tarragon were placed in the shoes before beginning long trips on foot in order to prevent tired feet.

- During the thirteenth century, tarragon was used by herbalists to sweeten the breath and promote sleep.

- The American Indians made a tea from the plant for diarrhea, colds, headaches, and difficult childbirths.

- The roots resemble a serpent and were, therefore, used as a treatment for snakebites.

- The plant yields 0.5 to 1 percent essential oil. Tarragon is used in perfumes, soaps, cosmetics, and to flavor foods and liqueurs.

Practical Uses

Improves mental clarity and alertness

Relieves aches, pains, and menstrual pain

Documented Properties

Analgesic, anthelmintic, antifungal, anti-inflammatory, antioxidant, antirheumatic, antiseptic, antispasmodic, antiviral, aperitive, carminative, cholagogue, digestive, diuretic, emmenagogue, hepatic, hypnotic, laxative, parasiticide, stimulant (circulatory system), stomachic, tonic, vermifuge

Aromatherapy Methods of Use

Application, aroma lamp, bath, diffusor, inhaler, lightbulb ring, massage, mist spray

Caution: Use in small amounts.

TEA TREE

Botanical Name: *Melaleuca alternifolia, Melaleuca linariifolia, Melaleuca uncinata*

Family: *Myrtaceae*

The essential oil is obtained from the leaves and twigs.

History and Information

- Tea tree is an evergreen tree native to Australia and is found in wet lowland locations.

- Melaleuca alternifolia grows to a height of about 10–25 feet (3–7.5 meters), has a papery white bark, dark-green needlelike leaves and purple, yellow, or white flowers.

- Melaleuca linariifolia grows to about 20–35 feet (6–10.5 meters) high, has papery bark, narrow leaves, and white flowers. The tree is also known as narrow-leaved paperbark and snow storm.

- Melaleuca uncinata grows to a height of about 10 feet (3 meters), has papery bark, needlelike leaves, and brush-like yellow flowers. The tree is also known as broom brush.

- Tea tree belongs to a family of approximately two hundred species of evergreen trees.

- Tea tree was discovered during the expedition of Captain Cook in 1770. The crew members brewed a tea from the leaves that they enjoyed drinking.

Practical Uses

Vapors open the sinus and breathing passages

Mood uplifting; reviving, improves mental clarity

Relieves pain

Disinfectant

Healing to the skin

Soothes insect bites

Documented Properties

Analgesic, antibacterial, antifungal, anti-inflammatory, antipruritic, antiseptic (strong), antiviral, balsamic, cicatrizant, cordial, decongestant, diaphoretic, expectorant, insecticide, parasiticide, refreshing, revitalizing, stimulant, sudorific, vulnerary

Aromatherapy Methods of Use

Application, aroma lamp, bath, diffusor, inhaler, lightbulb ring, massage, mist spray, steam inhalation, steam room and sauna

Caution: There have been reports of fatalities when a small amount of tea tree essential oil was used on cats.

TEA TREE *(Black)*

Botanical Name: *Melaleuca bracteata, Melaleuca lanceolata, Melaleuca pubescens*

Family: *Myrtaceae*

The essential oil is obtained from the leaves and branches.

History and Information

- Black tea tree is an evergreen tree native to Australia and is found along banks of creeks and rivers. The tree grows to a height of about 25 feet (7.5 meters), has a black trunk, pointed narrow leaves, and fluffy white flowers.

- Melaleuca bracteata is also known as river tea tree and white cloud.

- Melaleuca lanceolata is also known as moonah.

Practical Uses

Cooling

Calming, relaxing, reduces stress and tension; promotes a restful sleep

Encourages dreaming

Helps to breathe easier

Mood uplifting, euphoric; improves mental clarity

Documented Properties

Antimicrobial, carminative

Aromatherapy Methods of Use

Application, aroma lamps, bath, diffusor, inhaler, lightbulb ring, massage, mist spray, steam inhalation, steam room and sauna

Caution: There have been reports of fatalities when a small amount of tea tree essential oil was used on cats.

TEA TREE *(Lemon)*
TEA TREE *(Lemon-Scented)*

Botanical Name: *Leptospermum citratum, Leptospermum petersonii* (Lemon-scented tea tree), *Leptospermum liversidgei* (Lemon tea tree)

Family: *Myrtaceae*

The essential oil is obtained from the leaves and stems.

History and Information

- Lemon-scented tea tree is an evergreen shrub native to Australia, where it is found along creeks on the edge of the wet forest. The shrub grows to a height of about 12–20 feet (3.5–6 meters), has lanceolate, lemon-scented, light-green leaves and white or pink flowers.

- Leptospermum liversidgei is native to Australia, and is found in low-lying sandy, swampy soil. The shrub grows to a height of about 3–10 feet (1–3 meters), has narrow green leaves that are strongly lemon scented and small white or pink flowers. The tree is also known as swamp may.

Practical Uses

Warming

Improves digestion

Calming, reduces stress and tension, relaxes the nerves

Helpful for meditation

Vapors help open the sinus and breathing passages

Mood uplifting, euphoric; refreshing, improves mental clarity and alertness

Loosens tight muscles, relieves pain

Documented Properties

Antibacterial, antifungal, anti-inflammatory, antiseptic, antiviral, carminative, expectorant, sedative

Aromatherapy Methods of Use

Application, aroma lamp, bath, diffusor, inhaler, lightbulb ring, massage, mist spray, steam inhalation, steam room and sauna

TEA TREE *(Prickly Leaf)*

Botanical Name: *Melaleuca squamophloia*

Family: *Myrtaceae*

The essential oil is obtained from the leaves.

Practical Uses

Warming

Calming

Helps to breathe easier

Euphoric, aphrodisiac; improves mental clarity

Loosens tight muscles

Aromatherapy Methods of Use

Application, aroma lamp, bath, diffusor, inhaler, lightbulb ring, massage, mist spray, steam inhalation, steam room and sauna

Caution: There have been reports of fatalities when a small amount of tea tree essential oil was used on cats.

TEMPLE ORANGE

See Orange

TEREBINTH

Botanical Name: *Pinus maritimus, Pinus palustris, Pistacia terebinthus,* and other *Pinus species*

Family: *Anacardiaceae* (Pistacia species) and *Pinaceae* (Pinus species)

The essential oil is obtained from the sap of the tree bark.

History and Information

- Terebinth is native to the Mediterranean region. The resin is extracted from a large variety of trees, including Pistacia terebinthus and various pine trees. Pinus palustris reaches a height of about one hundred feet (30.5 meters), has green needlelike leaves, and brownish-red cones that contain seeds. Pistacia terebinthus grows to about 15 feet (4.5 meters) tall.

- The people of the Near East chewed terebinth to strengthen their teeth and gums.

- Terebinth was used as a treatment to get rid of lice, as an expectorant for breathing congestion, and made into an ointment for a chest rub.

- In Africa, the seeds are applied topically on tumors.

- In the Middle East, the gum is used to freshen the breath, and the resin is used on tumors.

Practical Uses

Vapors open the sinus and breathing passages

Refreshing, reviving, improves mental clarity

Lessens aches and pains

Disinfectant

Repels insects

Documented Properties

Analgesic, antidote, anti-inflammatory, antipruritic, antirheumatic, antiseptic, antispasmodic, antitussive, aphrodisiac, astringent, balsamic, carminative, cicatrizant, counterirritant, digestive, diuretic, emmenagogue, expectorant, febrifuge, healing, hemostatic, insecticide, laxative, parasiticide, rubefacient, sedative, stimulant, stomachic, tonic, vermifuge, vulnerary

Aromatherapy Methods of Use

Application, aroma lamp, bath, diffusor, inhaler, lightbulb ring, massage, mist spray, steam inhalation, steam room and sauna

THUJA *(Cedar Leaf)*

Botanical Name: *Thuja occidentalis*

Family: *Cupressaceae*

The essential oil is obtained from the leaves, bark, and twigs.

History and Information

- Thuja is an evergreen tree native to China and North America. The tree grows to a height of about 65 feet (20 meters), has dark-green leaves and cones. Thuja is also known as arbor vitae or northern white cedar.

- The Egyptians made coffins from the wood and used the oil for embalming.

- Native American Indians used thuja to remedy menstrual discomforts, headaches, fever, coughs, colds, breathing and heart problems. The twigs were also made into a tea for muscle and joint pain.

- Thuja was listed in the United States Pharmacopia in the nineteenth century.

Documented Properties

Abortifacient, anthelmintic, antirheumatic, antiseptic, antiviral, astringent, cicatrizant, counterirritant, diuretic, emmenagogue, expectorant, hemostatic, hypotensor, insect repellent, parasiticide (skin), rubefacient, stimulant (nerves; uterine), sudorific, tonic, vermifuge

Comments: The oil is approved for use in food, provided its toxic component, thujone, is removed.

Caution: Thuja oil is toxic due to the high content of thujone, which can interfere with brain and nervous system functions. It is not recommended for use in aromatherapy.

THYME

Botanical Name: *Thymus aestivus, Thymus citriodorus, Thymus ilerdensis, Thymus satureiodes, Thymus valentianus, Thymus vulgaris, Thymus vulgaris var. linalol, Thymus webbianus*

Family: *Lamiaceae*

The essential oil is obtained from the leaves and flowering tops.

The CO_2 extract is obtained from the leaves.

History and Information

- Thyme is an evergreen plant native to the Mediterranean region. The plant grows to a height of about 1 foot (.5 meter), has small leaves and pink or pale lilac-colored flowers. There are over one hundred varieties of thyme.

- The thymus gland was named after the botanical name thymus, because the gland's appearance resembled the thyme flower.

- Since ancient times, thyme has been used in Egypt, Greece, and Rome. The Greeks used thyme for nervous conditions and to invigorate the senses. Thyme was burned to repel insects and to preserve meats. The Roman soldiers would bathe in water with thyme added to gain vigor and courage. Thyme was associated with courage well into the Middle Ages.

- The Roman physician, Pliny the Elder, used thyme to treat melancholy and epilepsy.

- Herbalists of the Middle Ages recommended thyme for melancholy, epilepsy, nightmares, to help urination problems, strengthen the lungs, improve digestion, for coughs, muscle and joint discomforts, and female problems. The leaves were used to relieve toothaches.

- From the fifteenth to the seventeenth century, when the plague devastated the people of Europe, thyme was used as a germicide. Members of the nobility carried posies of aromatic herbs, including thyme, to protect themselves from the germs of the public.

- In World War I, thymol, derived from thyme, was used as an antiseptic to treat the wounds of the soldiers. In addition, thymol was used to purify the air in hospitals and sickrooms.

- Bees are attracted to thyme, and the honey they produce has been a longtime favorite in Europe.

- In Germany, thyme preparations are applied to clear chest congestion.

- The herb yields approximately 1 percent essential oil. The oil is extensively used in perfumery, cosmetics, liqueurs, and to flavor foods.

Practical Uses

Heating; increases circulation, induces perspiration

Improves digestion, cleanses the intestines

Purifying; removes cellulite, waste material and excessive fluids from the body

Relaxes the nerves

Vapors open the sinus and breathing passages

Mood uplifting; improves mental clarity and alertness, sharpens the senses

Stimulates the thyroid gland, increases physical endurance and energy

Loosens tight muscles, relieves aches, pains, inflammation, and spasms

Disinfectant

Repels insects and kills lice

Documented Properties

Analgesic, anthelmintic, antibacterial, antidepressant, antifungal, anti-inflammatory, antioxidant, antipruritic, antiputrid, antirheumatic, antiseptic (strong), antispasmodic, antitoxic, antitussive, antivenomous, antiviral, aperitif, aphrodisiac, astringent, balsamic, bronchodilator, cardiac, carminative, cicatrizant, counterirritant, cytophylactic, diaphoretic, digestive, diuretic, emmenagogue, expectorant, hypertensor,

insecticide, nervine, parasiticide, pectoral, rubefacient, sedative, stimulant, stomachic, sudorific, tonic, uplifting, vermifuge, warming

Aromatherapy Methods of Use

Application, aroma lamp, bath (only the linalol variety), diffusor, inhaler, lightbulb ring, massage, mist spray, steam inhalation

Comments: The varieties of lemon-scented thyme (*Thymus citriodorus*), *Thymus satureiodes,* and *Thymus linalol* (*Thymus vulgaris var. linalol*) are gentler and less irritating to the skin than common thyme.

Caution: People with dry or sensitive skin may require additional carrier oil when applying thyme essential oil topically. Use small amounts. Thyme should be avoided by people prone to epileptic seizures.

TOBACCO LEAF

Botanical Name: *Nicotiana tabacum*

Family: *Solanaceae*

The absolute and CO_2 extract are obtained from the leaves.

History and Information

- Tobacco is a flowering perennial plant native to the Americas and West Indies. The plant thrives in rich, moist soil and reaches a height of about 3–15 feet (1–4.5 meters). Depending on the variety, the flowers are pink, green, or white, and emit their fragrant scent after dark. There are nearly one hundred species of Nicotiana.

- In Europe, tobacco was used for joint pains, headaches, and for the plague.

- The American Indians were the first to grow and smoke tobacco. They believed the plant possessed medicinal properties and burned the leaves as incense during their ceremonies. Tobacco was used to ease childbirth delivery, relieve headaches and snake and insect bites, and as a parasite expeller.

- The genus Nicotiana was named in honor of Jean Nicot, a French ambassador to Portugal, who played a significant role in influencing the spread of tobacco use in Europe.

Practical Uses

Calms hysteria

Dulls the senses

Aphrodisiac

Documented Properties

Diuretic, emetic, laxative

Aromatherapy Methods of Use

Application

Caution: Tobacco leaf oil is toxic.

TOLU BALSAM

Botanical Name: *Myroxylon balsamum, Myroxylon toluiferum*

Family: *Fabaceae*

The resin and essential oil are obtained from the bark.

History and Information

- Tolu is an evergreen tree native to Central and South America. The tree grows to a maximum height of about 120 feet (36.5 meters), has glossy leaves and small, white, fragrant flowers that develop into fruits. The resin is obtained by making an incision in the tree.

- The use of tolu balsam dates back to the 1500s, when it was added to cough medicines for its expectorant effect.

- The sap has been valued to for its ability to help with headaches, colds, breathing problems, muscle and joint aches, sprains, skin infections, and wounds.

- Tolu balsam is used to flavor foods and soft drinks and to fragrance perfumes and soaps. Some of the

trees are grown for timber. The wood, resembling mahogany, is hard and strong, and used for making furniture.

Practical Uses

Mood uplifting

Deodorant

A fixative to hold the scent of a fragrance

Documented Properties

Antiseptic, expectorant, fixative

Aromatherapy Methods of Use

Application, massage, mist spray

TONKA BEAN
(Tonquin Bean)

Botanical Name: *Baryosma tongo, Coumarouna odorata, Dipteryx odorata*

Family: *Fabaceae*

The absolute and essential oil are obtained from the beans.

History and Information

- Tonka is native to South America. The tree grows to a height of about 100 feet (30.5 meters) and has red fragrant flowers, followed by yellow fruits that contain a few strongly fragrant black seeds called tonka beans. The fragrance of the beans intensifies during the drying process. The bark and the wood are odorless.

- Tonka bean is used for flavoring foods and as a vanilla substitute in perfumery. In Europe, an insecticide product is made from the beans.

- Tonka bean is used for the manufacture of coumarin, which is used by the perfume industry, and to flavor tobacco products. As synthetic coumarin began to be produced, the demand lessened for tonka bean.

Practical Uses

Calming

Mood uplifting

Fragrancing

A fixative to hold the scent of a fragrance

Documented Properties

Insecticide

Aromatherapy Methods of Use

Application, aroma lamp, fragrancing, lightbulb ring, mist spray

Caution: Tonka bean oil is toxic.

TUBEROSE

Botanical Name: *Polianthes tuberosa*

Family: *Agavaceae*

The absolute and essential oil are obtained from the flowers.

History and Information

- Tuberose is native to Asia and Central America. The plant grows to a height of about 4 feet (1.5 meters) and produces strongly fragrant white flowers that bloom in the summer. There are thirteen species of tuberose that belong to the agave family.

- Tuberose has long been a symbol of seductiveness. Early writers warned young girls to avoid smelling the fragrance of the flowers because the scent would make them vulnerable. The Malays called the fragrance "Mistress of the Night" because its scent intensifies after sunset.

Practical Uses

Fragrancing

Documented Properties

Nervine, uplifting

Aromatherapy Methods of Use

Aroma lamp, fragrancing, lightbulb ring

TURMERIC

Botanical Name:
Amomum curcuma,
Curcuma domestica,
Curcuma longa

Family: *Zingiberaceae*

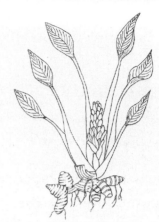

The essential oil and CO_2 extract are obtained from the roots.

History and Information

- Turmeric is native to Asia. The plant grows to a height of about 3 feet (1 meter) and has yellow flowers. The root is bright-orange with a thin brownish skin. The rhizomes provide the spice. Turmeric belongs to the same family as ginger and is also known as Indian saffron.

- Turmeric has been used as a spice and dye since biblical times.

- The plant was called Indian saffron during the Middle Ages because of its orange-yellow color. The dye is used to color cosmetics, foods, confectionary, fabrics, and paper.

- In folk medicine, turmeric was taken to strengthen the liver.

- In Chinese and Ayurvedic medicine, turmeric root has been used to stimulate circulation, improve digestion, lower blood pressure, ease menstrual problems, and relieve aches, pains, and inflammation.

- In Asia, a tea made from the rhizome is consumed to regulate blood sugar, as a tonic to the body, for liver conditions, urinary problems, stomach disorders, to promote menstruation, as a contraceptive, and to abort a fetus. It is also used to heal wounds and insect bites. The leaves are topically applied to reduce fevers.

- In Africa, the rhizome is used as a tonic, to aid digestion, and as a laxative.

- In Arabic countries, a tea is made from the rhizome to abort a fetus.

- Turmeric is added to Oriental-type perfumes, used to flavor food products, and is an ingredient in curry powder and various mustards.

Practical Uses

Warming; increases circulation

Calming, relaxing, reduces stress; promotes a restful sleep

Mood uplifting; improves mental clarity

Documented Properties

Abortifacient, analgesic, anthelmintic, antiarthritic, antibacterial, antidiabetic, antigalactagogue, anti-inflammatory, antioxidant (strong), antirheumatic, aphrodisiac, carminative, cholagogue, expectorant, digestive, diuretic, hepatic, hypotensive, insecticidal, laxative, rubefacient, stimulant

Aromatherapy Methods of Use

Application, massage, mist spray

Caution: Use small amounts.

VALERIAN

Botanical Name: *Valeriana officinalis*

Family: *Valerianaceae*

The essential oil and CO_2 extract are obtained from the roots.

History and Information

- Valerian is native to Europe and Asia. The plant grows to a height of about 4–5 feet (1–1.5 meters) and has clusters of fragrant small pink or white flowers. Valerian is also known as "all-heal."

- Since ancient times, valerian has been used as a medicinal herb in the treatment of epilepsy and as a calmative for nervous disorders and hysteria.

- American Indian warriors used valerian as an antiseptic for wounds.

- The oil is used in cosmetics, perfumery, and as a food flavoring. The herb is a leading over-the-counter tranquilizer in Europe.

Practical Uses

Calming; promotes a restful sleep

Relieves pain

Documented Properties

Analgesic, antibacterial, anticonvulsive, antidepressant, antidiuretic, antipyretic, antispasmodic, carminative, diuretic, febrifuge, hepatic, hypotensor, nervine, sedative (strong), stomachic, tonic (strong) (nerves), tranquilizer, vermifuge

Aromatherapy Methods of Use

Application, aroma lamp, inhaler, massage, mist spray

Caution: Due to the relaxing effect of the oil, valerian should not be used before driving or doing anything that requires full attention. Use small amounts.

VANILLA

Botanical Name:
Vanilla fragrans,
Vanilla planifolia

Family: *Orchidaceae*

The absolute is obtained from the unripe pods.

The CO_2 extract is obtained from the pods.

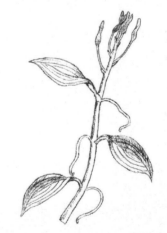

History and Information

- Vanilla is native to Mexico and Central America. The climbing plant reaches a height of about 12 feet (3.5 meters) and has clusters of green-yellow flowers that develop into aromatic brown seed pods with small seeds inside.

- In Mexico, vanilla was added to foods to enhance their flavor during the time of the Aztecs. The

Spaniards, learning that the Aztecs of Mexico flavored cocoa with vanilla, introduced its use into Europe.

- In Africa, healers used vanilla for stomach problems.

- European physicians used vanilla during the sixteenth and seventeenth centuries as an antidote for poisoning, stomach complaints, and as an aphrodisiac.

- Vanilla has been taken for congestion, muscle and joint pain, to relieve stress and anxiety, uplift the mood, and for better sleep.

- Vanilla is an ingredient in soaps, skin lotions, body and hair care products, massage oils, incense, baked goods, ice cream, and flavorings. Most perfumes contain vanilla.

Practical Uses

Calming, reduces stress; promotes a restful sleep

Encourages dreaming

Mood uplifting, aphrodisiac

Fragrancing

A fixative to hold the scent of a fragrance

Documented Properties

Antispasmodic, aphrodisiac, balsamic, calmative, emmenagogue, febrifuge

Aromatherapy Methods of Use

Application, aroma lamp, bath, fragrancing, inhaler, lightbulb ring, massage, mist spray

VETIVER

Botanical Name: *Andropogon muricatus, Vetiveria zizanoides*

Family: *Poaceae*

The essential oil is obtained from the roots.

History and Information

- Vetiver is native to Asia. The tropical grass grows to a height of about 4–8 feet (1–2.5 meters), has sharp edged leaves, tiny flowers, and aromatic roots. Since the strong roots reach deep below the soil it is often planted to protect steep hillsides and other areas vulnerable to soil erosion.

- In Asia, the grass has been smoked, the root used for tumors, and the oil for nausea and cholera.

- In India, the plant is known as khas. It is hung over windows and placed into clothing to repel insects. Vetiver is also used as a food flavoring.

- In Ayurvedic medicine, the roots are used for bad breath and fevers.

- In Latin America, the root tea is taken for digestive problems, headaches, muscle and joint aches, nerve pains, flu, and fevers.

- In Russia, the oil is placed in sachets and sewn into the linings of fur coats to protect against damage caused by moths.

- Vetiver oil is used extensively as a fixative in perfumery.

- The roots yield a small amount of oil; therefore, it is often adulterated with synthetics. In the 1970s, vetiver oil was restricted in many countries because of problems with adulteration.

Practical Uses

Improves digestion

Calms nervousness, relieves stress and tension; promotes a restful sleep

Mood uplifting

Strengthens the body

Loosens tight muscles, relieves pain

Repels insects

Healing to the skin

A fixative to hold the scent of a fragrance

Documented Properties

Abortifacient, analgesic, anthelmintic, antibacterial, anti-inflammatory, antiseptic, antispasmodic, anti-stress, aphrodisiac, astringent, calmative, cardiotonic, carminative, detoxifier, diaphoretic, diuretic, emetic, emmenagogue, insect repellent, insecticide, nervine, parasiticide, revitalizing, rubefacient, sedative, stimulant (immune system), stomachic, tonic, vermifuge

Aromatherapy Methods of Use

Application, aroma lamp, bath, inhaler, lightbulb ring, massage, mist spray

VIOLET

Botanical Name: *Viola odorata*

Family: *Violaceae*

The absolute and essential oil are obtained from the flowers.

History and Information

- Violet is native to Europe and Africa. The plant grows to a height of about 6 inches (20 centimeters), has heart-shaped leaves, and sweetly fragrant dark-violet flowers.

- Pliny, the Roman herbalist, recommended violets to relieve headaches, dizziness, and to calm and induce sleep.

- The Romans and Greeks used violet for beauty and aromatic purposes. They also enjoyed a wine made from the flowers. Roman women added violets to goat's milk and applied the mixture on their face to beautify their complexion. The Greeks regarded violet as the flower of fertility and frequently added it to love potions.

- In the nineteenth century, fragrances made with violets were the most popular in France and England.

- The aroma of violets can cause a temporary loss of smell.

- The flowers can be cooked or eaten raw in salads. In Europe, the flowers are candied and used in confectionery to decorate desserts.

Practical Uses

Calming; promotes a restful sleep

Mood uplifting

Fragrancing

Documented Properties

Analgesic, anti-inflammatory, antirheumatic, antiseptic, antispasmodic, aphrodisiac, calmative, demulcent, diaphoretic, diuretic, emetic, expectorant, febrifuge, hypnotic, laxative, liver decongestant, pectoral, sedative, stimulant (circulatory system), uplifting, vulnerary

Aromatherapy Methods of Use

Application, aroma lamps, bath, fragrancing, inhaler, lightbulb ring, massage, mist spray

VITEX *(Berry)*
VITEX *(Leaf)*

Botanical Name: *Vitex agnus castus*

Family: *Verbenaceae*

The essential oil is obtained from the berries.

The essential oil is obtained from the leaves.

History and Information

- Vitex is native to Africa, Asia, and Europe, where it is found around streams, but can also survive in dry areas. The shrub grows to a height of about 4–20 feet (1–6 meters) and has large, oblong bluish-green leaves. The small fragrant blue or purple flowers develop into brown to black berries with seeds. The berries have a pepperlike aroma and flavor. The tree is known as chaste tree.

- The berries have been used medicinally since about 500 B.C.

- Hippocrates recommended the berries be taken following childbirth and the herb be taken for inflammation.

- Dioscorides, the Greek physician, suggested taking the seeds for swellings.

- Pliny, the Roman physician, wrote that the plant was highly valued. He gave the herb for fevers, headaches, and to normalize menstruation and lactation. Roman women used the herb to reduce sexual drive.

- Vitex has been useful for female conditions, including menstrual cycle regulation, fibroids, and hormonal imbalances.

- The seeds were made into an infused drink to help relieve menstrual discomfort, relieve headaches and fever, and promote the flow of breast milk. The seeds and leaves were used for poisonous snake and spider bites.

- In the Middle East, the herb was taken for sleeping sickness and mental instability.

- In Unani medicine, pregnant women were advised to avoid the herb because of its likelihood to abort a fetus.

- In Asia, a mixture of leaves, fruit, and roots is used for colds, coughs, and bacterial infections. The leaves are smoked for headaches, and the juice from the leaves is taken for respiratory infections.

- In Europe, the seeds flavor foods as a substitute for pepper.

Practical Uses

Cooling

Calming, relaxing, reduces stress, relieves tension, promotes a peaceful state

Vapors open the sinus and breathing passages; deepens the breathing

Improves alertness

Loosens tight muscles, relieves pain and spasms

Balances female hormones, helps regulate menstrual problems

Increases breast milk

Documented Properties

Anaphrodisiac, diaphoretic, diuretic, emmenagogue, febrifuge, galactagogue, sedative, vulnerary

Aromatherapy Methods of Use

Application, bath, inhaler, massage, mist spray, steam inhalation

WINTERGREEN

Botanical Name: *Gaultheria procumbens*

Family: *Ericaceae*

The essential oil is obtained from the leaves.

History and Information

- Wintergreen is native to North America. The plant grows to a height of about 6 inches (15 centimeters), has deep-green, shiny, leathery leaves, and small white flowers that develop into red fruits.

- Native American Indians used the plant for aches, pains, headaches, colds, and stomachaches, and chewed the leaves to improve breathing.

- Early Americans chewed the roots to prevent tooth decay and used the berries as a tonic.

- A poultice made from the leaves was applied to aching, sore muscles and joints and nerve pain in the legs.

- Wintergreen contains high amounts of methyl salicylate, which is similar to salicylic acid in aspirin. Wintergreen yields approximately 0.5 percent essential oil; it is used in toothpaste, chewing gum, root beer, and other soft drinks.

Practical Uses

Warming; improves circulation

Purifying; helps in the reduction of cellulite

Calming, relaxes the nerves, reduces tension and stress; promotes a restful sleep

Mood uplifting

Relieves achy, tense, and sore muscles, reduces inflammation, lessens pain, especially in the joints

Documented Properties

Analgesic, antibacterial, anti-inflammatory, antirheumatic, antiseptic, antispasmodic, antitussive, astringent, carminative, decongestant, diuretic, emmenagogue, expectorant, galactagogue, hemostatic, hypotensor, rubefacient, stimulant, tonic, vulnerary

Comments: Wintergreen oil is often falsified with the synthetic chemical, methyl salicylate.

Caution: Wintergreen oil is toxic and can irritate the skin.

WORMWOOD

Botanical Name: *Artemisia absinthium*

Family: *Asteraceae*

The essential oil is obtained from the leaves and flowering tops.

History and Information

- Wormwood is native to Europe. The plant grows to a height of about 1–4 feet (.5–1 meter), has greyish-green aromatic leaves and clusters of small yellow flowers.

- In ancient times, the herb was favored by women because it helped to bring on the menstrual cycle.

- Wormwood was the main ingredient in an alcoholic drink known as absinthe, which was found to be toxic.

Documented Properties

Abortifacient, anthelmintic, antidote, anti-inflammatory, antipruritic, antiseptic, antispasmodic, aperitive, cardiac, carminative, cholagogue, choleretic, diaphoretic, digestive, disinfectant, diuretic, emmenagogue, febrifuge, hepatic, insect repellent, stimulant (digestive system), stomachic, tonic, vermifuge

Caution: Wormwood oil contains a component called thujone, which interferes with brain and nervous system functions. The oil is toxic and has been known to induce mental impairment.

YARROW

Botanical Name: *Achillea millefolium*

Family: *Asteraceae*

The essential oil is obtained from the flowering plant.

History and Information

- Yarrow is native to Europe and Asia. The plant grows to a height of about 1–3 feet (.5–1 meter) with white, yellow, lilac, or pink flower heads and feathery leaves. The plant is also known as staunch weed and wound wart.

- In ancient China, yarrow was believed to be a sacred plant.

- The American Indians used the root for pain relief, swellings, itching, and insect bites, and the leaves were taken to induce perspiration, reduce fevers, expel worms, clot the blood, and as a diuretic. The entire plant was used to heal burns and bruises, and for earaches.

- Early Americans chewed the leaves to relieve an upset stomach, regulate menstrual flow, for fever, chills, and rashes, and to promote dreaming. An infusion of the leaves was used for colds and a chest rub made from the flowers reduced congestion of the breathing passages.

- Nicholas Culpeper, an herbalist in the seventeenth century, recommended yarrow for wounds and to stop bleeding and inflammation.

- In Nordic countries, the plant was substituted for hops in the production of beer. In Germany, the seeds were used as a preservative in wine.

- Yarrow was listed in the United States Pharmacopoeia in the nineteenth century and was used to promote menstruation.

- In China, the herb is used for animal and snakebites.

- In Latin America, the plant is used for wounds, muscle and joint aches, and as a blood purifier.

- The plant contains proazulene, which, when distilled, produces the anti-inflammatory substance, azulene. Since the essential oil of yarrow is said to contain more azulene than chamomile, it is often added to chamomile to increase its azulene content.

- Yarrow yields 0.5 percent essential oil.

Practical Uses

Calming

Vapors open the sinus and breathing passages

Improves mental clarity

Lessens inflammation

Documented Properties

Abortifacient, analgesic, anthelmintic, anti-inflammatory, antiphlogistic, antiseptic, antispasmodic, aperitive, astringent, blood purifier, carminative, cholagogue, cicatrizant, diaphoretic, digestive, diuretic, emmenagogue, expectorant, febrifuge, healing, hemostatic, hepatic, hypotensor, insect repellent, laxative, stimulant (circulatory system), stomachic, sudorific, tonic, vulnerary (wounds)

Aromatherapy Methods of Use

Application, aroma lamp, bath, inhaler, lightbulb ring, massage, mist spray, steam inhalation, steam room and sauna

YLANG-YLANG

Botanical Name:
*Cananga odorata
var. genuina, Unona
odorantissimum*

Family: *Annonaceae*

The essential oil is obtained from the flowers.

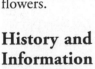

History and Information

- Ylang-ylang is an evergreen tree native to Asia. The tree grows to a height of about 80–100 feet (24–30.5 meters), has glossy leaves and large yellow fragrant flowers that develop into black fruit with many black seeds inside. Ylang-ylang is also known as perfume tree.

- The flowers are handpicked at dawn. If they are bruised, they spoil quickly and turn black.

- The name ylang-ylang in the Malayan language means "flower of flowers."

- In Indonesia, ylang-ylang flowers are placed on the bed of a newlywed couple on their wedding night.

- The leaves are rubbed on the skin to help reduce itching. The tree resin is used for aching muscles and joints and skin problems.

- The first distillation of the essential oil is called ylang-ylang extra and is considered in the industry to be the highest grade. As the distillation continues, the next grades are first, second, and third, in the order of quality. The higher grades are used in perfume formulations.

- Ylang-ylang is an ingredient in cosmetics, soaps, detergents, lotions, and perfumes. It is also extensively used in foods, alcoholic and regular beverages, dairy desserts, baked goods, and candy.

- Ylang-ylang mixed with coconut oil is known as macassar oil.

Practical Uses

Calming, relaxing, reduces stress; promotes a restful sleep

Mood uplifting, euphoric, aphrodisiac; brings out feelings, enhances communication

Loosens tight muscles, lessens pain

Disinfectant

Documented Properties

Antidepressant, antipruritic, antiseptic, aphrodisiac, calmative, carminative, emmenagogue, emollient, euphoriant, fixative, hypotensor, moisturizer, nervine, rejuvenator (skin and hair), relaxant, sedative, stimulant (circulatory system), tonic

Aromatherapy Methods of Use

Application, aroma lamp, bath, diffusor, fragrancing, inhaler, lightbulb ring, massage, mist spray

YUZU

Botanical Name: *Citrus junos*

Family: *Rutaceae*

The essential oil is obtained from the peel.

History and Information

- Yuzu is an evergreen tree native to Asia. The tree grows to a height of about 8–20 feet (2.5–6 meters), has dark-green leaves and white flowers that develop into yellow-orange fruit. Yuzu is a hybrid of bitter orange and citron and is also known as Japanese citron.

- In Japan, the citrus fruit is used to flavor foods and beverages.

- In the Shinto religion, the priests use yuzu during religious ceremonies.

- The essential oil is an ingredient in perfumes, soaps, and cosmetics.

Practical Uses

Purifying; helps in the reduction of cellulite

Reduces stress, tension, and anxiety

Mood uplifting; refreshing, energizing, improves mental clarity

Loosens tight muscles

Documented Properties

Analgesic, antibacterial, antidepressant, antifungal, antineuralgic, antiputrid, antiseptic, antistress, antiviral, calmative, depurative, nervine, sedative, stimulant, tonic

Aromatherapy Methods of Use

Application, aroma lamp, bath, diffusor, inhaler, lightbulb ring, massage, mist spray

Caution: People with dry or sensitive skin may require additional carrier oil when applying yuzu essential oil topically. Use small amounts.

ZANTHOXYLUM

Botanical Name: *Zanthoxylum alatum, Zanthoxylum americanum, Zanthoxylum rhesta*

Family: *Rutaceae*

The essential oil is obtained from the fruit.

History and Information

- Zanthoxylum is native to Asia and North America. The tree grows to a height of about 10–25 feet (3–7.5 meters) and has light-green flowers that develop into small berries. Zanthoxylum belongs to a species of about 250 trees and shrubs; it is in the same family as citrus. It is also known as prickly ash and toothache tree.

- The variety Zanthoxylum americanum is native to North America. The fruits and bark of the tree were used by the American Indians and early settlers to relieve muscle and joint pains, toothaches, and stomach disorders.

- In Africa, the root bark has been used to lessen pain, remove parasites, for wounds, and as an overall tonic.

- The Native American Indians applied a decoction of the roots topically to treat paralysis.

- Prickly ash was listed in the United States Pharmacopoeia in the nineteenth and twentieth centuries.

- The fruits are used for toothaches and to treat dental problems.

Practical Uses

Warming

Reduces stress and nervous tension; promotes a restful sleep

Vapors open the sinus and breathing passages

Mood uplifting, euphoric, aphrodisiac; improves mental clarity

Loosens tight muscles

Documented Properties

Analgesic, anthelmintic, antibacterial, anti-inflammatory, antiseptic, antispasmodic, astrigent, carminative, diaphoretic, disinfectant, emmenagogue, febrifuge, nervine, sedative, stimulant (circulation and immune systems), stomachic, tonic

Aromatherapy Methods of Use

Application, aroma lamp, bath, inhaler, lightbulb ring, massage, mist spray, steam inhalation, sauna and steam room

ZEDOARY

Botanical Name: *Curcuma zedoaria*

Family: *Zingiberaceae*

The essential oil is obtained from the rhizomes.

History and Information

- Zedoary is native to Asia. The plant reaches about 1 foot (.5 meter) high, has green leaves, yellow flowers, and a large rhizome. Zedoary is in the tumeric and ginger family, and is also known as white turmeric and wild turmeric.

- In ancient times, the plant was used in Japan and China to help digestion.

- In Asia, the rhizome and leaves are eaten.

- In China, zedoary is taken for tumors.

- A yellow dye is made from the root.

- The essential oil is used in perfumery.

Practical Uses

Cooling

Improves digestion

Reduces stress, relieves tension

Vapors opens the sinus and breathing passages; deepens the breathing

Mood uplifting, euphoric; energizing, improves mental clarity

Documented Properties

Antiemetic, astringent, carminative, cholagogue, febrifuge, stimulant (circulatory system)

Aromatherapy Methods of Use

Application, aroma lamp, bath, inhaler, lightbulb ring, massage, mist spray, steam inhalation, sauna and steam room

CHAPTER 4

Infused Oils

Infused oils are made from plant materials that are extracted into a carrier oil medium. Since they are already heavily diluted, these oils can be used without adding a carrier oil. This method is usually used for plants that yield a very small amount of essential oil.

The following infused oils are covered in this chapter:

Aloe Vera   Bladderwrack *(Seaweed)*

Aloe Vera Butter   Mullein

Arnica   Usnea Lichen

ALOE VERA

ALOE VERA BUTTER

Botanical Name: *Aloe barbadensis, Aloe vera*

Family: *Liliaceae*

The oil and butter are obtained from the leaves.

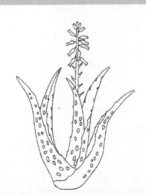

History and Information

- Aloe vera is native to Africa. The plant grows to a height of about 5 feet (1.5 meters), has swordlike leaves and orange-red flowers. There are 300 varieties of aloe, however, only a few are suitable for herbal medicine.

- The Arabs were thought to have been the first to master the art of pressing the juice from the plant, which was done with their bare feet.

- Clay tablets in Mesopotamia reveal the use of aloe vera in 1750 B.C.

- The Egyptian Ebers Papyrus from 1550 B.C. described the use of aloe vera for burns, skin ulcers, and infections.

- The Greeks, credited with the early research of aloe in 25 A.D., were already using it to regulate the bowels.

- In the first century, the Greek physician Dioscorides suggested that aloe vera be used to heal skin problems.

- The Greeks and Romans used aloe for wound healing.

- Alexander the Great and Aristotle were known to have enjoyed aloe's soothing and healing effects. It is said that Aristotle asked Alexander the Great to conquer the African island of Socotra in order to obtain a supply of aloe.

- Cleopatra used the gel of the aloe as a cosmetic and skin moisturizer. It is said that aloe vera was one of the main ingredients in her secret beauty cream.

- Aloe juice has been used to cleanse the intestines and lower fevers.

- In Mexican folk medicine, two tablespoons of aloe gel are taken to relieve stiff joints.

- In Africa, aloe is utilized as a purgative for internal systems and to eliminate strong body odors.

- In Asia, aloe is applied on the scalp to stimulate hair growth. Internally it is taken for colon inflammations.

- In the Amazon region, aloe juice is used for inflammation and toothaches. The mucilage is used to stop hair from falling out, soothe an irritated throat, ease coughs, and for gall bladder problems.

- In the United States, aloe is well known for its healing properties of skin tissue.

- A tea made from the plant is taken to regulate blood sugar levels, help menstrual problems, as a contraceptive, laxative, and to improve skin conditions.

Practical Uses

Soothing to the digestion

Lessens pain

Healing, moisturizing, and rejuvenating to the skin

Makes the hair more manageable, hydrates dry hair

Documented Properties

Abortifacient, analgesic, anthelmintic, antiaging, antibacterial, anti-inflammatory, antioxidant, antipruritic, antiseptic, antitumor, aphrodisiac, calmative, cholagogue, decongestant, demulcent, deodorant, depurative, digestive, emmenagogue, emollient, hypotensor, immunostimulant, insecticide, larvicide, laxative, moisturizer, purgative, regenerator (damaged tissues), stimulant (blood circulation), stomachic, tonic, vermifuge, vulnerary

Aromatherapy Methods of Use

Application, massage

Comments: Aloe vera is excellent for healing tissues of any kind.

ARNICA

Botanical Name:
Arnica montana

Family: *Asteraceae*

The infused oil and CO_2 extract are obtained from the flowers.

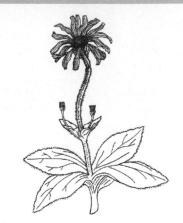

History and Information

- Arnica is native to Europe. The plant grows to a height of about 2 feet (.5 meter) and has daisylike yellow flowers.

- From the early 1800s to 1960, arnica was officially listed in the United States Pharmacopoeia for its ability to reduce pain and swelling.

- The oil is used to soothe muscle aches, sprains, and heal bruises and wounds. It was said to help promote the growth of hair when applied to the scalp.

Practical Uses

Lessens pain

Helps injured skin tissue heal faster, as well as wounds and black and blue bruises

Documented Properties

Analgesic, anti-inflammatory, antiseptic, antispasmodic, cardiac, counterirritant, diaphoretic, diuretic, emollient, expectorant, febrifuge, healing (sprains, dislocations, fractures), hypertensor, rubefacient, stimulant (circulatory system), tonic, vulnerary

Aromatherapy Methods of Use

Application

Caution: Arnica is not recommended to be used on an open cut or wound; use only on unbroken skin. The oil is toxic.

BLADDERWRACK *(Seaweed)*

Botanical Name:
Fucus vesiculosus

Family: *Fucaceae*

The infused oil is obtained from the seaweed plant.

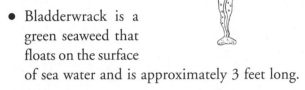

History and Information

- Bladderwrack is a green seaweed that floats on the surface of sea water and is approximately 3 feet long.

- Sea vegetables were perhaps the first sign of life on our planet.

- In ancient Chinese writings, seaweed was used for water retention, abscesses, and to reduce tumors.

- Tribesmen of the south seas used the herb for skin, stomach problems, and inflammations.

- In 1750, a jelly made from the plant was rubbed on the body to reduce obesity. Also in the eighteenth century, a British physician prescribed bladderwrack as a treatment for goiter, an enlargement of the thyroid gland.

- The extraction of iodine from kelp (derived from bladderwrack) was discovered by Professor Courtois in 1812 and used by overweight people who previously had been unsuccessful in reducing weight by other methods.

- In 1862, Dr. Duchesne-Dupart found that while treating patients with skin problems, bladderwrack not only improved the skin, but there was also a reduction in the person's weight.

- In 1867, a French physician named Bonnardiere coined the term thalassotherapy from the Greek word meaning "therapy from the sea." The therapy involves the use of various seaweeds added to the diet, in addition to bathing and being massaged with extracts from plants found in the sea. Thalassotherapy has been part of the European tradition for centuries with impressive results. Besides helping overweight individuals lose weight, the seaweeds produce other beneficial effects. Studies in Japan have shown improvement in goiters, high blood pressure, joint problems, and nervous disorders, and an increase in longevity for those who consume the sea vegetables regularly.

- Scientists at McGill University in Canada, found that after sea vegetables are eaten, they combine with radioactive strontium inside the body and help remove this harmful substance. This research was conducted in the 1960s and 1970s and was published in the *Canadian Medical Association Journal.*

- Sea vegetables provide an abundant source of all the minerals contained in sea water and a high concentration of iodine, which is necessary for the proper functioning of the thyroid gland to produce its hormone, thyroxin. Seaweeds are consumed daily by millions of people in Asia and parts of Europe.

Practical Uses

Stimulates the metabolism and the thyroid gland; improves circulation

Reduces cellulite and obesity

Encourages dreaming

Documented Properties

Alterative, antisclerotic, depurative, diuretic, emollient, hemostatic, laxative, stimulant (circulatory system; combats fatigue), tonic (immune system), rejuvenator (wrinkles and sagging skin, conditions the hair and leaves it silky looking)

Aromatherapy Methods of Use

Application, massage

MULLEIN

Botanical Name: *Verbascum thapsus*

Family: *Scrophulariaceae*

The infused oil is obtained from the flowers.

History and Information

- The infused flower oil has traditionally been used as ear drops for earaches, providing the ear drum is not punctured.

See Mullein in Chapter 3, page 143.

Practical Uses

Ear oil (Infused oil only)

Inflammation

Documented Properties

Anti-inflammatory, antiviral, expectorant

Aromatherapy Methods of Use

Application

USNEA LICHEN

Botanical Name: *Usnea barbata*

Family: *Usneaceae*

The infused CO_2 extract is obtained from lichen.

History and Information

- Usnea is a combination of algae and fungus and is also known as tree moss and beard moss.

- Usnea has been used throughout the world for infections and to enhance immune system function, help with breathing congestion, urinary tract problems, and kidney conditions.

- Usnea is used for infectious inflammatory conditions, sores, wounds, and to help stomach problems.

- Usnea lichen CO_2 extract is added to personal care products for its antimicrobial activity. It has been proven effective against various organisms.

- Lichens are a source of a red dye.

Practical Uses

Helps to breathe easier

Calming, reduces stress, relieves tension

Mood uplifting

Loosens tight muscles

Documented Properties

Analgesic, antibacterial, antifungal, anti-inflammatory, antimicrobial, astringent, deodorizer, product preservative

Aromatherapy Methods of Use

Application, massage

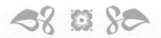

CHAPTER 5

Methods of Application, Dispersion, and Inhalation of Essential Oils

APPLICATION

The self-application method is used when another person isn't available to give a massage or when a massage is not necessary. The oils should be rubbed into the skin until they are fully absorbed. Then a small amount of cornstarch can be applied over the area so that the skin does not remain greasy.

AROMA LAMP

An aroma lamp has a small container that is heated after water and essential oils are added. When the water becomes hot, the aromatic vapors are dispersed into the air.

BATHS

The combination of a warm bath with essential oils can serve as a delightful therapeutic measure to either relax and calm or invigorate and refresh the body. An aromatherapy bath can be so pleasurable that it can become an anticipated and planned-for event.

Instructions: Close the bathroom door and window(s) to keep the essential oil vapors from escaping out of the room. Play soft music that you enjoy listening to. Fill the bathtub with water as warm as you like. Mix the essential oils in a carrier oil, and add the blend to the water when the tub is full. Swirl the water to distribute the oils evenly throughout the tub and enter the bath immediately.

DIFFUSORS

Diffusors disperse a mist of microparticles of essential oil, which creates an aromatic atmosphere for the indoors. There are different types of diffusors on the market. You can choose a smaller or larger unit depending on the size of the area to be fragranced.

INHALERS

This method is handy for quick results.

Instructions: Mix the essential oils in a small glass bottle and tighten the cap.

To use: Open the bottle and slowly inhale the vapors deeply, fifteen to twenty times. Cap the bottle immediately after use.

LIGHTBULB RING

A lightbulb ring is placed on the top of a cool lightbulb, and the essential oils are placed into the groove. When the light is turned on, the heated bulb disperses the aromatic vapors into the air.

MASSAGE

An aromatherapy massage can provide a means of counteracting the pressures of daily life. Only after receiving a massage do we realize how tight our muscles have been and the high amounts of tension stored in our bodies. Some people think of a massage as a luxury and utilize it only when in severe distress. But living under the strain of modern society, we should recognize massage as an extraordinarily beneficial measure for stressed individuals to receive on a regular basis.

For best results when giving or receiving a massage, please follow these guidelines:

- The room should be quiet, warm, and comfortable.

- Soft music can be played to promote relaxation.

- Mist a pleasant essential oil fragrance in the room before the treatment.

- Make sure to be in a calm state before giving the massage. Tension can be easily transferred from one person to another.

- Fingernails should be short to avoid scratching the skin.

- A firm cushion can be used if a massage table is unavailable. The recipient should be covered with a sheet or blanket for warmth.

- Choose the appropriate aromatherapy massage formula and place all oils nearby to avoid searching for them during the treatment.

- Wash hands with warm/hot water before and after giving the massage.

- Wear comfortable clothing.

- Warm the carrier/base oil by placing the small container in warm water. Pour an ample amount into the palm of your hand, and rub both hands together. Then apply the oil on the person's skin.

MIST SPRAYS

A convenient and effective way to disperse aromatic vapors into the air is through the use of a mist spray. As the aromas mature in the bottle, the fragrance improves and becomes stronger.

Instructions: Fill a two- or four-ounce fine-mist spray bottle with purified water and add the essential oils. Tighten the cap and shake well.

To use: Shake the bottle well. Sit comfortably in a chair. Close your eyes and begin to take slow deep breaths as you spray the mist approximately ten times over your head (two to three sprays at a time).

SKIN AND HAIR CARE

Many excellent and efficacious skin and hair care products can be easily made with unrefined vegetal oils and butters, pure essential oils, and resins. The vegetal oils and butters can be applied directly to the skin and hair for their moisturizing properties. However, only specific essential oils and resins diluted into a vegetal oil or butter can be used topically for facial applications and hair care.

STEAM INHALATION

This method is usually employed to open the breathing passages.

Instructions: Heat a small pot of water and pour into a bowl, then add the essential oils. Immediately drape a towel over your head, close your eyes, and lean over the vapors. Inhale slowly and deeply.

STEAM ROOM AND SAUNA

You can transform a steam or sauna room into a delightfully uplifting and refreshing atmosphere by utilizing essential oils.

Instructions for a Steam Room with Rocks as a Heat Source

Add a blend of essential oils to a container of water and toss it over the hot rocks. Be careful not to be splashed as the water hits the rocks.

Instructions for Other Steam Rooms and Saunas

Mist sprays made with a combination of vaporous essential oils and pure water are ideal to use in a steam or sauna.

Spray the mist away from your body and face to ensure that it does not come in direct contact with your skin or eyes, since the oils can become very irritating to the skin, especially in the hot steam room and sauna. Breathe in the vapors.

CHAPTER 6

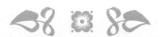

Category Listings of Oil Properties

The following categories serve as quick reference when a specific oil property is required.

BREATHING—OPENS/HELPS

Allspice
Angelica
Anise
Anise *(Star)*
Balm of Gilead
Bay *(Sweet)*
Bay *(West Indian)*
Benzoin
Blue Mountain Sage
Bluegrass *(African)*
Cabreuva
Cajeput
Camphor
Cape May
Cape Snowbush *(Wild Rosemary)*
Cape Verbena *(Lippia* or *Zinziba)*
Carrot Seed
Cascarilla Bark
Cedarwood
Champaca Flowers
Champaca Leaf

Clove
Copaiba
Cornmint
Cubeb
Cypress
Elecampane
Elemi
Eucalyptus
Eucalyptus Citriodora
Fennel
Fenugreek Seed
Fir Balsam Needles
Fir Needles
Fokienia
Frankincense
Ginger Lily
Gingergrass
Helichrysum
Helichrysum *(African)*
Hyssop
Kanuka
Katrafay
Khella *(Ammi Visnaga)*

Larch
Lavandin
Lavender
Lemongrass
Lovage
Magnolia *(Flowers)*
Manuka
Marjoram
Mastic
Monarda
Mullein
Myrtle
Myrtle *(Anise)*
Myrtle *(Lemon)*
Nerolina
Niaouli
Oregano
Peppermint
Perilla
Pine
Rambiazana
Ravensara Anisata

Ravensara Aromatica
Red Berry
Rhododendron
Rosalina
Rosemary
Savory
Schisandra
Spearmint
Spruce
St. John's Wort
Tana
Tea Tree
Tea Tree *(Black)*
Tea Tree *(Lemon)*
Tea Tree *(Prickly Leaf)*
Terebinth
Thyme
Usnea Lichen
Vitex
Yarrow
Zanthoxylum
Zedoary

CALMING/STRESS REDUCING

Allspice	Copaiba	Kunzea	Ravensara Aromatica
Ambrette Seed	Costus	Labdanum	Rhatany Root
Amyris	Cumin	Lantana	Rhododendron
Angelica	Cyperus	Lavandin	Rosalina
Anise	Cypress	Lavender	Rose
Anise *(Star)*	Davana	Ledum Groenlandicum	Sage
Arina	Desert Rosewood	Lemon	Sandalwood
Basil *(Sweet)*	Dill	Lemongrass	Saw Palmetto
Bay *(Sweet)*	Elemi	Lime	Schisandra
Bay *(West Indian)*	Eucalyptus Citriodora	Linaloe	Sea Buckthorn
Benzoin	Eucalyptus Staigeriana	Linden Blossom	Spikenard
Bergamot	Fennel	Litsea Cubeba	Spruce
Birch *(Sweet)*	Fenugreek Seed	Lovage	St. John's Wort
Bluegrass *(African)*	Feverfew	Mandarin	Styrax
Bois de Rose	Fir Balsam Needles	Manuka	Tana
Borage	Fir Balsam Resin	Marjoram	Tangelo
Cabreuva	Fir Needles	Massoia Bark	Tangerine
Cajeput	Fokienia	Mastic	Tea Tree *(Black)*
Calamint	Frankincense	Melissa	Tea Tree *(Lemon)*
Camphor Bush	Galangal	Monarda	Tea Tree *(Prickly Leaf)*
Cananga	Galbanum	Mugwort	Temple Orange
Cape Chamomile	Geranium	Mullein	Thyme
Cape Verbena *(Lippia* or *Zinziba)*	Ginger Lily	Myrrh	Tobacco
	Gingergrass	Myrtle	Tonka Bean
Carrot Seed	Goldenrod	Myrtle *(Anise)*	Turmeric
Cascarilla Bark	Grapefruit	Myrtle *(Lemon)*	Usnea Lichen
Cedarwood	Guaiacwood	Neroli	Valerian
Celery	Gurjun Balsam	Nerolina	Vanilla
Chamomile	Helichrysum	Nutmeg	Vetiver
Champaca Flower	Helichrysum *(African)*	Orange	Violet
Champaca Leaf	Hops	Osmanthus	Vitex
Chia Seed	Hyssop	Palmarosa	Wintergreen
Cinnamon	Juniper Berries	Parsley	Yarrow
Citronella	Kanuka	Peru Balsam	Ylang-Ylang
Clary Sage	Katrafay	Petitgrain	Yuzu
Clementine	Kava-Kava	Pomegranate	Zanthoxylum
Combava	Khella *(Ammi Visnaga)*	Ravensara Anisata	Zedoary

CELLULITE—REDUCES

Allspice
Basil *(Sweet)*
Bay *(Sweet)*
Bay *(West Indian)*
Benzoin
Bergamot
Birch *(Sweet)*
Birch *(White)*
Bladderwrack *(Seaweed)*
Cassia
Celery
Cinnamon
Clementine
Cumin
Cypress
Cypress *(Blue)*
Cypress *(Emerald)*
Cypress *(Jade)*
Fennel
Fir Balsam Needles
Fir Balsam Resin
Fir Needles
Geranium
Grapefruit
Juniper Berries
Lavandin
Lavender
Lemon
Lime
Lovage
Mandarin
Orange
Oregano
Pine
Rosemary
Sage
Sassafras
Savory
Styrax
Tangelo
Tangerine
Temple Orange
Thyme
Wintergreen
Yuzu

COOLING

Amyris
Angelica
Basil *(Sweet)*
Bergamot
Blue Mountain Sage
Cape May
Cedarwood *(Atlas)*
Celery
Citronella
Clementine
Combava
Cornmint
Costus
Cypress *(Blue)*
Cypress *(Emerald)*
Cypress *(Jade)*
Eucalyptus
Geranium
Grapefruit
Helichrysum
Lantana
Lemon
Lime
Litsea Cubeba
Mandarin
Myrrh
Nerolina
Orange
Peppermint
Perilla
Petitgrain
Rambiazana
Rose
Spearmint
St. John's Wort
Tana
Tangelo
Tangerine
Tea Tree *(Black)*
Temple Orange
Vitex
Zedoary

DIGESTION—IMPROVES

Allspice
Angelica
Anise
Anise *(Star)*
Basil *(Sweet)*
Bay *(Sweet)*
Bay *(West Indian)*
Caraway
Cardamom
Chamomile *(German)*
Chamomile *(Roman)*
Cinnamon
Clary Sage
Clove
Coriander
Cornmint
Cubeb
Cumin
Dill
Fennel
Fenugreek Seed
Galangal
Ginger
Lavandin
Lavender
Lemongrass
Litsea Cubeba
Marjoram
Melissa
Mullein
Myrtle *(Lemon)*
Nutmeg
Orange
Oregano
Parsley
Pepper *(Black)*
Peppermint
Perilla
Rosemary
Sage
Savory
Spearmint
Tangelo
Tea Tree *(Lemon)*
Temple Orange
Thyme
Vetiver
Zedoary

ENERGIZING, REFRESHING, REVIVING

Some oils can be reviving to one person and calming to another. This is due to an adaptogen property that the oil has to bring balance to the body.

Amyris
Bergamot
Bladderwrack *(Seaweed)*
Blue Mountain Sage
Camphor *(Borneol)*
Cape Verbena *(Lippia* or *Zinziba)*
Cardamom
Carrot Seed
Cassia
Cinnamon
Citronella
Clove
Coffee
Coriander
Cornmint

Cumin
Cypress
Cypress *(Blue)*
Cypress *(Emerald)*
Cypress *(Jade)*
Eucalyptus
Eucalyptus Citriodora
Eucalyptus Staigeriana
Fir Balsam Needles
Fir Needles
Galangal
Geranium
Ginger
Ginger Lily
Grapefruit
Helichrysum

Helichrysum *(African)*
Hyssop
Juniper Berries
Lemon
Lemon Verbena
Lemongrass
Lime
Litsea Cubeba
Massoia Bark
Mullein
Myrtle
Myrtle *(Lemon)*
Nutmeg
Oregano
Palmarosa
Patchouli

Pepper *(Black)*
Peppermint
Perilla
Pine
Ravensara Aromatica
Red Berry
Rhododendron
Rosemary
Spearmint
Tea Tree
Tea Tree *(Lemon)*
Terebinth
Thyme
Yuzu
Zedoary

INSECT BITES

Aloe Vera
Basil *(Sweet)*
Bluegrass *(African)*
Chamomile *(German)*

Chamomile *(Roman)*
Fir Balsam Resin
Geranium
Juniper Berries

Lavandin
Lavender
Lemon
Lime

Marigold *(Calendula)*
Savory
Tea Tree

INSECT REPELLENT

Bay *(Sweet)*
Bay *(West Indian)*
Cajeput
Camphor Bush
Cassia
Cedarwood *(Atlas)*
Cedarwood *(Himalayan/Deodar)*

Cedarwood *(Lebanon)*
Cinnamon
Citronella
Clove
Cornmint
Dill
Eucalyptus
Fennel

Geranium
Juniper Berries
Lavandin
Lavender
Lemongrass
Oregano
Patchouli
Pennyroyal

Peppermint
Rosemary
Savory
Spearmint
Terebinth
Thyme
Vetiver

CATEGORY LISTINGS OF OIL PROPERTIES

MENTAL CLARITY

Amyris
Angelica
Basil *(Sweet)*
Bay *(Sweet)*
Bay *(West Indian)*
Bergamot
Blue Mountain Sage
Bluegrass *(African)*
Cabreuva
Calamint
Cape Snowbush *(Wild Rosemary)*
Cape Verbena *(Lippia* or *Zinziba)*
Cardamom
Carrot Seed
Cedarwood *(Atlas)*
Cedarwood *(Himalayan/Deodar)*
Cedarwood *(Lebanon)*
Champaca Leaf
Chia Seed
Citronella
Clementine
Clove

Coffee
Combava
Copaiba
Coriander
Cornmint
Cypress
Cypress *(Blue)*
Cypress *(Emerald)*
Cypress *(Jade)*
Davana
Eucalyptus
Fir Balsam Needles
Fir Needles
Fokienia
Ginger
Ginger Lily
Gingergrass
Goldenrod
Grapefruit
Guaiacwood
Helichrysum
Hyssop
Juniper Berries
Kanuka
Khella *(Ammi Visnaga)*

Ledum Groenlandicum
Lemon
Lemon Verbena
Lime
Litsea Cubeba
Lovage
Mandarin
Manuka
Massoia Bark
Monarda
Mullein
Myrtle *(Anise)*
Myrtle *(Lemon)*
Nerolina
Nutmeg
Orange
Oregano
Pepper *(Black)*
Peppermint
Perilla
Petitgrain
Pine
Rambiazana
Ravensara Anisata
Ravensara Aromatica

Red Berry
Rhatany Root
Rhododendron
Rosalina
Rosemary
Schisandra
Spearmint
Spruce
St. John's Wort
Tangelo
Tangerine
Tarragon
Tea Tree
Tea Tree *(Black)*
Tea Tree *(Lemon)*
Tea Tree *(Prickly Leaf)*
Temple Orange
Terebinth
Thyme
Turmeric
Yarrow
Yuzu
Zanthoxylum
Zedoary

MOOD UPLIFTING

Allspice
Ambrette Seed
Anise
Anise *(Star)*
Basil *(Sweet)*
Benzoin
Bergamot
Birch *(Sweet)*
Bluegrass *(African)*
Bois de Rose
Cabreuva

Calamint
Camphor
Cananga
Cape Chamomile
Cape May
Cape Snowbush *(Wild Rosemary)*
Cape Verbena *(Lippia* or *Zinziba)*
Cardamom
Carnation

Carrot Seed
Cascarilla Bark
Cassia
Cassie
Chamomile *(German)*
Chamomile *(Roman)*
Champaca Flower
Cinnamon
Citronella
Clary Sage
Clementine

Clove
Coffee
Combava
Copaiba
Cornmint
Cumin
Cypress
Cypress *(Blue)*
Cypress *(Emerald)*
Cypress *(Jade)*
Davana

201

Elecampane	Jasmine	Myrrh	Spearmint
Elemi	Juniper Berries	Myrtle	Spikenard
Eucalyptus Citriodora	Kanuka	Myrtle (Anise)	Spruce
Eucalyptus Staigeriana	Katrafay	Myrtle (Lemon)	St. John's Wort
Feverfew	Khella (Ammi Visnaga)	Neroli	Styrax
Fir Balsam Needles	Labdanum	Nerolina	Tana
Fir Balsam Resin	Lantana	Nutmeg	Tangelo
Fir Needles	Larch	Orange	Tangerine
Fokienia	Lavandin	Oregano	Tea Tree
Frankincense	Lavender	Palmarosa	Tea Tree (Black)
Galangal	Lemon	Patchouli	Tea Tree (Lemon)
Galbanum	Lemon Verbena	Peppermint	Temple Orange
Gardenia	Lemongrass	Perilla	Thyme
Geranium	Lilac	Peru Balsam	Tolu Balsam
Ginger	Lime	Petitgrain	Tonka Bean
Ginger Lily	Litsea Cubeba	Pine	Turmeric
Gingergrass	Lovage	Ravensara Anisata	Usnea Lichen
Goldenrod	Magnolia (Flowers)	Ravensara Aromatica	Vanilla
Grapefruit	Mandarin	Rhatany Root	Vetiver
Guaiacwood	Manuka	Rhododendron	Violet
Helichrysum	Massoia Bark	Rosalina	Wintergreen
Helichrysum (African)	Melissa	Rose	Ylang-Ylang
Heliotrope	Mimosa	Rosemary	Yuzu
Honeysuckle	Monarda	Sandalwood	Zanthoxylum
Hyssop	Mullein	Sea Buckthorn	Zedoary

PAIN—LESSENS/RELIEVES

Allspice	Cabreuva	Clove	Ginger
Aloe Vera	Cade	Coriander	Goldenrod
Ambrette Seed	Cajeput	Cornmint	Helichrysum
Angelica	Calamint	Cubeb	Helichrysum (African)
Anise	Camphor Bush	Cumin	Honeysuckle
Anise (Star)	Cananga	Dill	Hops
Arnica	Caraway	Eucalyptus	Juniper Berries
Balm of Gilead	Cardamom	Fennel	Kanuka
Basil (Sweet)	Cassia	Fir Balsam Needles	Kava-Kava
Bay (Sweet)	Cedarwood	Fir Needles	Kunzea
Bay (West Indian)	Chamomile (German)	Fokenia	Lavandin
Birch (Sweet)	Chamomile (Roman)	Galangal	Lavender
Birch (White)	Cinnamon	Galbanum	Litsea Cubeba
Bois de Rose	Clary Sage	Geranium	Manuka

Marjoram	Palmarosa	Rue	Tea Tree (Lemon)
Melissa	Peppermint	Sage	Terebinth
Myrtle	Pine	Sassafras	Thyme
Myrtle (Anise)	Ravensara Anisata	Savory	Valerian
Myrtle (Lemon)	Ravensara Aromatica	Spearmint	Vetiver
Niaouli	Red Berry	St. John's Wort	Vitex
Nerolina	Rose	Tarragon	Wintergreen
Nutmeg	Rosemary	Tea Tree	Ylang-Ylang
Oregano			

RESTFUL SLEEP—PROMOTES

Ajowan	Clementine	Lantana	Petitgrain
Allspice	Combava	Lavandin	Ravensara Anisata
Anise	Copaiba	Lavender	Sandalwood
Anise (Star)	Costus	Lemon	Schisandra
Arina	Cyperus	Lemongrass	Spikenard
Basil (Sweet)	Cypress	Linden Blossom	Tangelo
Benzoin	Dill	Litsea Cubeba	Tangerine
Bergamot	Elemi	Mandarin	Tea Tree (Black)
Birch (Sweet)	Fennel	Marjoram	Temple Orange
Cajeput	Feverfew	Mastic	Turmeric
Cananga	Fir Balsam Resin	Melissa	Valerian
Cape Verbena (Lippia or Zinziba)	Frankincense	Myrrh	Vanilla
	Guaiacwood	Myrtle (Anise)	Vetiver
Cedarwood	Gurjun Balsam	Neroli	Violet
Celery	Hops	Nutmeg	Wintergreen
Chamomile (German)	Kava-Kava	Orange	Ylang-Ylang
Chamomile (Roman)	Labdanum	Peru Balsam	Zanthoxylum
Clary Sage			

SKIN—HEALING

Aloe Vera	Chamomile (Roman)	Mangosteen	Rose
Ambrette Seed	Combava	Manuka	Sandalwood
Arnica	Copaiba	Marigold (Calendula)	Schisandra
Balm of Gilead	Elemi	Myrrh	Tagetes
Benzoin	Frankincense	Palmarosa	Tea Tree
Bois de Rose	Guaiacwood	Patchouli	Vegetal/Carrier Oils & Butters
Cade	Kanuka	Peru Balsam	
Camphor Bush	Lavandin	Petitgrain	Vetiver
Chamomile (German)	Lavender		

TIGHT MUSCLES—LOOSENS/RELAXES

Ajowan
Allspice
Amyris
Arina
Balm of Gilead
Bay *(Sweet)*
Bay *(West India)*
Benzoin
Birch *(Sweet)*
Birch *(White)*
Blue Mountain Sage
Cabreuva
Cananga
Cape Chamomile
Cape Verbena *(Lippia* or *Zinziba)*

Carrot Seed
Cedarwood *(Atlas)*
Cedarwood *(Himalayan/ Deodar)*
Cedarwood *(Lebanon)*
Chia Seed
Cinnamon
Cypress
Desert Rosewood
Eucalyptus
Fenugreek Seed
Feverfew
Ginger Lily
Guaiacwood
Helichrysum *(African)*
Kanuka

Khella *(Ammi Visnaga)*
Labdanum
Lavandin
Lavender
Manuka
Marjoram
Mullein
Myrtle *(Anise)*
Myrtle *(Lemon)*
Nutmeg
Oregano
Pepper *(Black)*
Peru Balsam
Ravensara Anisata
Red Berry

Sage
Sassafras
Savory
Saw Palmetto
Sea Buckthorn
Tea Tree *(Lemon)*
Tea Tree *(Prickly Leaf)*
Thyme
Usnea Lichen
Vetiver
Vitex
Wintergreen
Ylang-Ylang
Yuzu
Zanthoxylum

WARMING/HEATING

Ajowan
Allspice
Arina
Bay *(Sweet)*
Bay *(West Indian)*
Benzoin
Birch *(Sweet)*
Cabreuva
Cajeput
Cape Chamomile
Cardamom
Carrot Seed
Cascarilla Bark
Cassia

Champaca Flower
Champaca Leaf
Cinnamon
Clove
Coffee
Copaiba
Cumin
Cyperus
Elemi
Fennel
Fenugreek Seed
Fir Balsam Resin
Ginger
Gingergrass

Goldenrod
Gurjun Balsam
Labdanum
Ledum Groenlandicum
Marjoram
Massoia Bark
Mullein
Myrtle *(Lemon)*
Nutmeg
Oregano
Palmarosa
Pepper *(Black)*
Pepper *(Red)*
Peru Balsam

Pomegranate
Ravensara Anisata
Red Berry
Rosemary
Savory
Saw Palmetto
Schisandra
Sea Buckthorn
Tea Tree *(Lemon)*
Tea Tree *(Prickly Leaf)*
Thyme
Turmeric
Wintergreen
Zanthoxylum

Cross-Reference of Botanical Names to Common Names

Abelmoschus esculentus—Okra

Abelmoschus moschatus—Ambrette Seed

Abies alba—Fir Needles, Silver Fir

Abies balsamea—Fir Balsam Needles, Fir Balsam Resin

Abies balsamifera—Fir Balsam Resin

Abies grandis—Grand Fir, Fir Needles

Acacia dealbata—Mimosa

Acacia decurrens—Mimosa

Acacia farnesiana—Cassie

Achillea millefolium—Yarrow

Acorus calamus—Calamus *(Sweet Flag)*

Acrocomia aculeata—Macauba

Acrocomia sclerocarpa—Macauba

Actinidia chinensis—Kiwifruit Seed

Adansonia digitata—Baobab

Adansonia grandidieri—Baobab

Agathosma betulina—Buchu

Aleurites moluccana—Kukui Nut

Allium cepa—Onion

Allium sativum—Garlic

Aloe barbadensis—Aloe Vera

Aloe vera—Aloe Vera

Aloysia citriodora—Lemon Verbena

Aloysia triphylla—Lemon Verbena

Alpinia galanga—Galangal

Alpinia officinarum—Galangal

Amaranthus candatus—Amaranth

Amaranthus cruentus—Amaranth

Amaranthus hypochondriacus—Amaranth

Ammi visnaga—Khella *(Ammi visnaga)*

Amomum curcuma—Turmeric

Amomum zingiber—Ginger

Amyris balsamifera—Amyris

Anacardium occidentale—Cashew Nut

Andropogon martinii—Palmarosa

Andropogon muricatus—Vetiver

Andropogon nardus—Citronella

Anethum foeniculum—Fennel

Anethum graveolens—Dill

Angelica archangelica—Angelica

Angelica levisticum—Lovage

Angelica officinalis—Angelica

Aniba rosaeodora—Bois de Rose *(Rosewood)*

Anisum officinalis—Anise

Anisum officinarum—Anise

Annona muricata—Guanabana

Anthemis mixta—Chamomile *(Moroccan)*

Anthemis nobilis—Chamomile *(Roman)*

Anthriscus cerefolium—Chervil

Apium carvi—Caraway

Apium graveolens—Celery

Apium petroselinum—Parsley

Arachis hypogaea—Peanut

Argania sideroxylon—Argan

Argania spinosa—Argan

Armeniaca vulgaris—Apricot Kernel

Arnica montana—Arnica

Artemisia absinthium—Wormwood

Artemisia dracunculus—Tarragon *(Estragon)*

Artemisia pallens—Davana

Artemisia vulgaris—Mugwort *(Armoise)*

Aster officinalis—Elecampane

Astrocaryum murumuru—Murumuru

Astrocaryum tucuma—Tucuma

Astrocaryum vulgare—Tucuma

Avena sativa—Oat

Azadirachta indica—Neem

Backhousia anisata—Anise Myrtle

Backhousia citriodora—Lemon Myrtle

Bactris globosa—Macauba

Balsam styracis—Styrax

Balsamodendron myrrha—Myrrh

Barosma betulina—Buchu

Baryosma tongo—Tonka Bean *(Tonquin Bean)*

Bassia latifolia—Mowrah Butter

Bertholletia excelsa—Brazil Nut

Betula alba—Birch *(White)*

Betula lenta—Birch *(Sweet)*

Bixa orellana—Annatto

Borago officinalis—Borage

Boswellia carteri—Frankincense *(Olibanum)*

Boswellia sacra—Frankincense *(Olibanum)*

Boswellia thurifera—Frankincense *(Olibanum)*

Brassica napus—Canola *(Rapeseed)*

Brassica nigra—Black Mustard

Brassica oleracea—Broccoli Seed

Bulnesia sarmienti—Guaiacwood

Bursera glabrifolia—Linaloe

Butyrospermum parkii—Shea, Shea Butter

Calamintha clinopodium—Calamint *(Catnip)*

Calamintha grandiflora—Calamint *(Catnip)*

Calamintha hortensis—Savory *(Summer)*

Calamintha montana—Savory *(Winter)*

Calamintha officinalis—Calamint *(Catnip)*

Calamus aromaticus—Calamus *(Sweet Flag)*

Calendula officinalis—Marigold *(Calendula)*

Callitris columellaris—Emerald Cypress

Callitris glaucophylla—Jade Cypress

Callitris intratropica—Blue Cypress

Calodendrum capense—Yangu

Calophyllum inophyllum—Calophyllum

Camelina sativa—Camelina

Camellia japonica—Camellia

Camellia sinensis—Camellia

Cananga odorata—Cananga

Cananga odorata var. genuina—Ylang-Ylang

Canarium commune—Elemi

Canarium luzonicum—Elemi

Cannabis indica—Hemp

Cannabis sativa—Hemp

Capsicum frutescens—Red Pepper

Carapa guianensis—Andiroba

Carica papaya—Papaya Seed

Carthamus tinctorius—Safflower

Carum carvi—Caraway

Carum petroselinum—Parsley

Carya illinoinensis—Pecan

Caryocar brasiliense—Pequi

Caryophyllus aromaticus—Clove

Cassia ancienne—Cassie

Cedrelopsis grevei—Katafray

Cedrus atlantica—Cedarwood *(Atlas)*

Cedrus deodara—Himalayan Cedar, Deodar Cedar

Cedrus libani—Lebanon Cedar, Cedar-Of-Lebanon

Ceiba pentandra—Kapok Seed

Ceratonia siliqua—Carob Pod

Chamaemelum nobile—Chamomile *(Roman)*

Chenopodium quinoa—Quinoa

Cinnamomum aromaticum—Cassia

Cinnamomum camphora—Camphor, Ravensara Anisata, Ravensara Aromatica

Cinnamomum cassia—Cassia

Cinnamomum vera—Cinnamon

Cinnamomum zeylanicum—Cinnamon

Cistus creticus—Labdanum (*Cistus* or *Rock Rose*)

Cistus incanus—Labdanum (*Cistus* or *Rock Rose*)

Cistus ladanifer—Labdanum (*Cistus* or *Rock Rose*)

Citrullus lanatus—Kalahari Melon

Citrullus vulgaris—Watermelon Seed

Citrus aurantiifolia—Lime

Citrus aurantiifolia var. swingle—Lime (*Key*)

Citrus aurantium—Neroli, Orange (*Bitter*)

Citrus bergamia—Bergamot

Citrus bigaradia—Petitgrain

Citrus clementine—Clementine

Citrus hystrix—Combava

Citrus junos—Yuzu

Citrus limetta—Lime

Citrus limon—Lemon

Citrus nobilis—Mandarin

Citrus paradisi—Grapefruit

Citrus reticulata—Clementine, Mandarin, Tangerine, Temple Orange

Citrus sinensis—Orange (*Blood*), Orange (*Sweet*)

Citrus tangelo—Tangelo

Cocos nucifera—Coconut

Coffea arabica—Coffee

Coleonema album—Cape May

Commiphora erythraea—Opopanax

Commiphora myrrha—Myrrh

Copaifera officinalis—Copaiba

Copernicia cerifera—Carnauba

Copernicia prunifera—Carnauba

Coriandrum sativum—Coriander

Corylus avellana—Hazelnut

Coumarouna odorata—Tonka Bean (*Tonquin Bean*)

Crocus sativus—Saffron

Croton eleuteria—Cascarilla Bark

Croton insularis—Cascarilla Bark

Croton lechieri—Dragon's Blood (*Sangre de Grado*)

Cryptocarya massoia—Massoia Bark

Cubeba officinalis—Cubeb

Cucumis sativus—Cucumber Seed

Cucurbita pepo—Pumpkinseed

Cuminum cyminum—Cumin

Cuminum odorum—Cumin

Cupressus sempervirens—Cypress

Curcuma domestica—Turmeric

Curcuma longa—Turmeric

Curcuma zedoaria—Zedoary

Cymbopogon citratus—Lemongrass

Cymbopogon flexuosus—Lemongrass

Cymbopogon martinii var. motia—Palmarosa

Cymbopogon martinii var. sofia—Gingergrass

Cymbopogon nardus—Citronella

Cymbopogon validus—African Bluegrass

Cynara cardunculus—Cardoon

Cyperus esculentus—Chufa

Cyperus scariosus—Cyperus (*Cypriol*)

Daucus carota—Carrot Root, Carrot Seed

Dianthus caryophyllus—Carnation (*Clove Pink*)

Dipterocarpus glandulosa—Gurjun balsam

Dipterocarpus gracilis—Gurjun balsam

Dipterocarpus griffithi—Gurjun balsam

Dipterocarpus jourdaninii—Gurjun balsam

Dipterocarpus palasus—Gurjun balsam

Dipterocarpus turbinatus—Gurjun balsam

Dipteryx odorata—Tonka Bean (*Tonquin Bean*)

Dryobalanops aromatica—Camphor (*Borneol*)

Dryobalanops camphora—Camphor (*Borneol*)

Echium plantagineum—Echium

Elaeis guineensis—Palm Fruit, Palm Kernel

Elettaria cardamomum—Cardamom

Eremophila mitchellii—Desert Rosewood

Eriocephalus africanus—Cape Snowbush *(Wild Rosemary)*

Eriocephalus punctulatus—Cape Chamomile

Erysimum officinale—Sisymbrium

Eucalyptus citriodora—Eucalyptus Citriodora

Eucalyptus dives—Eucalyptus Dives

Eucalyptus globulus—Eucalyptus

Eucalyptus macarthurii—Eucalyptus Macarthurii

Eucalyptus polybractea—Eucalyptus Blue Mallee

Eucalyptus radiata—Eucalyptus Radiata

Eucalytpus sideroxylon—Eucalytpus Sideroxylon

Eucalyptus smithii—Eucalyptus Smithii

Eucalyptus staigeriana—Eucalyptus Staigeriana

Eugenia aromatica—Clove

Eugenia caryophyllata—Clove

Eugenia caryophyllus—Clove

Euphorbia antisyphilitica—Candelilla Wax

Euphorbia cerifera—Candelilla Wax

Euterpe edulis—Acai Fruit, Acai Seed

Euterpe oleracea—Acai Fruit, Acai Seed

Fagus grandifolia—Beechnut

Fagus sylvatica—Beechnut

Ferula assafoetida—Asafoetida

Ferula galbaniflua—Galbanum

Ferula gumosa—Galbanum

Ferula rubricaulis—Galbanum

Foeniculum officinale—Fennel

Foeniculum vulgare—Fennel

Fokienia hodginsii—Fokienia

Fragaria ananassa—Strawberry Seed

Fragaria vesca—Strawberry Seed

Fructus anethi—Dill

Fucus vesiculosus—Bladderwrack *(Seaweed)*

Garcinia indica choisy—Mangosteen (Kokum Butter)

Garcinia mangostana—Mangosteen (Kokum Butter)

Gardenia grandiflora—Gardenia

Gaultheria procumbens—Wintergreen

Gossypium species—Cottonseed

Guaiacum officinale—Guaiacwood

Guizotia abyssinica—Ramtil

Hedychium spicatum—Ginger Lily

Helenium grandiflorum—Elecampane

Helianthus annuus—Sunflower

Helichrysum angustifolium—Helichrysum *(Everlasting* or *Immortelle)*

Helichrysum gymnocephalum—Rambiazana

Helichrysum italicum—Helichrysum *(Everlasting* or *Immortelle)*

Helichrysum splendidum—African Helichrysum

Heliotropium arborescens—Heliotrope

Hibiscus abelmoschus—Ambrette Seed

Hibiscus esculentus—Okra

Hippophae rhamnoides—Sea Buckthorn

Humulus lupulus—Hops

Hydnocarpus anthelmintica—Chaulmoogra

Hydnocarpus kurzii—Chaulmoogra

Hydnocarpus laurifolia—Chaulmoogra

Hydnocarpus wightiana—Chaulmoogra

Hypericum perforatum—St. John's Wort

Hyssopus officinalis—Hyssop

Hyssopus officinalis var. decumbens—Hyssop Decumbens

Illicium verum—Anise *(Star)*

Inula helenium—Elecampane

Iris florentina—Orris Root

Iris pallida—Orris Root

Isatis tinctoria—Pastel

Jasminum officinale—Jasmine

Jessenia bataua—Pataua Fruit, Pataua Seed

Jessenia polycarpa—Pataua Fruit, Pataua Seed

Juglans regia—Walnut

Juniperus communis—Juniper Berries

Juniperus oxycedrus—Cade

Juniperus virginiana—Cedarwood

Kadsura chinensis—Schisandra

Krameria lappacea—Rhatany

Krameria triandra—Rhatany

Kunzea ambigua—Kunzea

Kunzea ericoides—Kanuka

Languas officinarum—Galangal

Lantana camara—Lantana

Larix europaea—Larch

Laurus camphora—Camphor

Laurus cassia—Cassia

Laurus cinnamomum—Cinnamon

Laurus nobilis—Bay *(Sweet)*

Lavandula angustifolia—Lavender

Lavandula fragrans—Lavandin

Lavandula hortensis—Lavandin

Lavandula hybrida—Lavandin

Lavandula latifolia—Spike Lavender

Lavandula officinalis—Lavender

Lavandula spica—Spike Lavender

Lavandula taemina—Santolina

Lavandula vera—Lavender

Ledum groenlandicum—Ledum Groenlandicum

Leptospermum citratum—Lemon-Scented Tea Tree

Leptospermum ericoides—Kanuka

Leptospermum liversidgei—Lemon Tea Tree

Leptospermum petersonii—Lemon-Scented Tea Tree

Leptospermum phylicoides—Kunzea

Leptospermum scoparium—Manuka *(New Zealand Tea Tree)*

Levisticum officinale—Lovage

Ligusticum levisticum—Lovage

Limnanthes alba—Meadowfoam

Limnanthes douglasii—Meadowfoam

Linum usitatissimum—Flaxseed

Lippia citriodora—Lemon Verbena

Lippia javanica—Cape Verbena *(Lippia* or *Zinziba)*

Lippia triphylla—Lemon Verbena

Liquidambar orientalis—Styrax *(Asian)*

Liquidambar styraciflua—Styrax *(American)*

Lithospermum erythrorhizon—Gromwell Root

Litsea citrata—Litsea Cubeba

Litsea cubeba—Litsea Cubeba

Lonicera fragrantissims—Honeysuckle

Lonicera joponica—Honeysuckle

Lycium barbarum—Wolfberry

Lycium chinense—Wolfberry

Lycopersicon esculentum—Tomato Seed

Macadamia integrifolia—Macadamia Nut

Macadamia ternifolia—Macadamia Nut

Macadamia tetraphylla—Macadamia Nut

Madhuca indica—Mowrah Butter

Madhuca latifolia—Mowrah Butter

Magnolia grandiflora—Magnolia Flowers

Magnolia liliiflora—Magnolia Flowers

Magnolia officinalis—Magnolia Bark

Majorana hortensis—Marjoram *(Sweet)*

Mangifera indica—Mango

Matricaria chamomilla—Chamomile *(German)*

Matricaria recutita—Chamomile *(German)*

Mauritia flexuosa—Buriti Fruit, Buriti Kernel

Melaleuca alternifolia—Tea Tree

Melaleuca bracteata—Black Tea Tree *(White Cloud)*

Melaleuca cajuputi—Cajeput

Melaleuca ericifolia—Rosalina *(Lavender Tea Tree)*

Melaleuca lanceolata—Black Tea Tree

Melaleuca leucadendron—Cajeput

Melaleuca linariifolia—Tea Tree

Melaleuca minor—Cajeput

Melaleuca pubescens—Black Tea Tree

Melaleuca quinquenervia—Nerolina

Melaleuca quinquenervia—Niaouli

Melaleuca squamophloia—Prickly Leaf Tea Tree

Melaleuca uncinata—Tea Tree

Melaleuca viridiflora—Niaouli

Melissa officinalis—Melissa *(Lemon Balm)*

Mentha arvensis—Cornmint

Mentha piperita—Peppermint

Mentha pulegium—Pennyroyal

Mentha spicata—Spearmint

Mentha viridis—Spearmint

Michelia alba—Champaca

Michelia champaca—Champaca

Monarda fistulosa—Monarda

Morinda citrifolia—Noni Seed

Moringa oleifera—Moringa *(Ben* or *Behen)*

Moringa pterygosperma—Moringa *(Ben* or *Behen)*

Myrcia acris—Bay *(West Indian)*

Myristica aromata—Nutmeg

Myristica fragrans—Nutmeg

Myristica officinalis—Nutmeg

Myrocarpus fastigiatus—Cabreuva

Myrospermum pereirae—Peru Balsam

Myroxylon balsamum—Tolu Balsam

Myroxylon pereirae—Peru Balsam

Myroxylon toluiferum—Tolu Balsam

Myrtus communis—Myrtle

Nardostachys grandiflora—Spikenard

Nardostachys jatamansi—Spikenard

Nepeta cataria—Calamint *(Catnip)*

Nicotiana tabacum—Tobacco Leaf

Nigella sativa—Black Cumin

Ocimum basilicum—Basil *(Sweet)*

Oenocarpus bataua—Pataua Fruit, Pataua Seed

Oenothera biennis—Evening Primrose

Olea europaea—Olive

Oleum papaveris—Poppy Seed

Oncoba echinata—Chaulmoogra

Opuntia ficus-indica—Prickly Pear

Opuntia streptacantha—Prickly Pear

Orbignya barbosiana—Babassu

Origanum majorana—Marjoram *(Sweet)*

Origanum vulgare—Oregano

Ormenis mixta—Chamomile *(Moroccan)*

Ormenis multicaulis—Chamomile *(Moroccan)*

Oryza sativa—Rice Bran

Osmanthus fragrans—Osmanthus

Papaver somniferum—Poppy Seed

Parinari curatellifolia—Mobola Plum *(Parinari Kernel)*

Passiflora incarnata—Passion Fruit Seed

Pelargonium graveolens—Geranium

Pentaclethra filamentosa—Pracaxi

Pentaclethra macroloba—Pracaxi

Perilla frutescens—Perilla Seed

Perilla ocimoides—Perilla Seed

Persea americana—Avocado

Persea gratissima—Avocado

Petroselinum crispum—Parsley

Petroselinum hortense—Parsley

Petroselinum sativum—Parsley

Peucedanum graveolens—Dill

Peumus boldus—Boldo

Picea mariana—Spruce *(Black)*

Picea sitchensis—Spruce *(Sitka)*

Pimenta acris—Bay *(West Indian)*

Pimenta dioica—Allspice

Pimenta officinalis—Allspice

Pimenta racemosa—Bay *(West Indian)*

Pimpinella anisum—Anise

Pinus balsaamea—Fir Balsam Resin

Pinus edulis—Pine Nut

Pinus maritima—Terebinth

Pinus palustris—Terebinth

Pinus pinea—Pine Nut

Pinus sylvestris—Pine

Piper cubeba—Cubeb

Piper methysticum—Kava-Kava

Piper nigrum—Pepper *(Black)*

Pistacia lentiscus—Mastic

Pistacia officinarum—Pistachio Nut

Pistacia reticulata—Pistachio Nut

Pistacia terebinthus—Terebinth

Pistacia vera—Pistachio Nut

Platonia esculenta—Bacuri

Platonia insignis—Bacuri

Pogostemon cablin—Patchouli

Pogostemon patchouli—Patchouli

Polianthes tuberosa—Tuberose

Pongamia glabra—Karanja

Pongamia pinnata—Karanja

Populus balsamifera—Balm of Gilead

Populus candicans—Balm of Gilead

Populus deltoides—Balm of Gilead

Populus gileadensis—Balm of Gilead

Populus tacamahaca—Balm of Gilead

Pouteria sapota—Sapote

Prunus amygdalus—Almond *(Bitter)*, Almond *(Sweet)*

Prunus armeniaca—Apricot Kernel

Prunus avium—Cherry Kernel

Prunus domestica—Prunus Kernel

Prunus dulcis—Almond *(Bitter)*, Almond *(Sweet)*

Prunus persica—Peach Kernel

Prunus serotina—Cherry Kernel

Pseudotsuga menziesii—Douglas Fir

Psiadia altissima—Arina

Punica granatum—Pomegranate Seed

Ravensara anisata—Ravensara Anisata *(Havozo Bark)*

Ravensara aromatica—Ravensara Aromatica

Rhododendron anthopogon—Rhododendron

Rhus taratana—Tana

Ribes nigrum—Black Currant Seed

Ricinus communis—Castor

Rosa centifolia—Rose

Rosa damascena—Rose

Rosa eglanteria—Rose Hip Seed

Rosa rubiginosa—Rose Hip Seed

Rosmarinus officinalis—Rosemary

Rubus fruticosus—Blackberry Seed

Rubus idaeus—Raspberry Seed

Rubus occidentalis—Black Raspberry Seed

Rubus urisinus—Boysenberry Seed

Ruta graveolens—Rue

Sabel serulata—Saw Palmetto

Salvia chia—Chia Seed

Salvia hispanica—Chia Seed

Salvia lavandulifolia—Sage *(Spanish)*

Salvia officinalis—Sage

Salvia sclarea—Clary Sage

Salvia stenophylla—Blue Mountain Sage

Santalum album—Sandalwood

Santalum spicatum—Sandalwood *(Australian)*

Santolina chamaecyparissus—Santolina *(Lavender Cotton)*

Sassafras albidum—Sassafras

Sassafras officinale—Sassafras

Satureja calamintha—Calamint *(Catnip)*

Satureja hortensis—Savory *(Summer)*

Satureja montana—Savory *(Winter)*

Satureja obovata—Savory *(Winter)*

Saussurea costus—Costus

Saussurea lappa—Costus

Schimmelia oleifera—Amyris

Schinus molle—Red Berry

Schinus terebinthifolius—Red Berry

Schinziophyton rautanenii—Manketti

Schisandra chinensis—Schisandra

Schisandra japonica—Schisandra

Schisandra sphenanthera—Schisandra

Sclerocarya birrea—Marula

Sclerocarya caffra—Marula

Serenoa repens—Saw Palmetto

Serenoa serrulata—Saw Palmetto

Sesamum indicum—Sesame

Sesamum orientale—Sesame

Shorea robusta—Sal Butter *(Shorea Butter)*

Shorea stenoptera—Illipe Butter

Simmondsia chinensis—Jojoba

Sisymbrium officinale—Sisymbrium

Soja hispida—Soybean

Solidago canadensis—Goldenrod

Solidago odora—Goldenrod

Styrax benzoin—Benzoin

Styrax tonkinensis—Benzoin

Syringa vulgaris—Lilac

Syzygium aromaticum—Clove

Tagetes erecta—Tagetes

Tagetes minuta—Tagetes

Tagetes patula—Tagetes

Tamarindus indica—Tamarind Seed

Tanacetum parthenium—Feverfew

Tanacetum vulgare—Tansy

Taraktogenos kurzii—Chaulmoogra

Tarchonanthus camphoratus—Camphor Bush

Tarchonanthus minor—Camphor Bush

Theobroma cacao—Cocoa Butter

Theobroma grandiflorum—Cupuacu Butter

Thuja occidentalis—Thuja *(Cedar Leaf)*

Thymus aestivus—Thyme

Thymus citriodorus—Thyme

Thymus ilerdensis—Thyme

Thymus mastichina—Marjoram *(Spanish)*

Thymus satureiodes—Thyme

Thymus valentianus—Thyme

Thymus vulgaris—Thyme

Thymus vulgaris var. linalol—Thyme Linalol

Thymus webbianus—Thyme

Tilia europaea—Linden Blossom

Tilia vulgaris—Linden Blossom

Toluifera pereirae—Peru Balsam

Trachyspermum ammi—Ajowan

Trachyspermum copticum—Ajowan

Trichilia emetica—Mafura Butter

Trichilia roka—Mafura Butter

Trigonella foenum-graecum—Fenugreek Seed

Triticum vulgare—Wheat Germ

Tsuga canadensis—Spruce-Hemlock, White Spruce

Unona odorantissimum—Ylang-Ylang

Usnea barbata—Usnea Lichen

Vaccinium macrocarpon—Cranberry Seed

Vaccinium myrtillus—Blueberry Seed

Valeriana officinalis—Valerian

Vanilla fragrans—Vanilla

Vanilla planifolia—Vanilla

Verbascum thapsus—Mullein

Verbena triphylla—Lemon Verbena

Vetiveria zizanoides—Vetiver

Viola odorata—Violet

Virola sebifera—Ucuuba Butter

Vitex agnus castus—Vitex *(Berry)*, Vitex *(Leaf)*

Vitis vinifera—Grapeseed

Ximenia americana—Ximenia

Zanthoxylum alatum—Zanthoxylum

Zanthoxylum americanum—Zanthoxylum

Zanthoxylum rhesta—Zanthoxylum

Zea mays—Corn

Zingiber officinale—Ginger

Plant Family Name Classification

Actinidiaceae

Kiwifruit Seed—*Actinidia chinensis*

Agavaceae

Tuberose—*Polianthes tuberosa*

Amaranthaceae

Amaranth—*Amaranthus candatus, Amaranthus cruentus, Amaranthus hypochondriacus*

Anacardiaceae

Cashew Nut—*Anacardium occidentale*

Mango—*Mangifera indica*

Marula—*Sclerocarya birrea, Sclerocarya caffra*

Mastic—*Pistacia lentiscus*

Pataua—*Jessenia bataua, Jessenia polycarpa, Oenocarpus bataua*

Pistachio Nut—*Pistacia officinarum, Pistacia reticulata, Pistacia vera*

Red Berry *(Pepper Tree)*—*Schinus molle, Schinus terebinthifolius*

Tana—*Rhus taratana*

Terebinth—*Pistacia terebinthus*

Annonaceae

Cananga—*Cananga odorata*

Guanabana—*Annona muricata*

Ylang-Ylang—*Cananga odorata var. genuina, Unona odorantissimum*

Apiaceae

Ajowan—*Trachyspermum ammi, Trachyspermum copticum*

Angelica—*Angelica archangelica, Angelica officinalis*

Anise—*Anisum officinalis, Anisum officinarum, Pimpinella anisum*

Asafoetida—*Ferula assafoetida*

Caraway—*Apium carvi, Carum carvi*

Carrot—*Daucus carota*

Celery—*Apium graveolens*

Chervil—*Anthriscus cerefolium*

Coriander—*Coriandrum sativum*

Cumin—*Cuminum cyminum, Cuminum odorum*

Dill—*Anethum graveolens, Fructus anethi, Peucedanum graveolens*

Fennel—*Anethum foeniculum, Foeniculum officinale, Foeniculum vulgare*

Galbanum—*Ferula galbaniflua, Ferula gumosa, Ferula rubricaulis*

Khella—*Ammi visnaga*

Lovage—*Angelica levisticum, Levisticum officinale, Ligusticum levisticum*

Parsley—*Apium petroselinum, Carum petroselinum, Petroselinum crispum, Petroselinum hortense, Petroselinum sativum*

Araceae

Calamus *(Sweet Flag)*—*Acorus calamus, Calamus aromaticus*

Arecaceae

Acai—*Euterpe edulis, Euterpe oleracea*

Babassu—*Orbignya barbosiana*

Buriti—*Mauritia flexuosa*

Carnauba Wax—*Copernicia cerifera, Copernicia prunifera*

Coconut—*Cocos nucifera*

Macauba—*Acrocomia aculeata, Acrocomia sclerocarpa, Bactris globosa*

Murumuru Butter—*Astrocaryum murumuru*

Palm—*Elaeis guineensis*

Saw Palmetto—*Sabel serulata, Serenoa repens, Serenoa serrulata*

Asteraceae

Arina—*Psiadia altissima*

Arnica—*Arnica montana*

Camphor Bush—*Tarchonanthus camphoratus, Tarchonanthus minor*

Cape Chamomile—*Eriocephalus punctulatus*

Cape Snowbush *(Wild Rosemary)*—*Eriocephalus africanus*

Chamomile *(German)*—*Matricaria chamomilla, Matricaria recutita*

Chamomile *(Moroccan)*—*Anthemis mixta, Ormenis mixta, Ormenis multicaulis*

Chamomile *(Roman)*—*Anthemis nobilis, Chamaemelum nobile*

Costus—*Saussurea costus, Saussurea lappa*

Cynara—*Cynara cardunculus*

Davana—*Artemisia pallens*

Elecampane—*Aster officinalis, Helenium grandiflorum, Inula helenium*

Feverfew—*Tanacetum parthenium*

Goldenrod—*Solidago canadensis, Solidago odora*

Helichrysum *(Everlasting* or *Immortelle)*—*Helichrysum angustifolium, Helichrysum italicum*

Helichrysum *(African)*—*Helichrysum splendidum*

Marigold *(Calendula)*—*Calendula officinalis*

Mugwort *(Armoise)*—*Artemisia vulgaris*

Rambiazana *(Rambiaze)*—*Helichrysum gymnocephalum*

Ramtil—*Guizotia abyssinica, Guizotia oleifera*

Safflower—*Carthamus tinctorius*

Santolina *(Lavender Cotton)*—*Lavandula taemina, Santolina chamaecyparissus*

Sunflower—*Helianthus annuus*

Tagetes—*Tagetes erecta, Tagetes minuta, Tagetes patula*

Tansy—*Tanacetum vulgare*

Tarragon *(Estragon)*—*Artemisia dracunculus*

Wormwood—*Artemisia absinthium*

Yarrow—*Achillea millefolium*

Betulaceae

Birch *(Sweet)*—*Betula lenta*

Birch *(White)*—*Betula alba*

Hazelnut—*Corylus avellana*

Bixaceae

Annatto—*Bixa orellana*

Bombaceae

Baobab—*Adansonia digitata, Adansonia grandidieri*

Kapok Seed—*Ceiba pentandra*

Boraginaceae

Borage—*Borago officinalis*

Echium—*Echium plantagineum*

Gromwell Root—*Lithospermum erythrorhizon*

Heliotrope—*Heliotropium arborescens*

Shikonin Seed—*Lithospermum erythrorhizon*

Brassicaceae

Broccoli Seed—*Brassica oleracea*

Camelina—*Camelina sativa*

Canola *(Rapeseed)*—*Brassica napus*

Mustard *(Black)*—*Brassica nigra*

Pastel—*Isatis tinctoria*

Sisymbrium *(Hedge Mustard)*—*Erysimum officinale, Sisymbrium officinale*

Burseraceae

Elemi—*Canarium commune, Canarium luzonicum*

Frankincense *(Olibanum)*—*Boswellia carteri, Boswellia sacra, Boswellia thurifera*

Linaloe—*Bursera glabrifolia*

Myrrh—*Balsamodendron myrrha, Commiphora myrrha*

Opopanax—*Commiphora erythraea*

Buxaceae

Jojoba—*Simmondsia chinensis*

Cactaceae

Prickly Pear *(Opuntia)—Opuntia ficus-indica, Opuntia streptacantha*

Caesalpiniaceae

Carob Pod—*Ceratonia siliqua*

Tamarind Seed—*Tamarindus indica*

Cannabaceae

Hemp—*Cannabis indica, Cannabis sativa*

Caprifoliaceae

Honeysuckle—*Lonicera fragrantissims, Lonicera japonica*

Caricaceae

Papaya Seed—*Carica papaya*

Caryocaraceae

Pequi—*Caryocar brasiliense*

Caryophyllaceae

Carnation *(Clove Pink)—Dianthus caryophyllus*

Cistaceae

Labdanum *(Cistus* or *Rock Rose)—Cistus creticus, Cistus incanus, Cistus ladanifer*

Clusiaceae

Bacuri—*Platonia esculenta, Platonia insignis*

Mangosteen *(Kokum Butter)—Garcinia indica choisy, Garcinia mangostana*

Chenopodiaceae

Quinoa—*Chenopodium quinoa*

Chrysobalanaceae

Mobola Plum *(Parinari Kernel)—Parinari curatellifolia*

Cocoideae

Tucuma Butter—*Astrocaryum tucuma*

Cucurbitaceae

Cucumber Seed—*Cucumis sativus*

Kaluhari Melon Seed—*Citrullus lanatus, Citrullus vulgaris*

Pumpkinseed—*Cucurbita pepo*

Watermelon Seed—*Citrullus lanatus, Citrullus vulgaris*

Cupressaceae

Cade—*Juniperus oxycedrus*

Cedarwood—*Juniperus virginiana*

Cypress—*Cupressus sempervirens*

Cypress *(Blue)—Callitris intratropica*

Cypress *(Emerald)—Callitris columellaris*

Cypress *(Jade)—Callitris glaucophylla*

Fokienia *(Bois de Siam)—Fokienia hodginsii*

Juniper Berries—*Juniperus communis*

Thuja *(Cedar Leaf)—Thuja occidentalis*

Cyperaceae

Chufa—*Cyperus esculentus*

Cyperus *(Cypriol)—Cyperus scariosus*

Dipterocarpaceae

Camphor *(Borneol)—Dryobalanops aromatica, Dryobalanops camphora*

Gurjun Balsam—*Dipterocarpus gracilis, Dipterocarpus griffithi, Dipterocarpus jourdainii, Dipterocarpus palasus, Dipterocarpus turbinatus*

Illipe Butter—*Shorea stenoptera*

Sal Butter *(Shorea Butter)—Shorea robusta*

Elaeagnaceae

Sea Buckthorn—*Hippophae rhamnoides*

Ericaceae

Blueberry Seed—*Vaccinium myrtillus*

Cranberry Seed—*Vaccinium macrocarpon*

Ledum Groenlandicum—*Ledum groenlandicum*

Rhododendron—*Rhododendron anthopogon*

Wintergreen—*Gaultheria procumbens*

Euphorbiaceae

Dragon's Blood *(Sangre de Grado)—Croton lechieri*

Candelilla Wax—*Euphorbia antisyphilitica, Euphorbia cerifera*

Cascarilla Bark—*Croton eleuteria*

Castor—*Ricinus communis*

Kukui Nut—*Aleurites moluccana*

Manketti *(Mongongo Nut)—Schinziophyton rautanenii*

Fabaceae

Cabreuva—*Myrocarpus fastigiatus*

Carob Pod—*Ceratonia siliqua*

Copaiba—*Copaifera officinalis*

Fenugreek Seed—*Trigonella foenum-graecum*

Karanja—*Pongamia glabra, Pongamia pinnata*

Peanut—*Arachis hypogaea*

Peru Balsam—*Myrospermum pereirae, Myroxylon pereirae, Toluifera pereirae*

Pracaxi—*Pentaclethra filamentosa, Pentaclethra macroloba*

Soybean—*Soja hispida*

Tolu Balsam—*Myroxylon balsamum, Myroxylon toluiferum*

Tonka Bean *(Tonquin Bean)—Baryosma tongo, Coumarouna odorata, Dipteryx odorata*

Fagaceae

Beechnut—*Fagus grandifolia, Fagus sylvatica*

Flacourtiaceae

Chaulmoogra—*Hydnocarpus anthelmintica, Hydnocarpus kurzii, Hydnocarpus laurifolia, Hydnocarpus wightiana, Oncoba echinata, Taraktogenos kurzii*

Fucaceae

Bladderwrack *(Seaweed)—Fucus vesiculosus*

Geraniaceae

Geranium—*Pelargonium graveolens*

Gramineae

Oat—*Avena sativa*

Grossulariaceae

Black Currant Seed—*Ribes nigrum*

Guttiferae

Bacuri—*Platonia esculenta, Platonia insignis*

Calophyllum—*Calophyllum inophyllum*

Mangosteen *(Kokum Butter)—Garcinia indica choisy, Garcinia mangostana*

St. John's Wort—*Hypericum perforatum*

Hamamelidaceae

Styrax *(American)—Liquidambar styraciflua*

Styrax *(Asian)—Balsam styracis, Liquidambar orientalis*

Illiciaceae

Anise *(Star)—Illicium verum*

Iridaceae

Orris Root—*Iris florentina, Iris pallida*

Saffron—*Crocus sativus*

Juglandaceae

Pecan—*Carya illinoinensis*

Walnut—*Juglans regia*

Krameriaceae

Rhatany Root—*Krameria lappacea, Krameria triandra*

Lamiaceae

Basil *(Sweet)—Ocimum basilicum*

Blue Mountain Sage—*Salvia stenophylla*

Calamint *(Catnip)—Calamintha clinopodium, Calamintha grandiflora, Calamintha officinalis, Nepeta cataria, Satureja calamintha*

Chia Seed—*Salvia chia, Salvia hispanica*

Clary Sage—*Salvia sclarea*

Cornmint—*Mentha arvensis*

Hyssop—*Hyssopus officinalis*

Hyssop Decumbens—*Hyssopus officinalis var. decumbens*

Lavandin—*Lavandula fragrans, Lavandula hortensis, Lavandula hybrida*

Lavender—*Lavandula angustifolia, Lavandula officinalis, Lavandula vera*

Lavender *(Spike)*—*Lavandula latifolia, Lavandula spica*

Marjoram *(Spanish)*—*Thymus mastichina*

Marjoram *(Sweet)*—*Majorana hortensis, Origanum majorana*

Melissa *(Lemon Balm)*—*Melissa officinalis*

Monarda—*Monarda fistulosa*

Oregano—*Origanum vulgare*

Patchouli—*Pogostemon cablin, Pogostemon patchouli*

Pennyroyal—*Mentha pulegium*

Peppermint—*Mentha piperita*

Perilla—*Perilla frutescens, Perilla ocimoides*

Rosemary—*Rosmarinus officinalis*

Sage—*Salvia officinalis*

Sage *(Spanish)*—*Salvia lavandulifolia*

Savory—*Calamintha montana, Satureja montana, Satureja obovata* (Winter Savory*); Calamintha hortensis, Satureja hortensis* (Summer Savory*)*

Spearmint—*Mentha spicata, Mentha viridis*

Thyme—*Thymus aestivus, Thymus citriodorus, Thymus ilerdensis, Thymus satureiodes, Thymus valentianus, Thymus vulgaris, Thymus vulgaris var. linalol, Thymus webbianus*

Lauraceae

Avocado—*Persea americana, Persea gratissima*

Bay *(Sweet)*—*Laurus nobilis*

Bois de Rose *(Rosewood)*—*Aniba rosaeodora*

Camphor—*Cinnamomum camphora, Laurus camphora*

Cassia—*Cinnamomum aromaticum, Cinnamomum cassia, Laurus cassia*

Cinnamon—*Cinnamomum verum, Cinnamomum zeylanicum, Laurus cinnamomum*

Litsea Cubeba—*Litsea citrata, Litsea cubeba*

Massoia Bark—*Cryptocarya massoia*

Ravensara Anisata *(Havozo Bark)*—*Cinnamonum camphora, Ravensara anisata*

Ravensara Aromatica—*Cinnamonum camphora, Ravensara aromatica*

Sassafras—*Sassafras albidum, Sassafras officinale*

Lecythidaceae

Brazil Nut—*Bertholletia excelsa*

Liliaceae

Aloe Vera—*Aloe barbadensis, Aloe vera*

Garlic—*Allium sativum*

Onion—*Allium cepa*

Limnanthaceae

Meadowfoam—*Limnanthes alba, Limnanthes douglasii*

Linaceae

Flaxseed—*Linum usitatissimum*

Magnoliaceae

Champaca—*Michelia alba, Michelia champaca*

Magnolia *(Bark)*—*Magnolia officinalis*

Magnolia *(Flowers)*—*Magnolia grandiflora, Magnolia liliiflora*

Malvaceae

Ambrette Seed—*Abelmoschus moschatus, Hibiscus abelmoschus*

Baobab—*Adansonia digitata, Adansonia grandidieri*

Cottonseed—*Gossypium species*

Kapok Seed—*Ceiba pentandra*

Okra—*Abelmoschus esculentus, Hibiscus esculentus*

Meliaceae

Andiroba—*Carapa guianensis*

Mafura Butter—*Trichilia emetica, Trichilia roka*

Neem—*Azadirachta indica*

Mimosaceae

Cassie—*Acacia farnesiana, Cassia ancienne*

Mimosa—*Acacia dealbata, Acacia decurrens*

Monimiaceae

Boldo—*Peumus boldus*

Moraceae

Hops—*Humulus lupulus*

Moringaceae

Moringa *(Ben* or *Behen)—Moringa oleifera, Moringa pterygosperma*

Myoporaceae

Desert Rosewood—*Eremophila mitchellii*

Myristicaceae

Nutmeg—*Myristica aromata, Myristica fragrans, Myristica officinalis*

Ucuuba Butter—*Virola sebifera*

Myrtaceae

Allspice *(Pimento)—Pimenta dioica, Pimenta officinalis*

Bay *(West Indian)—Myrcia acris, Pimenta acris, Pimenta racemosa*

Cajeput—*Melaleuca cajuputi, Melaleuca leucadendron, Melaleuca minor*

Clove—*Caryophyllus aromaticus, Eugenia aromatica, Eugenia caryophyllata, Eugenia caryophyllus, Syzygium aromaticum*

Eucalyptus—*Eucalyptus globulus*

Eucalyptus Blue Mallee—*Eucalyptus polybractea*

Eucalyptus Citriodora—*Eucalyptus citriodora*

Eucalyptus Dives—*Eucalyptus dives*

Eucalyptus Macarthurii—*Eucalyptus macarthurii*

Eucalyptus Radiata—*Eucalyptus radiata*

Eucalyptus Sideroxylon—*Eucalyptus sideroxylon*

Eucalyptus Smithii—*Eucalyptus smithii*

Eucalyptus Staigeriana—*Eucalyptus staigeriana*

Kanuka—*Kunzea ericoides, Leptospermum ericoides*

Kunzea—*Kunzea ambigua*

Leptospermum *(New Zealand Tea Tree)—Leptospermum scoparium*

Myrtle—*Myrtus communis*

Myrtle *(Anise)—Backhousia anisata*

Myrtle *(Lemon)—Backhousia citriodora*

Nerolina—*Melaleuca quinquenervia* (chemotype nerolidol*)*

Niaouli—*Melaleuca quinquenervia, Melaleuca viridiflora*

Rosalina *(Lavender Tea Tree)—Melaleuca ericifolia*

Tea Tree—*Melaleuca alternifolia, Melaleuca linariifolia, Melaleuca uncinata*

Tea Tree *(Black)—Melaleuca bracteata, Melaleuca lanceolata, Melaleuca pubescens*

Tea Tree *(Lemon)—Leptospermum liversidgei*

Tea Tree *(Lemon-Scented)—Leptospermum citratum, Leptospermum petersonii*

Tea Tree *(Prickly Leaf)—Melaleuca squamophloia*

Olacaceae

Ximenia Seed—*Ximenia americana*

Oleaceae

Jasmine—*Jasminum officinale*

Lilac—*Syringia vulgaris*

Olive—*Olea europaea*

Osmanthus—*Osmanthus fragrans*

Onagraceae

Evening Primrose—*Oenothera biennis*

Orchidaceae

Vanilla—*Vanilla fragrans, Vanilla planifolia*

Papaveraceae

Poppy Seed—*Papaver somniferum*

Passifloraceae

Passionflower—*Passiflora incarnata*

Pedaliaceae

Sesame—*Sesamum indicum, Sesamum orientale*

Pinaceae

Cedarwood *(Atlas)—Cedrus atlantica*

Cedarwood *(Himalayan/Deodar)—Cedrus deodara*

Cedarwood *(Lebanon)—Cedrus libani*

Fir Balsam Needles—*Abies balsamea*

Fir Balsam Resin—*Abies balsamea, Abies balsamifera, Pinus balsaamea*

Fir Needles—*Abies alba, Abies grandis, Pseudotsuga menziesii*

Larch—*Larix europaea*

Pine—*Pinus sylvestris*
Pine Nut—*Pinus edulis, Pinus pinea*
Spruce *(Black)*—*Picea mariana*
Spruce *(Sitka)*—*Picea sitchensis*
Spruce *(White)*—*Tsuga canadensis*
Spruce-Hemlock—*Tsuga canadensis*
Terebinth—*Pinus maritima, Pinus palustris*

Piperaceae

Cubeb—*Cubeba officinalis, Piper cubeba*
Kava-Kava—*Piper methysticum*
Pepper *(Black)*—*Piper nigrum*

Poaceae

African Bluegrass—*Cymbopogon validus*
Citronella—*Andropogon nardus, Cymbopogon nardus*
Corn—*Zea mays*
Gingergrass—*Cymbopogon martinii var. sofia*
Lemongrass—*Cymbopogon citratus, Cymbopogon flexuosus*
Palmarosa—*Andropogon martinii, Cymbopogon martinii var. motia*
Rice Bran—*Oryza sativa*
Vetiver—*Andropogon muricatus, Vetiveria zizanoides*
Wheat Germ—*Triticum vulgare*

Polygolaceae

Rhatany Root—*Krameria lappacea, Krameria triandra*

Proteaceae

Macadamia Nut—*Macadamia integrifolia, Macadamia ternifolia, Macadamia tetraphylla*

Ptaeroxylaceae

Katrafay—*Cedrelopsis grevei*

Punicaceae

Pomegranate—*Punica granatum*

Ranunculaceae

Black Cumin—*Nigella sativa*

Rosaceae

Almond *(Bitter)*—*Prunus amygdalus, Prunus dulcis*
Almond *(Sweet)*—*Prunus amygdalus, Prunus dulcis*
Apricot Kernel—*Armeniaca vulgaris, Prunus armeniaca*
Black Raspberry Seed—*Rubus occidentalis*
Blackberry Seed—*Rubus fruticosus*
Boysenberry Seed—*Rubus urisinus*
Cherry Kernel—*Prunus avium, Prunus serotina*
Peach Kernel—*Prunus persica*
Prunus Kernel—*Prunus domestica*
Raspberry Seed—*Rubus idaeus*
Rose—*Rosa centifolia, Rosa damascena*
Rose Hip Seed—*Rosa eglanteria, Rosa rubiginosa*
Strawberry Seed—*Fragaria ananassa, Fragaria vesca*

Rubiaceae

Coffee—*Coffea arabica*
Gardenia—*Gardenia grandiflora*
Noni Seed—*Morinda citrifolia*

Rutaceae

Amyris—*Amyris balsamifera, Schimmelia oleifera*
Bergamot—*Citrus bergamia*
Buchu—*Agathosma betulina, Barosma betulina*
Cape May—*Coleonema album*
Clementine—*Citrus clementine, Citrus reticulata*
Combava—*Citrus hystrix*
Grapefruit—*Citrus paradisi*
Lemon—*Citrus limon*
Lime—*Citrus aurantiifolia, Citrus limetta*
Lime *(Key)*—*Citrus aurantiifolia var. swingle*
Mandarin—*Citrus nobilis, Citrus reticulata*
Neroli—*Citrus aurantium*
Orange *(Bitter)*—*Citrus aurantium*
Orange *(Blood)*—*Citrus sinensis*
Orange *(Sweet)*—*Citrus sinensis*
Petitgrain—*Citrus bigaradia*
Rue—*Ruta graveolens*
Tangelo—*Citrus tangelo*

Tangerine—*Citrus reticulata*

Temple Orange—*Citrus reticulata*

Yangu—*Calodendrom capense*

Yuzu—*Citrus junos*

Zanthoxylum—*Zanthoxylum alatum, Zanthoxylum americanum, Zanthoxylum rhesta*

Salicaceae

Balm of Gilead—*Populus balsamifera, Populus candicans, Populus deltoides, Populus gileadensis, Populus tacamahaca*

Santalaceae

Sandalwood—*Santalum album*

Sandalwood *(Australian)*—*Santalum spicatum*

Sapotaceae

Argan—*Argania sideroxylon, Argania spinosa*

Mowrah Butter—*Bassia latifolia, Madhuca indica, Madhuca latifolia*

Sapote—*Pouteria sapota*

Shea—*Butyrospermum parkii*

Schisandraceae

Schisandra—*Kadsura chinensis, Schisandra chinensis, Schisandra japonica, Schisandra sphenanthera*

Scrophulariaceae

Mullein—*Verbascum thapsus*

Simmondsaceae

Jojoba—*Simmondsia chinensis*

Solanaceae

Pepper *(Red) (Cayenne Pepper)*—*Capsicum frutescens*

Tobacco Leaf—*Nicotiana tabacum*

Tomato Seed—*Lycopersicon esculentum*

Wolfberry Seed—*Lycium barbarum, Lycium chinese*

Sterculiaceae

Cocoa Butter—*Theobroma cacao*

Cupuacu Butter—*Theobroma grandiflorum*

Styracaceae

Benzoin—*Styrax benzoin, Styrax tonkinensis*

Theaceae

Camellia—*Camellia japonica, Camellia sinensis*

Tiliaceae

Linden Blossom—*Tilia europaea, Tilia vulgaris*

Usneaceae

Usnea Lichen—*Usnea barbata*

Valerianaceae

Spikenard—*Nardostachys grandiflora, Nardostachys jatamansi*

Valerian—*Valeriana officinalis*

Verbenaceae

Cape Verbena *(Lippia* or *Zinziba)*—*Lippia javanica*

Lantana—*Lantana camara*

Lemon Verbena—*Aloysia citriodora, Aloysia triphylla, Lippia citriodora, Lippia triphylla, Verbena triphylla*

Vitex—*Vitex agnus castus*

Violaceae

Violet—*Viola odorata*

Vitaceae

Grapeseed—*Vitis vinifera*

Zingiberaceae

Cardamom—*Elettaria cardamomum*

Galangal—*Alpinia galanga, Alpinia officinarum, Languas officinarum*

Ginger—*Amomum zingiber, Zingiber officinale*

Ginger Lily—*Hedychium spicatum*

Turmeric—*Amomum curcuma, Curcuma domestica, Curcuma longa*

Zedoary—*Curcuma zedoaria*

Zygophyllaceae

Guaiacwood—*Bulnesia sarmienti, Guaiacum officinale*

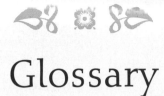

Glossary

Abortifacient. Abortion inducing. Causes childbirth or premature labor.

Adaptogen. Increases the body's ability to handle stress.

Aerophagy. A buildup of air in the body that is relieved through burping or flatulence.

Alterative. Produces a gradual improvement in the nutritional state of the body.

Analgesic. Relieves or reduces pain.

Anaphrodisiac. Reduces sexual desire.

Anesthetic. Numbs the nerves and causes a loss of sensation.

Anthelmintic. Expels or kills intestinal worms.

Antibacterial. Prevents the growth of and kills bacteria.

Anticoagulant. Prevents clotting of the blood.

Antidepressant. Alleviates or prevents depression.

Antidiarrhoeic. Relieves diarrhea.

Antidote. A remedy to counteract a poison.

Antiemetic. Counteracts nausea and stops vomiting.

Antifungal. Kills fungal infections.

Antigalactagogue. Lessens the production of milk secretion of nursing mothers.

Anti-inflammatory. Reduces inflammation.

Antilithic. Prevents formation of stones or calculus.

Antimicrobial. Inhibits the growth of micro-organisms.

Antimutagenic. The ability to protect against the effects of a mutagenic substance.

Antineuralgic. Stops nerve pain.

Antiphlogistic. Counteracts, reduces, or prevents inflammation.

Antipruritic. Relieves or prevents itching.

Antiputrid. Stops putrefaction.

Antisclerotic. Removes deposits from circulatory vessels and the body.

Antiscorbutic. Preventative for scurvy.

Antiseptic. Inhibits the growth of and kills bacteria.

Antispasmodic. Relieves or prevents spasms, cramps, and convulsions.

Antisudorific. Stops perspiration.

Antitoxic. Counteracts poisons.

Antitussive. Relieves coughs.

Antiviral. Weakens and kills viruses.

Aperient. A gentle purgative of the bowels.

Aperitif. An alcoholic drink taken to stimulate the appetite before a meal.

Aperitive. Stimulates the appetite.

Aphrodisiac. Arouses sexual desires.

Astringent. Contracts tissue and reduces secretions.

Balsamic. Softens phlegm.

Bronchodilator. Dilates the spastic bronchial tube.

Calmative. Mild sedative or tranquilizer.

Cardiac. Stimulates or affects the heart.

Cardiotonic. Tones the heart muscle.

Carminative. Expels gas from the intestines.

Caustic. Can damage skin tissue through chemical action.

Cephalic. Problems relating to the head.

Cholagogue. Increases the flow of bile.

Choleretic. Stimulates the production of bile.

Cicatrizant. Helps the formation of scar tissue; healing.

Coagulant. Clots the blood.

Cordial. Stimulant and tonic.

Counterirritant. An irritant used to counteract irritation or inflammation in another part of the body.

Cytophylactic. Protects the cells of the organism.

Decongestant. Relieves congestion.

Demulcent. Soothes irritated tissue, particularly mucous membranes.

Deodorant. Deodorizer. Eliminates offensive odors.

Depurative. Cleanses and purifies the blood and internal organs.

Detersive. Detergent. Cleanses wounds and sores, and promotes the formation of scar tissue.

Diaphoretic. Causes perspiration.

Digestive. Promotes and aids digestion.

Disinfectant. Kills infections and disease-producing micro-organisms.

Diuretic. Increases the secretion and elimination of urine.

Emetic. Induces vomiting.

Emmenagogue. Promotes and regulates menstruation.

Emollient. Softens the skin and soothes inflamed and irritated tissues.

Estrogenic. Similar to estrogen.

Euphoriant. Brings on an exaggerated sense of physical and emotional well-being.

Expectorant. Promotes the discharge of mucous from the lungs and bronchial tubes.

Febrifuge. Reduces or prevents fevers.

Fixative. Holds the scent of a fragrance.

Galactagogue. Promotes or increases the secretion of milk in nursing mothers.

Germicide. Kills germs.

Hallucinogen. Induces hallucinations—an imagined or false sense of perception.

Hemostatic. Stops hemorrhaging.

Hepatic. Acts on the liver.

Hypertensor. Raises the blood pressure.

Hypnotic. Induces sleep.

Hyoglycemient. Lowers blood sugar levels.

Hypotensor. Lowers the blood pressure.

Intoxicant. An intoxicating substance.

Insect Repellent. Repels insects.

Insecticide. Kills insects.

Larvicide. Kills the larvae of insects.

Laxative. Promotes the evacuation of the bowels; a mild purgative.

Narcotic. Relieves pain and induces a deep state of sleep. Large amounts can cause a feeling of stupor or coma.

Nervine. Calming and soothing to the nervous system.

Parasiticide. Kills parasites, especially those living on or in the skin.

Parturient. Facilitates labor and childbirth.

Pectoral. Having an effect on the respiratory system.

Purgative. Promotes a vigorous evacuation of the bowels.

Refrigerant. Cools and lowers the body temperature.

Regenerator. Promotes new growth or repair of structures or tissues lost by disease or injury.

Rejuvenator. To make young again and bring back a youthful appearance.

Relaxant. Lessens or reduces tension, and produces relaxation.

Resolvent. Disperses swellings.

Restorative. Restores consciousness and/or normal physiological activity.

Rubefacient. A local irritant that reddens the skin.

Sedative. Calms anxiety and promotes drowsiness.

Stimulant. Excites or quickens an activity in the body.

Stomachic. Strengthens, stimulates, and tones the stomach.

Styptic. Reduces or stops external bleeding by contracting the blood vessels.

Sudorific. Promotes or increases perspiration.

Tonic. Strengthens and invigorates the entire body or specific organs.

Tranquilizer. Calms the nerves and brings on a state of peacefulness without inducing sleep.

Vasoconstrictor. Constricts the blood vessels, which raises the blood pressure.

Vasodilator. Dilates the blood vessels.

Vermifuge. Expels intestinal worms.

Vulnerary. Heals wounds and sores by external application.

Bibliography

Aihara, Herman. *Basic Macrobiotics*. Tokyo, Japan: Japan Publications, 1985.

Angier, Bradford. *Field Guide to Medicinal Wild Plants*. Harrisburg, PA: Stackpole Books, 1978.

Arasaki, Seiban, and Teruko Arasaki. *Vegetables from the Sea*. Tokyo, Japan: Japan Publications.

Ayensu, Edward S. *Our Green and Living World*. New York, NY: Cambridge University Press, 1984.

Barwick, Margaret. *Tropical and Subtropical Trees*. Portland, OR: Timber Press, 2004.

Bianchini, Francesco. *Health Plants of the World*. New York, NY: Newsweek Books, 1975.

Bircher, Alfred G., and Warda H. Bircher. *Encyclopedia of Fruit Trees and Edible Flowering Plants*. Cairo, Egypt: The American University in Cairo Press, 2000.

Blakely, W.F. *A Key to the Eucalyptus*. Camberra, AU: Forestry and Timber Bureau Camberra, 1955.

Bose, T.K. *Trees of the World*. Orrisa, India: Regional Plant Resource Centre, 1998.

Bown, Deni. *Encyclopedia of Herbs & Their Uses*. London, UK: Dorling Kindersley, 1995.

Bremness, Lesley. *The Complete Book of Herbs*. New York, NY: Viking Penguin, 1988.

Bremness, Lesley. *Herbs*. London, UK: Dorling Kindersley, 1994.

Brooker, M.I.H., and D.A. Kleinig. *Field Guide to Eucalyptus*. Melbourne, AU: Inkata Press, 1983.

Carper, Jean. *The Food Pharmacy*. Toronto, CAN: Bantam Books, 1988.

Carroll, Anstice. *The Health Food Dictionary*. New York, NY: Weathervane Books, 1973.

Castner, James, and James Duke. *A Field Guide to Medicinal and Useful Plants of the Upper Amazon*. Gainesville, FL: Feline Press, 1998.

Chiej, Roberto. *The MacDonald Encyclopedia of Medicinal Plants*. London, UK: MacDonald & Co. Publishers Ltd., 1984.

Cunningham, Donna. *Flower Remedies Handbook: Emotional Healing & Growth with Bach & Other Flower Essences*. New York, NY: Sterling Publishing Company, 1992.

Dorfler, Dr. Hans-Peter, and Prof. Gerhard Roselt. *The Dictionary of Healing Plants*. London, UK: Blandford Press, 1989.

Duff, Gail. *A Book of Herbs and Spices*. Topsfield, MA: Salem House Pub., 1987.

Duke, James A. *Amazonian Ethnobotanical Dictionary*. Boca Raton, FL: CRC Press, 1994.

Duke, James A. *Handbook of Medicinal Plants*. Boca Raton, FL: CRC Press, 1985.

Duke, James A. *Handbook of NorthEastern Indian Medicinal Plants*. Lincoln, MA: Quarterman Pub., 1986.

Duke, James A. *Handbook of Nuts*. Boca Raton, FL: CRC Press, 1989.

Duke, James A. *Herbs of the Bible*. Loveland, CO: Interweave Press, 1999.

Erasmus, Udo. *Fats and Oils*. Vancouver, CAN: Alive, 1986.

Erdmann, Robert, and Jones Meirion. *Fats, Health and Nutrition*. Wellingborough Northamp Tonshire, UK: Thorsons Publishing Group, 1990.

Farrell, Kenneth T. *Spices, Condiments and Seasonings*. Westport, CT: Avi Publishing, 1985.

Fischer-Rizzi, Susanne. *Complete Aromatherapy Handbook:*

Essential Oils for Radiant Health. New York, NY: Sterling Publishing Company, 1990.

Foster, Steven, and Christopher Hobbs. *A Field Guide To Western Medicinal Plants and Herbs.* Boston, MA: Houghton Mifflin Co., 2002.

Foster, Steven, and James A. Duke. *A Field Guide to Medicinal Plants.* Boston, MA: Houghton Mifflin, 1990.

Fox, Francis William, and Marion Emma Norwood Young. *Food from the Veld.* Johannesburg, SA: Delta Books Ltd., 1982.

Franchomme, Pierre, and Daniel Pénoël. *L'Aromathérapie Exactement.* Roger Jollois (Editeur). Limoges, France: 1995.

Genders, Roy. *Cosmetics from the Earth.* New York, NY: Alfred van der Mark Editions, 1986.

Graham, Judy. *Evening Primrose Oil.* New York, NY: Thorsons Publishers Inc., 1984.

Griffith, Mark. *Index of Garden Plants.* Portland, OR: Timber Press, 1992.

Groom, Nigel. *The Perfume Handbook.* London, UK: Chapman and Hall, 1992.

Gurib-Fakim, Ameenah, and Thomas Brendler. *Medicinal and Aromatic Plants of Indian Ocean Islands.* Stuttgart, Germany: Medpharm, 2004.

Gurudas. *Flower Essences and Vibrational Healing.* Albuquerque, NM: Brotherhood of Life, 1983.

Hageneder, Fred. *The Meaning of Trees.* San Francisco, CA: Chronicle Books, 2005.

Hampton, Aubrey. *Natural Organic Hair and Skin Care.* Tampa, FL: Organica Press, 1987.

Harrison, S.G. *The Oxford Book of Food Plants.* London, UK: Oxford University Press, 1969.

Heaven, Ross, and Howard Charing. *Plant Spirit Shamanism.* Rochester, VT: Destiny Books, 2006.

Hemphill, Ian. *The Spice and Herb Bible.* Toronto, CAN: Robert Rose, 2006.

Holliday, Ivan. *A Field Guide to Australian Trees.* Adelade, AU: Rigby Ltd., 1969.

Holliday, Ivan. *A Field Guide to Melaleucas.* Port Melbourne Victoria, AU: Hamlyn, 1989.

Huang, Kee Chang. *The Pharmacology of Chinese Herbs.* Boca Raton, FL: CRC Press, 1993.

Hurley, Judith Benn. *The Good Herb.* New York, NY: William Morrow Company, 1995.

Hutchens, Alma. *Indian Herbalogy of North America.* Ann Arbor, MI: Merco, 1973.

Iwu, Maurice. *Handbook of African Medicinal Plants.* Boca Raton, FL: CRC Press, 1993.

Keville, Kathi. *The Illustrated Herb Encyclopedia.* New York, NY: Mallard Press, 1991.

Kushi, Michio. *Macrobiotic Home Remedies.* Tokyo, Japan: Japan Publications, 1985.

Lavabre, Marcel. *Aromatherapy Workbook.* Rochester, VT: Healing Arts Press, 1990.

Lawless, Julia. *The Encyclopedia of Essential Oils.* Rockport, MA: Element Books, 1992.

Leung, Albert Y. *Chinese Herbal Remedies.* New York, NY: Phaidon Universe, 1984.

Leung, Albert Y. *Encyclopedia of Common Natural Ingredients.* New York, NY: John Wiley & Sons, 1980.

Lewington, Anna, and Edward Parker. *Ancient Trees.* London, UK: Collins and Brown, 1999.

Levy, Juliette de Bairacli. *Common Herbs for Natural Health.* New York, NY: Schocken Books, 1971.

Loewenfeld, Claire, and Philippa Back. *The Complete Book of Herbs and Spices.* New York, NY: G.P. Putnams, 1974.

Lust, John. *The Herb Book.* New York, NY: Bantam Books, 1974.

Lyle, Susanna. *Fruit & Nuts.* Portand, OR: Timber Press, 2006.

Mabberley, D.J. *The Plant Book.* New York, NY: Cambridge University Press, 1987.

Mairesse, Michelle. *Health Secrets of Medicinal Herbs.* New York, NY: Arco Pub., 1981.

Mars, Brigitte. *The Desktop Guide to Herbal Medicine.* Laguna Beach, CA: Basic Health Publications, 2007.

Martin, Laura C. *Wildflower Folklore.* Charlotte, NC: East Woods Press, 1984.

McKenna, Dennis J. *Botanical Medicines.* New York, NY: Haworth Herbal Press, 2002.

Menninger, Edwin A. *Edible Nuts of the World.* Stuart, FL: Horticulture Books, 1977.

Morton, Julia F. *Atlas of Medicinal Plants of Middle America.* Springfield, IL: Charles C. Thomas Publisher, 1980.

Morton, Julia F. *Fruits of Warm Climates.* Miami, FL: Julia F. Morton, 1987.

National Academy Press. *Neem, A Tree for Solving Global Problems*. Washington D.C.: National Academy Press, 1992.

Ody, Penelope. *The Complete Medicinal Herbal*. London, UK: Dorling Kindersly, 1993.

Price, Shirley. *Aromatherapy for Common Ailments*. London, UK: Gaia Books Limited, 1991.

Price, Shirley. *Aromatherapy Workbook*. London, UK: Thorsons, 1993.

Reader's Digest. *Magic and Medicine of Plants*. Pleasantville, NY: Reader's Digest, 1986.

Riffle, Robert Lee, and Paul Craft. *The Encyclopedia of Cultivated Palms*. Portland, OR: Timber Press 2003.

Roberts, Margaret. *Indigenous Healing Plants*. Cape Town, SA: Southern Book Publishers, 1990.

Rosengarten, Frederic, Jr. *The Book of Spices*. New York, NY: Pyramid Books, 1973.

Rosengarten, Frederic, Jr. *The Book of Edible Nuts*. New York, NY: Walker and Company, 1984.

Ross, Ivan A. *Medicinal Plants of the World*. Totowa, NJ: Humana Press, 1999.

Ryman, Daniele. *The Complete Guide to Plants and Flower Essences for Health and Beauty*. New York, NY: Bantam Books, 1993.

Sadler, Julie. *Aromatherapy: Family Matters*. New York, NY: Sterling Publishing Company, 1991.

Salmon, J.T. *Native Trees of New Zealand*. Sidney, AU: A.H. & A.W. Reed Ltd., 1980.

Sanecki, Kay N. *The Complete Book of Herbs*. New York, NY: Macmillan, 1974.

Santillo, Humbart. *Natural Healing with Herbs*. Prescott Valley, AZ: Hohn Press, 1984.

Schiller, Carol, and David Schiller. *500 Formulas for Aromatherapy*. New York, NY: Sterling Publishing Company, 1994.

Schiller, Carol, and David Schiller. *Aromatherapy for Mind and Body*. New York, NY: Sterling Publishing Company, 1996.

Sellar, Wanda. *The Directory of Essential Oils*. Saffron Waldon, UK: C.W. Daniel Company Limited 1992.

Sofowora, Abayomi. *Medicinal Plants and Traditional Medicine in Africa*. Chichester West Sussex, UK: John Wiley and Sons, 1982.

Taylor, Leslie. *Herbal Secrets of the Rainforest*. Rocklin, CA: Prima Publishing, 1998.

Tenney, Louise. *Today's Herbal Health, Sixth Edition*. Orem, UT: Woodland Publishing, 2007.

Thomson, William A.R., MD. *Medicines from the Earth*. New York, NY: McGraw Hill, 1978.

Tierra, Michael. *The Way of Herbs*. Santa Cruz, CA: Unity Press, 1980.

Tierra, Michael. *Planetary Herbology*. Twin Lakes, WI: Lotus Press, 1988.

Tisserand, Robert. *The Art of Aromatherapy*. Rochester, VT: Healing Arts Press, 1975.

Toussaint-Samat, Maguelonne. *History of Food*. Cambridge, MA: Blackwell Publishers, 1992.

Uphof, J.C., Th. *Dictionary of Economic Plants*. Tampa, FL: Verlag Von J. Cramer, 1968.

Valnet, Jean. *Organic Garden Medicine*. New Paltz, NY: Erbonia Books, 1975.

Valnet, Jean. *The Practice of Aromatherapy*. New York, NY: Destiny Books, 1982.

Vaughan, J.G., and P.A. Judd. *The Oxford Book of Health Foods*. Oxford, UK: Oxford University Press, 2003.

Venter, Fanie, and Julye-Ann Venter. *Making the Most of Indigenous Trees*. Pretoria, SA: Briza Publications, 1996.

Wasson, Ernie. *The Complete Encyclopedia of Trees and Shrubs*. San Diego, CA: Thunder Bay Press, 2003.

Weiner, Michael A. *The People's Herbal*. New York, NY: Putnam Publishing, 1984.

Weiss, Gaea and Shandor Weiss. *Growing and Using the Healing Herbs*. Emmaus, PA: Rodale Press, 1985.

Westland, Pamela. *The Encyclopedia of Spices*. Secaucus, NJ: Chartwell Books, 1979.

Worwood, Valerie Ann. *The Complete Book of Essential Oils and Aromatherapy*. San Rafael, CA: New World Library, 1991.

Wrigley, John W. *Australian Native Plants*. Sydney, AU: William Collins Publishers, 1979.

Yu, He-Ci. *Perilla*. Amsterdam, Netherlands: Harwood Academic Publishers, 1997.

Index

Abortifacient, 15, 46, 51, 55, 62, 73, 76, 77, 88, 92, 93, 98, 100, 103, 112, 114, 125, 133, 142, 148, 152, 153, 154, 165, 172, 174, 178, 182, 183, 186, 187, 192

Acai fruit and seed, 9

Adaptogen, 169

Ajowan, 69

Alcohol, 3

Alexander the Great, 89, 191

Allspice Berry *(Pimento Berry)*, 69

Allspice Leaf *(Pimento Leaf)*, 69

Allspice, 69

Almond *(Bitter)*, 70

Almond *(Sweet)*, 9–10

Aloe Vera Butter, 191–192

Aloe Vera, 191–192

Alteratives, 10, 30, 115, 122, 154, 157, 168, 172, 193

Amaranth, 10

Ambrette seed, 70

Ammi visnaga. *See* Khella.

Amyris. 5, 71

Analgesic, 10, 11, 15, 18, 19, 23, 30, 33, 40, 43, 46, 47, 49, 50, 51, 56, 58, 64, 69, 70, 72, 73, 75, 76, 77, 78, 79, 80, 81, 83, 84, 85, 86, 88, 91, 93, 94, 96, 97, 98, 100, 102, 103, 105, 107, 108, 109, 113, 114, 115, 116, 118, 119, 121, 123, 124, 125, 126, 127, 128, 129, 130, 131, 133, 137, 138, 139, 140, 141, 142, 144, 146, 147, 148, 149, 150, 151, 152, 154, 155, 156, 157, 159, 161, 164, 165, 167, 169, 170, 171, 172, 175, 176, 177, 179, 182, 183, 184, 185, 187, 188, 189, 192, 194

Anaphrodisiac, 139, 150, 185

Anesthetic, 15, 33, 78, 91, 96, 98, 98, 100, 103, 127, 157

Angelica root, 71–72

Angelica seed, 71–72

Angelica, 71

Anise *(Star)*, 73–74

Anise, 72–73

Annatto, 11

Anthelmintic, 11, 13, 15, 21, 22, 25, 28, 30, 33, 35, 38, 39, 40, 51, 53, 62, 64, 65, 78, 79, 83, 85, 90, 96, 98, 100, 102, 103, 107, 109, 115, 142, 147, 150, 151, 152, 165, 168, 171, 174, 175, 178, 179, 182, 183, 186, 187, 189, 192

Antiaging, 19, 24, 44, 51, 58, 65, 192

Antianemic, 94, 131, 153

Antianxiety, 127

Antiarthritic, 30, 93, 128, 182

Antiatheroslerotic, 30

Antibacterial, 11, 13, 15, 16, 20, 25, 28, 32, 35, 40, 42, 43, 46, 51, 52, 55, 58, 59, 63, 64, 69, 72, 76, 77, 78, 80, 81, 83, 84, 85, 86, 88, 91, 93, 94, 96, 97, 98, 100, 101, 102, 103, 105, 106, 107, 108, 109, 110, 111, 114, 115, 116, 118, 120, 121, 122, 123, 124, 126, 127, 130, 131, 133, 134, 135, 136, 138, 139, 141, 142, 145, 146, 147, 148, 149, 150, 152, 153, 154, 155, 156, 157, 158, 159, 160, 161, 162, 164, 166, 167, 169, 171, 172, 173, 174, 176, 177, 179, 182, 183, 185, 188, 189, 192, 194

Anticholeric, 155

Anticoagulant, 50, 58, 74, 77, 116, 118, 121, 128, 150

Anticongestive, 135

Anticonvulsant, 15, 47, 77, 81, 84, 86, 93, 94, 96, 97, 115, 123, 129, 130, 134, 141, 155, 157, 162, 169, 171, 182

Antidepressant, 17, 44, 47, 64, 69, 76, 78, 81, 85, 86, 87, 88, 89, 93, 94, 96, 97, 98, 99, 110, 114, 115, 116, 120, 121, 124, 127, 129, 130, 131, 132, 133, 134, 135, 137, 138, 141, 146, 150, 151, 154, 157, 158, 163, 164, 166, 167, 169, 170, 172, 179, 182, 187, 188

Antidiabetic, 15, 22, 30, 38, 43, 96, 103, 109, 116, 133, 144, 134, 166, 169, 182

Antidiarrhoeic, 16, 51, 55, 96, 157

Antidiuretic, 182

Antidote, 13, 17, 25, 42, 46, 83, 96, 109, 111, 155, 165, 168, 177, 186

Antidysentery, 103

Antiedema, 15

Antiemetic, 33, 73, 91, 94, 96, 98, 111, 118, 137, 148, 150, 154, 189

Antifertility, 51, 91

Antifungal, 14, 32, 40, 43, 46, 52, 59, 69, 72, 75, 77, 80, 81, 86, 91, 93, 94, 97, 98, 107, 108, 109, 110, 116, 118, 121, 125, 127, 130, 131, 132, 136, 137, 139, 142, 144, 145, 146, 150, 152, 153, 154, 158, 159, 160, 161, 162, 164, 166, 167, 168, 169, 171, 172, 174, 175, 176, 177, 179, 188, 194

Antigalactagogue, 64, 93, 95, 153, 157, 166, 168, 170, 182

Anti-inflammatories, 10, 11, 15, 17, 18, 22, 23, 24, 28, 29, 30, 31, 32, 33, 34, 37, 40, 42, 43, 46, 47, 49, 51, 52, 53, 55, 57, 58, 59, 64, 72, 75, 78, 79, 80, 81, 82, 83, 84, 85, 86, 91, 94, 95, 96, 97, 100, 102, 103, 105, 106, 107, 109, 110, 112, 114, 115, 116, 118, 120, 121, 122, 123, 124, 125, 126, 127, 130, 131, 134, 135, 138, 141, 142, 143, 144, 145, 147, 149, 150, 153, 154, 156, 157, 158, 163, 166, 167, 169, 171, 172, 173, 174, 175, 176, 177, 179, 182, 183, 184, 185, 186, 187, 189, 192, 194

Antilithic, 10, 16, 21, 33, 64, 90, 93, 95, 116, 123, 125, 131, 134, 153

Antimicrobial, 14, 15, 19, 27, 33, 36, 37, 39, 42, 46, 55, 58, 74, 103, 121, 122, 145, 156, 160, 174, 176, 194

THE AROMATHERAPY ENCYCLOPEDIA

Antimutagenic, 32, 54, 57, 78, 91, 100, 103, 106, 169
Antineuralgic, 77, 83, 94, 98, 109, 117, 131, 135, 157, 159, 164, 165, 188
Antioxidants, 9, 11, 15, 16, 17, 19, 20, 21, 23, 24, 25, 27, 28, 29, 30, 32, 36, 40, 42, 43, 44, 46, 47, 49, 51, 52, 54, 55, 58, 61, 64, 66, 69, 77, 78, 80, 90, 91, 93, 96, 98, 100, 102, 103, 106, 114, 118, 128, 131, 132, 134, 136, 139, 140, 141, 145, 148, 153, 162, 164, 166, 169, 171, 175, 179, 182, 192
Antiphlogistic, 71, 93, 111, 154, 157, 159, 163, 167, 168, 174, 187
Antipruritic, 10, 21, 45, 77, 78, 83, 88, 90, 92, 94, 109, 123, 124, 131, 154, 157, 158, 170, 176, 177, 179, 186, 187, 192
Antiputrid, 93, 96, 109, 116, 141, 144, 169, 179, 188
Antipyorrhea, 150
Antipyretic, 59, 91, 182
Antirheumatics, 11, 16, 17, 29, 31, 37, 72, 75, 77, 79, 82, 83, 84, 85, 91, 93, 94, 96, 98, 100, 104, 109, 110, 118, 120, 124, 125, 126, 129, 130, 131, 134, 142, 144, 147, 148, 149, 150, 153, 159, 161, 164, 166, 175, 177, 178, 179, 182, 184, 185
Antisclerotic, 16, 21, 62, 90, 116, 131, 134, 149, 193
Antiscorbutic, 16, 30, 36, 39, 75, 93, 113, 118, 125, 131, 134, 149, 150, 159
Antiseptic, 10, 11, 13, 15, 20, 25, 28, 30, 31, 34, 40, 42, 43, 49, 50, 51, 57, 62, 64, 65, 69, 71, 72, 73, 74, 75, 76, 77, 78, 79, 80, 81, 82, 83, 84, 85, 86, 87, 88, 89, 90, 91, 92, 93, 94, 95, 96, 97, 98, 99, 101, 102, 103, 104, 106, 107, 108, 109, 110, 111, 112, 113, 114, 115, 116, 117, 118, 120, 121, 122, 124, 125, 126, 127, 128, 129, 130, 131, 132, 133, 134, 135, 136, 137, 138, 139, 140, 141, 142, 144, 145, 146, 147, 148, 149, 150, 152, 153, 154, 155, 156, 157, 158, 159, 160, 161, 163, 164, 165, 166, 167, 168, 169, 170, 171, 172, 173, 174, 175, 176, 177, 178, 179, 180, 183, 184, 185, 186, 187, 188, 189, 192
Antispasmodic, 11, 15, 30, 32, 33, 40, 42, 44, 47, 49, 51, 57, 64, 70, 71, 72, 73, 74, 76, 77, 78, 82, 83, 84, 85, 86, 87, 88, 89, 91, 92, 93, 94, 96, 97, 98, 99, 100, 101, 102, 103, 104, 106, 107, 109, 111, 112, 114, 115, 116, 117, 118, 121, 122, 123, 124, 125, 127, 128, 130, 131, 132, 133, 134, 135, 136, 137, 139, 140, 141, 142, 144, 145, 146, 147, 148, 149, 150, 152, 153, 154, 155, 156, 157, 158, 159, 160, 161, 163, 164, 165, 166, 167, 168, 169, 170, 171, 172, 173, 174, 175, 177, 179, 182, 183, 184, 185, 186, 187, 189, 192
Antistress, 76, 78, 89, 94, 97, 98, 99, 102, 117, 120, 121, 124, 130, 132, 135, 137, 139, 141, 146, 150, 152, 154, 158, 163, 167, 183, 188
Antisudorific, 97, 104, 166
Antitoxic, 30, 50, 78, 79, 94, 103, 111, 118, 120, 125, 129, 130, 132, 134, 150, 154, 155, 161, 164, 165, 168, 170, 179
Antitumor, 10, 11, 15, 20, 30, 31, 51, 59, 64, 65, 91, 100, 103, 106, 140, 145, 157, 165, 192
Antitussive, 11, 15, 20, 22, 23, 31, 49, 51, 55, 70, 78, 96, 104, 107, 113, 114, 118, 121, 128, 130, 132, 135, 137, 139, 140, 144, 150, 155, 157, 158, 159, 161, 164, 165, 169, 172, 173, 177, 179, 185
Anti-ulcer, 100, 102
Antivenomous, 76, 109, 130, 179
Antiviral, 18, 30, 40, 51, 55, 69, 72, 77, 78, 81, 85, 86, 91, 96, 98, 102, 105, 106, 108, 109, 110, 116, 118, 121, 122, 124, 130, 134, 139, 141, 142, 143, 146, 147, 150, 152, 154, 157, 159, 160, 161, 163, 164, 165, 166, 167, 169, 172, 175, 176, 177, 178, 179, 188, 194
Antiwrinkle, 29, 58
Aperient, 13, 17, 25, 30, 40, 57, 77, 124, 153, 163
Aperitif, 89, 96, 98, 100, 111, 118, 120, 134, 142, 150, 166, 171, 179
Aperitive, 21, 22, 64, 72, 73, 76, 77, 78, 82, 84, 88, 89, 90, 93, 94, 95, 100, 103, 106, 116, 118, 120, 123, 130, 132, 133, 135, 137, 141, 142, 144, 148, 150, 152, 153, 155, 156, 157, 165, 166, 169, 170, 175, 186, 187
Aphrodisiac, 11, 13, 25, 30, 33, 46, 50, 51, 62, 69, 70, 71, 72, 73, 76, 78, 81, 82, 84, 86, 89, 91, 93, 95, 96, 97, 98, 101, 102, 103, 114, 115, 118, 120, 123, 124, 125, 127, 132, 136, 140, 146, 148, 149, 152, 153, 154, 155, 157, 163, 164, 165, 167, 169, 170, 177, 179, 182, 183, 184, 187, 192
Appetite, 111
Application of essential oils, 195–196
Apricot kernel, 11
Argan, 12
Arina, 74
Aristotle, 191
Arnica, 192
Aroma lamps, 195
Aromatherapy, 1–2
history, 1–2
Asafoetida, 74
Astringents, 10, 11, 13, 17, 19, 20, 21, 22, 23, 25, 27, 30, 31, 33, 35, 36, 38, 39, 40, 43, 50, 51, 52, 54, 55, 61, 64, 69, 77, 78, 79, 81, 84, 88, 90, 91, 92, 93, 94, 97, 99, 102, 103, 104, 106, 107, 109, 111, 113, 114, 117, 118, 119, 120, 121, 123, 124, 125, 128, 129, 132, 133, 134, 135, 137, 140, 141, 143, 144, 145, 146, 148, 150, 152, 154, 156, 157, 158, 160, 161, 163, 164, 166, 167, 169, 170, 172, 173, 177, 178, 179, 183, 185, 187, 189, 194
Atlas of Medicinal Plants of Middle America, 65
Avicenna, 1, 140
Avocado, 12–13

Bacuri *(Bukuri),* 13
Balancing (skin), 63, 120
Balm of Gilead, 74–75
Balsamic, 71, 82, 83, 87, 91, 92, 97, 100, 108, 109, 114, 115, 120, 124, 128, 144, 145, 147, 150, 158, 159, 161, 173, 175, 176, 177, 179, 183
Baobab, 13–15
Basil *(Sweet),* 75–76
Baths, 195
Bay *(Sweet),* 76–77
Bay *(West Indian),* 77
Beechnut, 14
Benzoin, 77–78
Bergamot, 78–79
Bibliography, 224–226
Birch *(Sweet),* 79
Birch *(White),* 79
Black Cumin, 15, 80
Black currant seed, 15–16
Black raspberry seed. *See* Raspberry seed.
Blackberry seed. *See* Raspberry seed.
Bladderwrack *(Seaweed),* 193
Blood builder, 153
Blood purifier, 40, 76, 121, 123, 125, 132, 146, 153, 154, 166, 168, 172, 187

Blue Mountain Sage, 80
Blueberry seed, 16
Bluegrass (African), 81
Bois de Rose (Rosewood), 81
Boldo, 81–82
Bonnardiere, Dr., 193
Borage, 16–17
Botanical names cross-
    referenced to common
    names, 205–212
Boysenberry seed. See
    Raspberry seed.
Braly, James, 65
Brazil nut, 17
Breathing, oils to help, 197
Broccoli seed, 17
Bronchodilator, 135, 179
Buchu, 82
Budwig, Johanna, 31
Buriti seed & kernel, 17–18

Cabreuva, 82
Cade, 82
Cajeput, 83
Calamint (Catnip), 83
Calamus (Sweet Flag), 84
Calmative, 17, 30, 51, 73,
    78, 81, 83, 89, 94, 97,
    99, 101, 104, 106, 110,
    111, 115, 116, 123, 125,
    130, 132, 133, 134, 135,
    136, 137, 139, 141, 146,
    148, 150, 151, 152, 153,
    154, 158, 163, 167, 171,
    172, 183, 184, 187, 188,
    192
Calming, oils to help, 198
Calophyllum, 18
Camelina, 18
Camellia, 19
Camphor (Borneol), 85
Camphor Bush, 85
Camphor, 74
Canadian Medical Association
    Journal, 193
Cananga, 5, 86
Candelilla wax, 19
Canola (Rapeseed), 19–20
Cape Chamomile, 86
Cape May, 87
Cape Snowbush (Wild
    Rosemary), 87
Cape Verbena (Lippia or
    Zinziba), 87–88
Caraway, 88
Cardamom, 89

Cardiac, 73, 85, 88, 96, 103,
    134, 148, 155, 179, 186,
    192
Cardiotonic, 15, 19, 29, 30,
    31, 32, 39, 40, 46, 47,
    51, 54, 58, 59, 64, 91,
    101, 102, 128, 140, 162,
    169, 171, 183
Cardiovascular protection, 36
Carminative, 10, 15, 21, 24,
    30, 35, 40, 46, 49, 51, 64,
    69, 70, 72, 73, 74, 76, 77,
    78, 79, 82, 83, 84, 85, 87,
    88, 89, 90, 91, 93, 94, 95,
    96, 97, 98, 101, 102,
    103, 106, 107, 111, 112,
    114, 115, 116, 118, 119,
    123, 125, 129, 130, 132,
    133, 135, 136, 137, 139,
    140, 141, 142, 144, 145,
    146, 148, 150, 152, 153,
    154, 155, 156, 157, 160,
    161, 162, 163, 164, 165,
    166, 167, 168, 169, 170,
    171, 172, 174, 175, 176,
    177, 179, 182, 183, 185,
    186, 187, 189
Carnation (Clove Pink), 89
Carnauba wax, 20
Carob pod, 20
Carrier oils. See Vegetal oils.
Carrot,
    root, 21
    seed, 90
Cascarilla Bark, 90
Cashew nut, 21–22
Cassia bark, 90–91
Cassia, 90
Cassie, 91
Castor, 22–23
Category listings of oil
    properties, 197–204
Caustic, 98
Cayce, Edgar, 23
Cedarwood (Atlas), 92–93
Cedarwood (Himalayan or
    Deodar), 92–93
Cedarwood (Lebanon), 92–93
Cedarwood, 91–92
Celery, 93
Cellulite, oils to help reduce,
    199
Cephalic, 72, 76, 78, 81, 87,
    89, 109, 114, 120, 121,
    130, 132, 135, 139, 141,
    157, 163, 164, 165, 170

Chamomile (German), 93–94
Chamomile (Moroccan), 94
Chamomile (Roman), 93–94
Champaca flower, 95
Champaca leaf, 95
Charlemagne, Emperor, 30,
    31, 106, 110, 140, 152,
    166
Charles V, King of France,
    140
Chaulmoogra, 23
Cherry kernel, 23
Chervil, 95
Chia seed, 24
Cholagogue, 29, 33, 40, 42,
    45, 64, 77, 80, 82, 86,
    93, 94, 95, 107, 116,
    120, 121, 125, 129, 130,
    132, 137, 142, 150, 157,
    159, 160, 161, 163, 164,
    165, 166, 170, 175, 182,
    186, 187, 189, 192
Choleretic, 115, 129, 141,
    150, 159, 160, 161, 163,
    164, 186
Chufa, 24
Cicatrizant, 78, 79, 82, 83,
    94, 95, 98, 104, 108,
    109, 113, 114, 115, 116,
    117, 121, 124, 125, 128,
    129, 130, 132, 144, 146,
    147, 152, 154, 163, 164,
    166, 167, 169, 176, 177,
    178, 179, 187
Cinnamon bark, 95–97
Cinnamon leaf, 95–97
Citronella, 97
Clary Sage, 97–98
Classification of plant family
    names, 213–220
Clement VIII, Pope, 26
Clement, P'ere, 137
Clementine. See Mandarin.
Cleopatra, 162, 191
Clove, 5
    bud, 98
    leaf, 98
    stem, 98
Coagulent, 132
Cocoa butter, 24–25
Coconut Cures, 25
Coconut, 25
Coffee, 26, 99
Columbus, Christopher, 25
Combava, 99
Contraceptive, 30, 51, 102

Cook, Captain, 138, 175
Cooling, 10, 66, 109, 132,
    134, 144, 153
    oils to help, 199
Copaiba, 99–100
Cordial, 78, 79, 129, 130,
    139, 141, 146, 157, 164,
    176
Coriander, 100–101
Corn, 26–27
Cornmint, 5, 101
Costus, 101–102
Counterirritant, 83, 85, 98,
    177, 178, 179, 192
Courtois, Professor, 193
Cranberry seed, 27
Cubeb, 102
Cucumber seed, 28
Culpepper, Nicholas, 112,
    152, 186
Cumin, 102–103
Cupuacu butter, 28
Cyanide, 10, 11, 48
Cynara (Cardoon), 28–29
Cyperus (Cypriol), 103
Cypress (Blue), 104–105
Cypress (Emerald), 104–105
Cypress (Jade), 104–105
Cypress, 103–104
Cytophylactic, 114, 117, 121,
    129, 130, 137, 141, 146,
    150, 152, 154, 163, 164,
    174, 179

Dangerous Grains, 65
Daniel, Kaayla, 60
Davana, 105
Decongestant, 17, 43, 46, 51,
    57, 60, 83, 87, 100, 103,
    109, 111, 116, 125, 130,
    131, 132, 135, 137, 139,
    145, 147, 154, 157, 159,
    162, 164, 167, 170, 174,
    176, 185, 192
Demulcent, 10, 11, 17, 19,
    20, 28, 30, 31, 33, 39,
    44, 45, 50, 51, 59, 65,
    143, 184, 192
Deodorant, 78, 79, 81, 97,
    99, 101, 104, 109, 117,
    130, 133, 135, 144, 145,
    146, 154, 158, 159, 167,
    171, 192
Deodorizer, 97, 104, 109,
    130, 133, 135, 136,
    194

Depurative, 11, 13, 17, 25, 30, 35, 40, 42, 43, 55, 56, 59, 64, 72, 79, 88, 93, 95, 101, 102, 103, 109, 111, 112, 117, 120, 124, 125, 128, 132, 133, 134, 136, 137, 144, 150, 153, 156, 157, 159, 163, 166, 168, 171, 188, 192, 193

Desert Rosewood, 105

Detersive, 79, 106

Detoxifier, 61, 93, 101, 111, 120, 121, 125, 130, 132, 135, 136, 139, 155, 164, 165, 183

Diaphoretic, 15, 16, 17, 40, 44, 46, 49, 51, 56, 72, 76, 77, 80, 83, 84, 85, 91, 93, 94, 95, 97, 101, 103, 106, 107, 109, 111, 116, 118, 119, 120, 122, 124, 127, 131, 132, 133, 135, 136, 137, 139, 141, 142, 147, 150, 154, 155, 157, 165, 164, 167, 168, 170, 172, 173, 174, 176, 179, 183, 184, 185, 186, 187, 189, 192

Diffusors, 195

Digestion, oils to improve, 199

Digestives, 15, 20, 29, 30, 31, 40, 43, 46, 50, 56, 57, 64, 69, 72, 73, 76, 77, 79, 82, 84, 87, 88, 89, 90, 91, 93, 94, 95, 96, 97, 99, 100, 102, 103, 106, 107, 111, 114, 116, 118, 120, 123, 124, 125, 131, 132, 133, 135, 136, 137, 139, 141, 142, 145, 146, 148, 149, 150, 152, 153, 154, 155, 156, 157, 158, 163, 164, 165, 166, 168, 169, 170, 171, 174, 175, 177, 179, 182, 186, 187, 192

Dilator, 127, 174

Dill seed, 105–106

Dill weed, 105–106

Dioscorides, 20, 30, 76, 88, 94, 102, 106, 110, 112, 116, 117, 122, 124, 132, 139, 143, 145, 148, 150, 151, 163, 184, 191

Disinfectant, 73, 78, 79, 83, 88, 97, 98, 100, 103, 106, 109, 116, 120, 121, 125, 130, 132, 133, 134, 135, 137, 144, 150, 159, 166, 169, 186, 189

Diuretics, 10, 11, 13, 15, 16, 17, 18, 19, 21, 22, 25, 26, 27, 28, 29, 30, 33, 35, 39, 40, 42, 44, 46, 47, 48, 51, 53, 55, 56, 57, 59, 60, 61, 62, 64, 65, 70, 72, 73, 75, 77, 78, 79, 80, 82, 85, 86, 87, 88, 89, 90, 91, 92, 93, 94, 95, 97, 99, 100, 101, 102, 103, 104, 106, 107, 109, 111, 113, 114, 115, 116, 117, 118, 119, 120, 121, 122, 123, 124, 125, 127, 128, 129, 130, 131, 132, 133, 135, 136, 137, 139, 140, 142, 143, 144, 145, 149, 150, 151, 153, 154, 155, 161, 163, 164, 165, 166, 167, 168, 170, 171, 172, 173, 175, 177, 178, 179, 180, 182, 183, 184, 185, 186, 187, 192, 193

Dragon's Blood *(Sangre de Grado),* 106

Drying, 78, 128, 144, 155, 159, 160

Duchesne-Dupart, Dr., 193

Duke, James A., 56

Ebers Papyrus, 102, 105, 127, 144, 191

Echium, 29

Edward I, King, 72, 111

Elecampane, 107

Elemi, 107–108

Emetic, 11, 42, 77, 144, 165, 180, 183, 184

Emmenagogue, 15, 18, 21, 24, 25, 30, 31, 33, 40, 46, 51, 59, 72, 76, 77, 84, 86, 88, 90, 91, 92, 93, 94, 96, 97, 98, 101, 102, 103, 106, 107, 111, 112, 114, 115, 118, 123, 124, 125, 128, 130, 131, 133, 136, 139, 140, 141, 142, 144, 145, 148, 150, 152, 153, 154, 157, 160, 161, 163, 164, 165, 166, 168, 169, 170, 171, 172, 174, 175, 177, 178, 179, 183, 184, 185, 186, 187, 189, 192

Emollients, 10, 11, 13, 17, 19, 25, 28, 30, 31, 33, 34, 38, 39, 41, 42, 44, 45, 51, 59, 62, 63, 64, 65, 81, 83, 86, 88, 92, 94, 95, 96, 97, 106, 114, 121, 123, 124, 125, 132, 135, 137, 146, 149, 152, 158, 163, 167, 174, 187, 192, 193

Energizing, oils for, 200

Essential oils, 1–2, 67–189
adulteration of, 5
alcohol and, 3
allergies to, 3
application of, 195
dispersion of, 195–196
extraction of, 4–5
history, 1–2
infused, 191–194
inhalation of, 195–196
medications and, 3
practical uses of, 197–204
pregnancy and, 3
safety and handling, 3–4
selection of, 5–6
storage of, 4

Estrogenic, 30, 52, 61, 72, 73, 76, 83, 96, 97, 103, 106, 111, 123, 148, 153, 160, 166

Eucalyptus Blue Mallee, 108–109

Eucalyptus Citriodora, 110

Eucalyptus Dives, 108–109

Eucalyptus Macarthurii, 108–109

Eucalyptus Radiata, 108–109

Eucalyptus Sideroxylon, 108–109

Eucalyptus Smithii, 108–109

Eucalyptus Staigeriana, 110

Eucalyptus, 5, 108–109

Euphoriant, 78, 81, 86, 97, 125, 146, 166, 167, 172, 187

Evening primrose, 29–30

Expectorant, 11, 17, 19, 30, 42, 46, 48, 49, 51, 57, 60, 62, 64, 71, 72, 73, 74, 75, 76, 77, 78, 79, 82, 83, 84, 85, 88, 89, 90, 91, 92, 93, 95, 96, 98, 100, 101, 102, 107, 108, 109, 110, 111, 113, 114, 115, 116, 118, 121, 122, 124, 125, 128, 130, 131, 132, 133, 135, 136, 139, 140, 142, 143, 144, 145, 147, 148, 149, 150, 151, 153, 154, 156, 157, 158, 159, 161, 164, 165, 166, 167, 169, 170, 172, 173, 176, 177, 178, 179, 180, 182, 184, 185, 187, 192, 194

Extraction of oils, 4–5
carbon dioxide gas extraction, 4
cold pressed oils, 4, 5
maceration, 4
solvent extraction, 4–5
steam distillation, 4

Febrifuge, 10, 11, 17, 22, 28, 30, 33, 35, 40, 43, 44, 49, 51, 56, 59, 61, 62, 65, 66, 72, 75, 76, 77, 79, 80, 83, 84, 85, 86, 87, 88, 91, 94, 95, 96, 97, 101, 102, 104, 109, 110, 112, 115, 116, 118, 122, 123, 124, 131, 132, 133, 134, 136, 137, 139, 141, 142, 144, 147, 150, 154, 155, 156, 157, 161, 165, 166, 167, 168, 170, 171, 172, 174, 177, 182, 183, 184, 185, 186, 187, 189, 192

Fennel, 110–111

Fenugreek seed, 30, 111

Feverfew, 111

Fife, Bruce, 25, 45

Fir *(Douglas),* 112

Fir *(Grand),* 112

Fir *(Silver),* 112

Fir Balsam Needles, 112–113

Fir Balsam Resin, 113

Fir Needles, 112–113

Fixative, 71, 78, 82, 86, 93, 97, 99, 115, 128, 144, 151, 152, 153, 154, 158, 167, 180, 187

Flaxseed, 31

Fokienia *(Bois de Siam),* 113

Frankincense *(Olibanum)*, 113–114

Galactagogue, 10, 15, 17, 19, 21, 23, 30, 32, 42, 46, 48, 57, 59, 61, 65, 73, 76, 88, 90, 103, 106, 111, 123, 125, 132, 133, 135, 139, 141, 160, 185
Galangal, 114–115
Galbanum, 115
Galen, 94, 124, 152, 170
Gardenia, 115
Garlic, 115–116
Gattefosse, René-Maurice, 1
Geranium, 116–117
Germicide, 83, 109
Ginger Lily, 118–119
Ginger, 117–118
Gingergrass, 118–119
Glossary, 221–223
Goldenrod, 119
Good Herb, The, 168
Grapefruit *(Pink)*, 119–120
Grapefruit *(Red)*, 119–120
Grapefruit, 119–120
Grapeseed, 31–32
Gromwell root, 32, 59
Guaiacwood, 120
Guanabana, 32
Gurjun Balsam, 5, 120–121

Hair care, 196
Hallucinogen, 33
Hazelnut, 32–33
Healing, 40, 72, 78, 81, 83, 92, 94, 97, 117, 124, 125, 130, 135, 144, 158, 166, 167, 177, 187, 192
Heating, 155, 156
oils for, 204
Helichrysum *(African)*, 121–122
Helichrysum *(Everlasting or Immortelle)*, 121
Helichrysum, 121
Heliotrope, 122
Hemostatic, 13, 21, 25, 35, 40, 48, 50, 51, 64, 74, 88, 90, 96, 104, 106, 109, 115, 117, 120, 125, 128, 129, 132, 134, 140, 144, 145, 150, 156, 163, 166, 172, 177, 178, 185, 187, 193
Hemp, 33

Henry VIII, King, 117
Hepatic, 11, 15, 16, 17, 21, 29, 30, 32, 40, 43, 50, 58, 66, 72, 73, 77, 86, 90, 91, 93, 94, 95, 96, 101, 103, 104, 111, 115, 119, 121, 123, 131, 132, 134, 140, 150, 153, 157, 163, 164, 165, 166, 168, 169, 170, 171, 175, 182, 186, 187
Hippocrates, 31, 32, 110, 115, 124, 155, 162, 166, 170, 184
Honeysuckle, 122
Hops, 123
Hurley, Judith Benn, 168
Hydrating (skin), 28, 40, 44
Hypertensive, 77, 85, 124, 159, 164, 166, 179, 192
Hypnotic, 84, 115, 123, 127, 137, 146, 149, 150, 151, 175, 184
Hypoglycemient, 149
Hypotensive, 11, 17, 22, 30, 43, 51, 55, 56, 65, 66, 71, 74, 77, 84, 86, 91, 93, 94, 97, 102, 114, 115, 116, 130, 132, 133, 135, 136, 139, 140, 141, 146, 147, 149, 150, 165, 168, 174, 178, 182, 185, 187, 192
Hyssop Decumbens, 123–124
Hyssop, 123–124

Illipe butter, 34
Immunostimulant, 15, 30, 64, 91, 162, 192
Infused oils, 191–194
Inhalers, 195
Insect bites, oils to help with, 200
Insect repellents, 76, 77, 79, 84, 85, 92, 93, 97, 98, 103, 104, 109, 110, 111, 117, 130, 132, 133, 141, 142, 145, 149, 153, 154, 155, 157, 166, 167, 168, 174, 178, 184, 186, 187
oils for, 200
Insecticides, 18, 35, 43, 62, 73, 76, 78, 79, 81, 83, 85, 87, 88, 91, 96, 97, 98, 104, 109, 111, 116, 117, 118, 125, 128, 131,

132, 133, 134, 135, 147, 154, 155, 159, 164, 165, 174, 176, 178, 179, 181, 182, 184, 192
Intoxicant, 33
Invigorating, 109, 132, 144, 148, 157, 164
Irritant, 156, 169

Jasmine, 124–125
Jojoba, 34
Juniper Berries, 125–126

Kalahari melon seed. *See* Watermelon seed.
Kanuka, 126
Kapok seed, 34–35
Karanja, 35
Katafray, 126
Kava-Kava, 126–127
Khella *(Ammi Visnaga)*, 127
Kiwifruit seed, 35–36
Kukui nut, 36
Kunzea, 127–128

Labdanum *(Cistus or Rock Rose)*, 128
Lantana, 128–129
Larch, 129
Larvicide, 103, 192
Lavandin, 5, 129–130
Lavender *(Spike)*, 130
Lavender, 5, 130
Laxative, 10, 11, 13, 15, 18, 20, 21, 23, 25, 31, 33, 38, 40, 43, 44, 45, 46, 48, 52, 54, 59, 60, 62, 64, 66, 70, 73, 76, 77, 78, 79, 82, 85, 90, 91, 94, 95, 106, 111, 112, 116, 118, 119, 120, 122, 124, 129, 132, 136, 139, 144, 145, 148, 150, 151, 153, 154, 155, 159, 163, 164, 166, 171, 175, 178, 180, 182, 184, 187, 192, 193
Ledum Groenlandicum, 131
Lemon Verbena, 132
Lemon, 131–132
Lemongrass, 132–133
Lightbulb ring, 195
Lilac, 133
Lime *(Key)*, 134
Lime, 134
Linaloe, 134

Linden Blossom, 135
Lithotriptic, 153
Litsea Cubeba, 135–136
Liver decongestant, 184
Lovage, 136
Lymphatic decongestant, 71

Macadamia nut, 36–37
Macauba & macauba seed, 37
Mafura butter, 37
Magnol, Pierre, 137
Magnolia *(Bark)*, 136
Magnolia *(Flowers)*, 137
Mandarin, 137–138
Mango & mango butter, 38
Mangosteen butter *(Kokum butter)*, 38–39
Manketti *(Mongongo nut)*, 39
Manuka *(New Zealand Tea Tree)*, 138
Marigold *(Calendula)*, 39–40
Marjoram, 138
Marjoram *(Spanish)*, 138–139
Marjoram *(Sweet)*, 138–139
Mark Anthony, Emperor, 162
Marula, 40
Massage oil blends, 8
Massage, 195–196
Massoia Bark, 139
Mastic, 139–140
Maury, Marguerite, 2
McGill University, 193
Meadowfoam, 40–41
Measurement equivalents, 8
Medications, 3
Medicinal Plants of China, 56
Melissa *(Lemon Balm)*, 140–141
Mental clarity, oils for, 201
Mimosa, 141
Mist sprays, 196
Mobola plum *(Parinari kernel)*, 41
Moisturizing, 13, 25, 33, 38, 42, 44, 47, 63, 64, 65, 125, 141, 144, 152, 187, 192
Monarda, 141–142
Mood uplifting, oils for, 201–202. *See also* Uplifting.
Moringa *(Ben* or *Behen)*, 41–42
Morton, Julia F., 65
Mowrah butter, 42
Mugwort *(Armoise)*, 142–143

Mullein, 143, 194
Murumuru butter, 42
Muscle relaxant, 127
Muscles, oils for, 204
Mustard *(Black)*, 143–144
Myrrh, 144
Myrtle *(Anise)*, 145
Myrtle *(Lemon)*, 146
Myrtle, 144–145

Narcotic, 51, 70
Neem, 42–43
Neroli, 5, 146–147
Nerolina, 147
Nervine, 10, 17, 19, 30, 44,
    47, 51, 70, 72, 76, 77,
    84, 86, 93, 94, 97, 99,
    101, 103, 108, 114, 115,
    121, 123, 124, 125, 127,
    130, 132, 133, 135, 139,
    141, 142, 145, 150, 152,
    154, 157, 158, 163, 164,
    165, 166, 169, 170, 171,
    172, 173, 174, 179, 181,
    182, 184, 187, 188, 189
Niaouli, 147
Noni seed, 43
Nourishing (skin), 11, 63
Nutmeg, 148
Nutritive, 30, 44, 57, 163

Oat, 43–44
Okra, 44
Olive, 44–45
Onion, 148–149
Opopanax, 149
Orange *(Bitter)*, 149–150
Orange *(Blood)*, 149–150
Orange *(Sweet)*, 149–150
Orange, 149–150
Oregano, 150–151
Orris Root, 151
Osmanthus, 151

Pain, oils for, 202–203
Palm & Palm kernel, 45–46
Palm Oil Miracle, The, 45
Palmarosa, 5, 152
Papaya seed, 46
Paracelsus, 140
Parasiticide, 10, 11, 21, 33,
    64, 69, 73, 77, 79, 81, 83,
    88, 90, 91, 94, 96, 97, 98,
    99, 103, 106, 107, 109,
    111, 116, 117, 124, 125,
    130, 132, 133, 136, 145,

151, 153, 154, 157, 158,
    164, 168, 169, 172, 174,
    175, 176, 178, 179, 184
Parsley, 152–153
Parturient, 153
Passion fruit seed, 46–47
Pastel, 47
Pataua fruit & seed, 47
Patchouli, 5, 153–154
Peach kernel, 47–48
Peanut, 48
Pecan, 48
Pectoral, 11, 52, 73, 78, 83,
    84, 109, 110, 113, 114,
    124, 132, 144, 159, 163,
    164, 179, 184
Pennyroyal, 154
Pepper *(Black)*, 154–155
Pepper *(Red) (Cayenne
    Pepper)*, 155–156
Peppermint, 5, 156–157
Pequi, 48–49
Perilla (book), 49
Perilla, 157
    seed, 49
Peru Balsam, 157–158
Petitgrain, 5, 158–159
Pimento berry, 5
Pine nut, 49
Pine, 159
Pistachio nut, 50
Plague, Great, 1
Plant name classification,
    213–220
Pliny, 9, 14, 16, 17, 72, 95,
    110, 115, 116, 132, 143,
    151, 164, 167, 170, 175,
    184
Pomegranate, 50–51
Poppy seed, 51
Pracaxi, 52
*Practice of Aromatherapy,
    The*, 2
Pregnancy, 3
Preservative, 78
Prickly pear seed *(Opuntia)*,
    52
Prickly pear, 52
Product preservative, 194
Protectant, 117
Prunus kernel, 52–53
Pumpkinseed, 53
Purgative, 11, 13, 20, 22, 25,
    28, 31, 37, 42, 50, 61,
    65, 91, 113, 114, 142,
    151, 153, 161, 192

Purifying, 109

Quinoa, 53

Rambiazana *(Rambiaze)*,
    159–160
Ramtil, 53–54
Raspberry seed, 54
Ravensara Anisata *(Havozo
    Bark)*, 160
Ravensara Aromatica,
    160–161
Red Berry *(Pepper Tree)*, 161
Refreshing, 76, 79, 84, 89,
    97, 99, 101, 104, 117,
    125, 132, 134, 150, 152,
    157, 158, 159, 168, 170,
    176
    oils for, 200
Refrigerant, 13, 17, 101, 122,
    157, 170
Regenerator (skin), 12, 17,
    18, 36, 56, 58, 81, 88,
    93, 94, 97, 101, 109,
    121, 130, 147, 152, 154,
    163, 192
Regulator (menstrual), 17,
    78, 111, 117, 124, 133,
    142, 156
Rejuvenator (skin), 13, 14,
    21, 22, 29, 34, 39, 41,
    47, 51, 55, 57, 78, 90,
    114, 117, 125, 144, 164,
    169, 187, 193
Relaxant, 45, 86, 97, 107,
    127, 167, 169, 187
Resolvent, 106, 111, 115,
    116, 120, 124, 149, 164,
    169
Restorative, 23, 30, 44, 57,
    76, 84, 104, 114, 115,
    120, 130, 134, 139, 156,
    157, 159, 169, 170
Revitalizing, 72, 101, 103,
    111, 114, 135, 136, 138,
    144, 169, 176, 184
Reviving, 120, 130, 133, 147,
    148, 159, 164, 170
    oils for, 200
Rhatany Root, 55–56
Rhododendron, 161–162
Rice bran, 55
Ricin, 22
Rosalina *(Lavender Tea Tree)*,
    162
Rose hip seed, 55

Rose, 5, 162–163
Rosemary, 5, 163–164
Rubefacient, 42, 69, 79, 85,
    109, 118, 125, 132, 151,
    155, 156, 158, 159, 164,
    165, 169, 172, 178, 179,
    182, 184, 185, 192
Rue, 164–165

Safflower, 56
Saffron, 165
Sage *(Spanish)*, 165–166
Sage, 165–166
Sal butter *(Shorea butter)*, 56
Sandalwood *(Australian)*, 167
Sandalwood, 5, 167
Santolina *(Lavender Cotton)*,
    167–168
Sapote, 56–57
Sassafras, 168
Saunas, 196
Savory, 168–169
Saw Palmetto, 57
Schisandra, 169
Sea Buckthorn fruit & seed,
    57–58
Sedative, 11, 17, 23, 32, 33,
    40, 43, 47, 48, 49, 50,
    51, 57, 70, 71, 76, 77,
    78, 79, 82, 84, 85, 86,
    87, 89, 91, 92, 93, 94,
    97, 98, 99, 103, 104,
    106, 107, 110, 112, 113,
    114, 115, 117, 121, 123,
    125, 127, 128, 130, 132,
    133, 135, 138, 139, 140,
    141, 142, 144, 145, 146,
    147, 148, 150, 151, 153,
    154, 155, 157, 158, 161,
    162, 163, 165, 167, 169,
    171, 172, 174, 177, 178,
    179, 182, 184, 185, 187,
    188, 189
Seductive, 106
Sesame, 58–59
Shea, 59
    butter, 59
Shikonin seed, 59
Sisymbrium, 60
Skin care, 196
Skin protectant, 39
Skin, oils for, 203
Sleep, oils for, 203
Solomon, King, 92
Soothing, 78
Soybean, 60–61

Spearmint, 170
Spikenard, 170–171
Spruce (Black), 171–172
Spruce (Sitka), 171–172
Spruce (White), 171–172
Spruce, 171
Spruce-Hemlock, 171–172
St. John's Wort, 172–173
Steam inhalation, 196
Steam rooms, 196
Stimulant, 17, 19, 21, 25, 26, 30, 40, 42, 44, 56, 61, 64, 70, 72, 73, 75, 76, 77, 78, 79, 81, 82, 83, 84, 85, 86, 88, 89, 90, 91, 92, 93, 94, 95, 96, 97, 99, 100, 101, 102, 103, 107, 108, 109, 111, 113, 114, 115, 116, 117, 118, 120, 121, 124, 125, 130, 131, 132, 133, 134, 135, 136, 137, 138, 140, 142, 144, 147, 148, 149, 150, 151, 152, 153, 154, 155, 156, 157, 158, 159, 161, 163, 164, 165, 166, 167, 168, 168, 169, 170, 173, 174, 175, 176, 178, 179, 182, 184, 185, 186, 187, 188, 189, 192, 193
Stomachic, 11, 13, 19, 22, 25, 33, 40, 46, 49, 51, 53, 60, 69, 70, 72, 73, 76, 77, 79, 84, 86, 87, 88, 89, 90, 93, 94, 95, 96, 97, 98, 99, 101, 102, 106, 107, 108, 111, 112, 114, 115, 116, 118, 124, 125, 130, 131, 132, 133, 135, 136, 138, 139, 140, 141, 144, 148, 150, 151, 153, 154, 155, 156, 157, 158, 160, 163, 164, 165, 166, 167, 168, 170, 172, 174, 175, 178, 179, 182, 184, 186, 187, 189, 192
Strawberry seed, 61
Stress reduction, oils to help, 198
Styptic, 35, 40, 55, 87
Styrax (American), 173

Styrax (Asian), 173
Sudorific, 17, 40, 51, 62, 72, 76, 83, 84, 85, 86, 87, 94, 107, 120, 123, 124, 125, 130, 132, 135, 142, 144, 151, 152, 156, 157, 159, 164, 176, 178, 179, 187
Sun protectant, 59
Sunflower, 61–62

Tagetes, 173–174
Tamarind seed, 62
Tana, 174
Tangelo, 149–150
Tangerine, 137–138
Tansy, 174
Tarragon (Estragon), 175
Tea Tree (Black), 176
Tea Tree (Lemon), 176–177
Tea Tree (Lemon-Scented), 176–177
Tea Tree (Prickly Leaf), 177
Tea Tree, 175–176
Temple Orange. See Orange.
Temple, William Chace, 149
Terebinth, 177–178
Theophrastus, 24, 72, 140, 151, 152
Thuja (Cedar Leaf), 178
Thyme, 178–179
Tobacco, 179
Tobacco Leaf, 179–180
Tolu Balsam, 180
Tomato seed, 62–63
Tonic, 10, 17, 21, 22, 25, 27, 30, 33, 35, 40, 42, 43, 44, 46, 49, 50, 51, 53, 55, 56, 57, 59, 60, 61, 64, 65, 66, 69, 71, 72, 73, 74, 75, 76, 77, 78, 79, 80, 81, 82, 83, 84, 85, 86, 87, 88, 89, 90, 91, 93, 94, 95, 96, 97, 98, 99, 101, 102, 103, 104, 106, 107, 108, 109, 110, 111, 113, 114, 115, 116, 117, 118, 119, 120, 121, 123, 124, 125, 127, 128, 130, 132, 133, 134, 135, 136, 137, 138, 139,

141, 142, 144, 145, 147, 148, 150, 151, 152, 153, 154, 155, 156, 157, 158, 159, 161, 163, 164, 165, 166, 167, 168, 169, 170, 171, 172, 174, 175, 178, 179, 182, 184, 185, 186, 187, 188, 189, 192, 193
Tonifying, 40, 97, 114, 116, 117, 118, 120, 125, 132, 133, 144, 155, 163
Tonka Bean (Tonquin Bean), 180–181
Tranquilizer, 51, 69, 70, 123, 127, 138, 171, 172, 174, 182
Tuberose, 181
Tucuma butter, 63
Tucuma, 63
Turmeric, 181–182

Ucuuba butter, 63
United States Agriculture Department, 149
Uplifting, 30, 76, 78, 79, 81, 88, 89, 97, 99, 101, 109, 114, 115, 117, 122, 124, 132, 134, 135, 137, 141, 148, 152, 157, 158, 163, 179, 181, 184. See also Mood uplifting.
Usnea Lichen, 194

Valerian, 182
Valnet, Jean, 2
Vanilla, 182–183
Vasoconstrictor, 64, 85, 86, 104, 117, 150, 157
Vasodilator, 21, 90, 91, 102, 106, 116, 139, 153, 155, 165
Vegetal oils, butters, waxes, 3, 5, 7–66
  combining with essential oils, 8
  extraction of, 5
  refining process for, 5
Vermifuge, 10, 13, 21, 23, 25, 28, 33, 38, 40, 42, 46, 47, 52, 53, 64, 65, 66, 76, 78, 79, 83, 84,

85, 86, 88, 90, 94, 96, 97, 98, 107, 109, 111, 112, 116, 117, 118, 123, 124, 125, 130, 132, 141, 142, 147, 149, 152, 153, 157, 159, 165, 166, 168, 169, 172, 174, 175, 178, 179, 182, 184, 186, 192
Vetiver, 183–184
Violet, 184
Vitex, 184
Vitex (Berry), 184–185
Vitex (Leaf), 184–185
Vulnerary, 10, 11, 21, 27, 30, 35, 37, 40, 44, 45, 46, 53, 59, 64, 75, 78, 79, 85, 87, 90, 93, 94, 106, 108, 109, 110, 113, 114, 115, 117, 121, 124, 125, 128, 129, 130, 135, 138, 139, 141, 143, 144, 147, 149, 150, 151, 158, 159, 161, 164, 166, 168, 172, 176, 178, 184, 185, 187, 192

Walnut, 63–64
Warming, 73, 97, 101, 104, 107, 113, 114, 116, 136, 139, 148, 151, 154, 164, 166, 168, 172, 179
  oils for, 204
Watermelon seed, 64–65
Wheat germ, 65
Whole Soy Story, The, 60
Wintergreen, 185–186
Wolfberry seed, 65–66
World War I, 116, 152, 179
World War II, 2, 116, 164
Wormwood, 186

Ximenia seed, 66

Yangu, 66
Yarrow, 186–187
Ylang-Ylang, 5, 187
Yu, He-Ci, 49
Yuzu, 188

Zanthoxylum, 188–189
Zedoary, 189

About the Authors

Carol Schiller and **David Schiller** are the authors of five internationally published books on the use of essential oils, and cofounders of the International Aromatherapy and Herb Association (IAHA). They are contributing writers to *Making Scents Magazine,* the association's publication. Carol and David have spent over twenty years studying and researching the benefits of plant oils, and determining their practical uses and applications. They have been instructing classes and training workshops for companies, colleges and other educational organizations since 1989. Carol has been a featured presenter at international conferences.

Jeffrey Schiller, the illustrator of this book, is a cofounder and president of the International Aromatherapy and Herb Association (IAHA), and publisher/editor/photographer of *Making Scents Magazine.* Jeffrey instructs classes on aromatherapy for educational organizations and colleges. He was also an organizer and speaker for seven years at the AromaHerb Conference and Trade Show.

The International Aromatherapy and Herb Association offers a complimentary digital back issue, sent by e-mail, of *Making Scents Magazine*, the organization's publication. If you'd like a copy, please contact us: MakingScentsMag@aol.com or call (602) 938-4439.